T0298668

SAYING GOODBYE

A Casebook of Termination in Child and Adolescent Analysis and Therapy

SAYING GOODBYE

A Casebook of Termination
in Child and Adolescent
Analysis and Therapy

edited by

Anita G. Schmukler

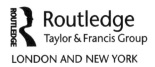

Routledge
Taylor & Francis Group

LONDON AND NEW YORK

First published 1991 by The Analytic Press, Inc.

Published 2018 by Routledge
2 Park Square, Milton Park, Abingdon, Oxon, OX14 4RN
52 Vanderbilt Avenue, New York, NY 10017

Routledge is an imprint of the Taylor & Francis Group, an informa business

Library of Congress Cataloging-in-Publication Data

Saying goodbye : a casebook of termination in child and adolescent
  analysis and therapy / edited by Anita G. Schmukler.
    p. cm.
  Includes bibliographical references and indexes.
  ISBN 0-88163-106-X
  1. Child psychotherapy—Termination. 2. Adolescent psychotherapy-
-Termination. 3. Transference (Psychology) 4. Psychotherapist and
patient. 5. Child analysis. 6. Adolescent analysis.
I. Schmukler, Anita G., 1941-
  [DNLM: 1. Latency Period (Psychology). 2. Physician-Patient
Relations. 3. Psychoanalytic Therapy—in adolescence—case studies.
4. Psychoanalytic Therapy—in infancy & childhood. 5. Transference
(Psychology) WS 463 S274]
RJ505.T47S28 1991
618.92'8914—dc20
DNLM/DLC
for Library of Congress   91-4575
                                          CIP

ISBN 13: 978-0-88163-106-7 (hbk)
ISBN 13: 978-1-138-87230-1 (pbk)

Contents

Early Adolescence

Midadolescence

Late Adolescence

II
Theoretical Papers

Acknowledgments

The idea of preparing a book on termination in child and adolescent analysis grew out of a conference held by The Association for Child Psychoanalysis in Philadelphia in March 1989. Initially, Dr. Martin Silverman made many helpful suggestions in the preparation of a paper I presented at that conference, and questions stirred by conversations with him first stimulated my interest in collecting this material.

Dr. Walter Troffkin was most helpful in reading sections of the manuscript and making suggestions related to analytic content. Dr. Naomi Myrvaagnes also read several chapters and added significantly to their clarity of expression.

Toby Troffkin's line editing was superb.

Many thanks to Dr. Paul Stepansky, Editor-in-Chief of The Analytic Press, who encouraged this project from the start and was gracious in answering questions at each stage of the work, and to his Managing Editor, Eleanor Starke Kobrin, for her helpful suggestions and ready availability.

Marian Cichetti, my secretary, deserves special thanks for her attention to detail and unstinting efforts; and Debbie Kaplan's help with editorial details has been invaluable in the final phase of this project.

I am grateful to The Psychoanalytic Study of the Child and Yale University Press for permission to reprint Chused's pivotal paper.

Finally, I wish to thank my many friends and colleagues whose eagerness to discuss both analytic and editorial matters and whose continuous encouragement and enthusiasm transformed a potentially arduous task into one of sheer pleasure.

Contributors

Paul M. Brinich, PhD—Clinical Associate Professor of Psychology, University of North Carolina, Chapel Hill; Director of Psychological Services, Children's Psychiatric Institute, John Umstead Hospital, Butler, North Carolina.

Marion Burgner—Training and Supervising Analyst, British Psychoanalytic Society; private practice, child analyst.

Judith Fingert Chused, MD—Clinical Professor of Psychiatry and Behavioral Sciences, George Washington University School of Medicine; Supervising and Training Analyst, Washington Psychoanalytic Institute.

Rhoda S. Frenkel, MD—Training and Supervising Analyst, Dallas Psychoanalytic Institute; Clinical Professor of Psychiatry, University of Texas Southwestern Medical Center at Dallas.

Robert D. Gillman, MD—Supervising Analyst and Emeritus Training Analyst, Baltimore-Washington Institute for Psychoanalysis; Past President, Association for Child Psychoanalysis.

Remigio G. Gonzalez, MD—Clinical Professor of Psychiatry, Tulane University; Training and Supervising Analyst in Adult, Child, and Adolescence, New Orleans Psychoanalytic Institute.

Calvin H. Haber, MD—Faculty, The Psychoanalytic Institute, Department of Psychiatry, New York University Medical Center; Attending Psychiatrist, Schneider Children's Hospital, Long Island Jewish Medical Center, New Hyde Park, New York.

Leon Hoffman, MD—Faculty, New York Psychoanalytic Institute; Assistant Clinical Professor, Cornell University School of Medicine.

Paul Kay, MD—Clinical Associate Professor of Psychiatry, New York University Medical Center; Faculty, The Psychoanalytic Institute, New York University Medical Center.

Paulina F. Kernberg, MD—Associate Professor of Psychiatry, Cornell University Medical College; Director, Child and Adolescent Psychiatry, The New York Hospital-Cornell Medical Center, Westchester Division.

Jack Novick, PhD—Supervising Analyst, Michigan Psychoanalytic Institute; Clinical Associate Professor of Psychiatry, University of Michigan and Wayne State University.

Kerry Kelly Novick—Faculty, Michigan Psychoanalytic Institute; private practice, child and adolescent psychoanalysis.

Lilo Plaschkes, MSW—Supervising Analyst, Child and Adolescent Analysis, New York Freudian Society; Member, Association for Child Psychoanalysis.

Anita Schmukler, DO (editor)—Faculty and Supervising Analyst, Child and Adolescent Analysis, Philadelphia Association for Psychoanalysis; Clinical Assistant Professor of Psychiatry, University of Pennsylvania.

Alan Sugarman, PhD—Faculty, San Diego Psychoanalytic Institute; Associate Clinical Professor of Psychiatry, University of California, San Diego.

Samuel Weiss, MD—Training and Supervising Analyst, Chicago Institute for Psychoanalysis; Clinical Associate Professor, University of Illinois College of Medicine.

Jaap Ubbels, MD—Member, Dutch Psychoanalysis Society; Coordinator, Child Department, Psychoanalytic Institute of the Dutch Psychoanalytic Society.

Judith A. Yanof, MD—Training and Supervising Analyst, Boston Psychoanalytic Society and Institute.

Preface

This is a book about attachment, separation, loss, and mourning, and about young patients' creative responses to these phenomena. While individual chapters inform us of these processes in the framework of ending treatment, implicitly we are observing them in a wider context, that of enhancing our understanding of normal development. The rich clinical material in this collection enables us to examine the type and depth of the child or adolescent's continually evolving relationship with the analyst, and the transformations that occur as the transference relationship undergoes various phases of relinquishment. Also, there is ample material for the reader to explain the various ways in which parents become attached to, and separate them from, the child's analyst and for us to examine the analyst's countertransference responses and counterreactions.

In collecting clinical material for this volume, my aim has been to present descriptions of the termination phase in child and adolescent analysis. Some of the cases demonstrate specific developmental conflicts with particular clarity. Others document the vicissitudes of transference/countertransference that we encounter with some frequency but do not typically find represented in the literature. Still others demonstrate the use of an analytic method with patients whose pathology is severe. In these cases, the termination phase may be attenuated, stormy, or especially burdensome to the analyst yet may reveal a good deal about the wide range of possibilities for analytic interventions.

Issues of the child's capacity to separate from the analyst at the conclusion of treatment are presented not simply from a theoretical perspective, but from careful delineation of clinical process during the final phase of treatment. Themes include conflict and developmental delay in the process of termination of analysis; the degree to which children and adolescents of varying levels of pathology are capable of resolving the transference neurosis; and the extent to which the analysts' interventions reflect their experience as a transference object, a real object, or both. This material also provides an opportunity to investigate the manner in which an analysis of countertransference during the termination phase of working with children can enrich our understanding of analytic process.

In our lifetimes as analysts we are exposed to relatively few patients. We hear presentations at clinical conferences but frequently we cannot explore them in depth. The cases included in this volume represent a wide range of psychopathology, varying developmental levels, and a broad scope of technical perspectives. As a result, we have access to interventions that may differ considerably from what our own might have been. Thus, this collection provides us with akind of workbook from which we can examine interventions and responses at leisure, consider alternatives, and refine our theory and practice.

In some of the clinical papers in this volume, process is presented directly. In others it must be inferred. Yet it is clear that each analyst has wrestled in some way with the meaning of ending treatment possibly because of the challenge of a particularly difficult case or in response to a particular personal experience.

Opinions vary about the manner in which the date of the final meeting is determined in work with children. Approaches range from giving the child complete liberty, calendar in hand, to choose a date several months hence to a gradual reduction in frequency of sessions.

An examination of criteria for ending analysis can be helpful in understanding how analysts, child patients, and parents respond to material that signals an approaching end to treatment; such an examination may also be useful for purposes of research. At issue is the question of using criteria to provide general guidelines, to understand dynamics, and as tools for research, rather than for defensive purposes, such as permitting a treatment to conclude because particular criteria have been met even though significant analytic work remains to be completed.

Some criteria for termination of analysis have evolved specifically with reference to work with child and adolescent patients. One set of criteria for these young patients highlights "restoring the child to the path of normal development, . . . the resolution of the transference, and the child's developmentally appropriate adaptation in his life outside the treatment setting . . . "(Sandler, Kennedy, and Tyson, 1980, p. 241).

Paulina Kernberg and her co-workers, and members of the child department of the Dutch Psychoanalytic Institute, are among those engaged in defining criteria for ending treatment with children and adolescents. Pooled research data from the international community will be helpful in examining different theoretical and technical perspectives and may underscore what remains unchanged in the analysis of material from the termination phase.

Dividing the work of termination into the pretermination phase, the termination phase proper, and the extended conscious and unconscious work accomplished by the former analysand following treatment, we will be more able to assess the ways in which the analytic process dovetails with normal development and affects progressive growth.

Samuel Abrams (1978, cited by several contributors to this volume) has a pivotal position in the study of the termination phase in child analysis. Abrams raises four crucial questions. "Are the dynamic issues engaged?". That is, "Have positive and negative oedipal matters been confronted and linked with specific references to the past? Are the preoedipal anlagen delineated?" "Have specific drive-derivatives become manifest?" (p. 462) To paraphrase Abrams, have the "passionate love" and "venomous destructiveness" of the oedipal drama been represented, delineated, and worked through in the analysis? "What is the direction of restructuring?" (p. 463) "Have the defenses, availability of signal affects, and general functioning demonstrated progression to the appropriate developmental level?" And finally, "Has the resolution of past conflicts found a more fortunate pathway?" (p. 463).

Is the transference neurosis present in children? Chused's comprehensive chapter underscores the fact that the development of transference neurosis in children may have been inhibited by the stance that pioneering child analysts assumed to be necessary to maintain an analytic situation; that is, benevolence superseded analytic neutrality. Earlier references to transference neurosis in children occur in the work of Weiss and his colleagues (1968) and Harley (1967).

Given the existence of transference neurosis in children, we are led to wonder about its fate during the termination phase and following termination. While "resolution of the *transference neu-*

rosis is not a reliable indicator with children'' (Abrams, 1978, p. 468), when termination of analysis is considered, the importance of working assiduously with this phenomenon cannot be underestimated. For example, the effect of an unresolved transference neurosis in a child or adolescent upon character development deserves substantial study and might well be a project for those involved with assessment at the conclusion of treatment and in succeeding developmental phases.

To what extent does the parent's attachment to the child's analyst hinder the resolution of the transference for the child patient? In chapter 4, John's mother responded with intense dismay to the announcement that her son's treatment was about to end. Conflictual responses to the ending of their children's analyses also occurred for parents in the cases reported by Sugarman, Gonzalez, and Ubbels.

Any study of a termination phase in children and in some adolescents ideally ought to take into account the attachment of the parents to the analyst and how that might affect the children's further integration of their gains during treatment.

The question of whether termination is even possible in child analysis is based partly on the idea that child analysis, whenever it ends, remains incomplete, since ultimate goals, as defined for adults, have not been attained: mature object relations, genital primacy, and the ability to work efficiently. Weiss addresses this matter in an astute, probing examination of whether termination exists or is simply a fictive construction. In our work with children, we assess, rather, the developmental level that has been attained and look for evidence of progressive development. And we analyze the child's wishes both to leave and to remain in treatment. Each developmental stage has unique tasks to complete. The delineation of these tasks permits us to evaluate the sufficiency of a particular termination phase. We have completed our analytic work when anticipated progression is able to occur without the hindrance of inhibition and developmental delays.

We must remind ourselves that *all* treatments remain, to some extent, incomplete and are subject both to the patient's ability to integrate the work of the analysis after it has ended and to the later vicissitudes of life, which can either support and strengthen our previous psychological work or subject it to severe tests. I propose that we view the termination of an analysis in children and adolescents as *complete* with respect to analytic function, when we have ''secured the best possible conditions for the ego'' (Freud, 1937), even though a particular child's *development* remains incomplete.

The papers in this volume offer us an opportunity to examine *process* during the termination phase. Clearly, ending treatment is a unique experience for each patient. Arlow and Brenner (1969, p. 29) underscore the fact that "patients do not react in a stereotyped way to the relatively uniform set of conditions which we call the psychoanalytic situation" (p. 29). And Abend (1988) reminds us that "the sole task of the termination phase is to analyze the analysand's reactions to termination . . ." (p. 164) and thus avoid obfuscating material at termination because of our preconceived notions of what is to be anticipated.

For many patients, the termination phase is an opportunity to seek fulfillment of unconscious wishes (Nunberg, 1926) and Arlow (1990, personal communication) has pointed out that these include "unfulfilled wishes of childhood and those that form the core of the neurotic conflict and the transference." Each child and adolescent patient experiences unique fantasies at termination. John (Ubbel's patient) had to acknowledge that his wish for narcissistic perfection in the form of great artistic talent would not be gratified. Since John's parents had harbored a similar hope, John, at 16, bore considerable burden in his efforts to analyze infantile wishes for omnipotence.

In my work with children, I find it valuable to pay particular attention to the patient's immediate response to the setting of the termination date. Sarah (Sugarman's patient) at not yet seven years old, responded to the establishment of a specific date for ending treatment, and to the associated negotiations, by asking permission to leave the room so she could wash her pierced ears to prevent infection. What stirred this specific fantasy in an early latency girl whose early history included masochistic behavior? When her treatment began, Sarah would plead for punishment in an effort to find relief from guilt and anxiety. When a definite date for ending treatment was established for eight-year-old Stanley (Haber's patient) after a lengthy analysis that involved gender reorganization, the child told his analyst that he felt as if he were being discharged from the Army. Stanley then asserted, in play, that "Dr. Stanley" could treat sexual problems. Immediately following his verbalization of his identification with his analyst, Stanley strode to the waiting room to tell his mother of the good news. Each patient has a distinctive assortment of fantasies and affect-laden responses to the setting of a final date of treatment, and Sarah, Stanley, and all the other children presented in this volume exemplify the multidetermined factors that shape these responses. Arlow (1990, personal communication) has mentioned a set of fantasies that may appear in the termination phase and express a fear of leaving treatment. These include the notion that the patient can "achieve maturity or true status as a parent only through the analyst's death. Accordingly, successfully completing the analysis means that they have killed the analyst and therefore cannot leave treatment."

Examination of fantasies at termination of treatment must include attention to metaphors, which are distinctive for each patient. Cindy (Yanof's patient) at 19, referred to her feeling at leaving treatment as "singing harmony," indicating that her own voice had meaning and value and could comfortably maintain a separate position that is in direct relation to others but need not join them. As we explore our patients' distinctive fantasies of terminating analysis with respect to their conflicts, we observe that each patient also presents a characteristic constellation of *feelings* that unfold progressively during the final phase of analysis.

Anna (Plaschkes's case) grappled with feelings about a sibling who had died and wondered if her parents had subsequently adopted a boy because they preferred males. Predictions of future events played a significant role in Anna's fantasies from the onset of treatment to the final day. She wanted her analyst to preserve her diary, which she imagined would assume special value for her analyst when Anna's accomplishments were recognized. During childhood Anna longed for recognition by parents, who, she believed, preferred sons. In early adolescence Anna wanted to anticipate that her analyst would "someday" acknowledge her accomplishments and feel honored to have known her; thus Anna would assume a preferential position. Sarah, (Sugarman's patient), Paul (Gonzalez's patient), John L. (Brinich's patient), and John (Ubbels's patients) all struggled with feelings about the divorce of their parents, and each patient had unique developmental difficulties involving separation. These were among the factors that affected the conflictual and developmental expressions of their efforts to disengage from the analyst.

The intense and sometimes overwhelming feelings that children experience over separation, coupled with a sometimes limited ability to articulate conflicts, may impede their ability to analyze material related to efforts to disengage from the analyst and thus result instead in defensive denial. Van Dam, Heinicke, and Shane (1975) point out that "even more than adults, children from prelatency throughout early adolescence find it difficult to tolerate painful aspects of this separation" (p. 469). The manner of wrestling with conflicts that arise from feelings and fantasies related to ending analysis delineates the unique attributes of each termination phase.

Fantasies, metaphors, dreams, and feelings that signal an approaching end to treatment are evaluated in the context of structural changes anticipated at the conclusion of treatment. In spite of specified guidelines that have been proposed by experienced clinicians for ending treatment, analysts frequently wonder if the child is *really* ready to conclude the work. Several of these cases included in this volume, both in complete clinical presentations and in vignettes set forth in theoretical papers, give clear evidence of the uncertainty stirred in analysts as termination approaches. The interplay of feelings over ending treatment in the child patient, in the parent, and in the analyst must be analyzed with meticulous care if an ending is to proceed in which gains can be sustained.

A study of children's fantasies during the termination phase of analysis can elucidate some aspects of normal development, as reflected in play, metaphor, fairy tales, nursery rhymes, and other creative phenomena. These fantasies also add to our understanding of a child's response to the divorce of the parents or to the death of a parent or sibling. Additionally it can help us to understand the profound affective responses to forward thrusts in development that necessitate the relinquishment of some aspect of an internalized object. At the same time, a study of normal child development can add enormously to analysts' grasp of nuances that occur as the end to treatment approaches for patients of any age.

With respect to factors that arise in the termination of analysis with young children, a prominent issue is that of amnesia for the entire analytic experience. Van Dam et al. (1975) discuss the relative amnesia "which in part serves to deal with the object loss of the analyst" and also is a factor in the child's relinquishing "the constant self-analysis and uncovering" so that he can resume "his ordinary childhood pursuits" (p. 471). Children's amnesia for their analyses may serve a function similar to that which object removal performs for the early adolescent. That is, the amnesia is a form of repudiation of incestuous bonds, the analysis of which remains incomplete because of the developmental immaturity of the child, and the analyst is represented in one vertex of the oedipal triangle.

A central purpose of the child's amnesia for the analytic experience is to avoid the painful separations to which van Dam et al. (p. 469) refer. I am reminded of a five-year-old girl who moved to the East Coast during the summer that preceded her entry to first grade. Immediately following the move, she asked each morning when the family would return to San Diego, although she had been well prepared for the move and had expressed enthusiasm about it. When the wish to return was no longer articulated and she became actively involved with new friends, yet still exhibited momentary sadness, she was asked about her feelings about the change. Her immediate reply to her astonished parents was, "Oh, I think it will take *my whole life* to get used to this move." While this example occurred in a prelatency child who exhibited healthy functioning in most areas, it illustrates the intensity of feeling that can be experienced and against which sufficient defenses must be erected.

Technical issues in working with young children at the conclusion of analysis include the amount of latitude one allows the child in selecting a termination date, that is, the degree to which a young child is able to deal with conflict over a specific termination date; postponing the date until sufficient material is analyzed; and the degree to which the analyst is comfortable with the uncertainty that arises. Assessing the importance of both structural and developmental factors in work with children during the termination phase and deciding when to leave structural factors for development that is expected to occur following the ending of analysis (Brinich, 1990, personal communication) are also significant considerations.

The difficulties prominent during the concluding phase of a psychoanalysis have been compared (Novick, 1976, p. 412) to developmental conflicts that arise as part of the typical adolescent process. For Eissler (1958), "adolescence appears to afford the individual a second chance; it is a kind of lease permitting revision of the solutions found during latency which had been formed in direct reaction to the oedipal conflict" (p. 250). In an analogous, although much more circumscribed, manner, the analysis itself provides an additional opportunity to rework conflicts. To continue along this line, a distinctive task of the termination phase of an analysis is to provide still another opportunity to rework and revise earlier solutions and to examine regressive impulses and fresh symptoms in the context of that material which characterizes the termination phase. Arlow (1990, personal communication) takes the position that as termination approaches "hitherto concealed anticipations and expectations come to the fore." It is in response to that which is anticipated and may or may not be gratified that new (or altered) symptoms and defenses emerge as disengagement from the analyst proceeds.

With respect to reworking earlier solutions, Burgner (1988) explores the idea that in some cases the adolescent process has been subjected to closure prematurely and needs to be reopened if further development is to take place and if closure is to occur at a later and more appropriate phase.

Does examination of the terminal phase in work with children and adolescents have application for analysts who analyze adults exclusively? Novick and Novick address this subject incisively, with rich clinical material to support their hypotheses. And many of the questions assessing termination that were raised by Firestein (1978) are clearly applicable to work with children.

Gillman presents rich clinical examples of termination in psychotherapy. A careful examination of this material reveals that, although it lacks the associative links we find in analysis, analytically oriented psychotherapists who are aware of process during termination of analysis may discover derivatives that can contribute significantly to their understanding of otherwise enigmatic clinical material and thus expand the breadth and depth of the experience of ending psychotherapy.

An interdisciplinary view may expand our theoretical and clinical perspectives on termination in the analysis of young patients. We can compare the conflicts that arise in our adolescents as they try to detach from infantile objects with the reactions of postpubertal children in societies, in which, for example, puberty rites are a significant factor in the step from childhood to adulthood. We find that what is experienced as intrapsychic conflict in industrialized societies is addressed in less developed areas in prescribed rituals, in which the entire community participates. Muensterberger (1975) outlines that course of initiation rites: The young person who has reached the appropriate age "must observe food restrictions" (p. 17). A period of enforced seclusion (p. 18) follows, and during this time "the neophyte is indoctrinated with certain tribal traditions, customs, mythology, secret ceremonies, and beliefs" (p. 18). The youth is subjected to "sexual rites, frequently painful, including circumcision, flagellations, tooth extractions"; is informed of adult secrets, such as the identity of "masked ghosts" (p. 18); shares a ritual meal; and undergoes transformation from child status to that of an adult. Thus, the transition to adulthood is a communal matter, and ambivalence at every phase of psychosexual development is addressed by ritualistic behavior. Our adolescents engage in a struggle to resolve ambivalence toward parental figures in a process, largely unconscious, that involves transformation and gradual relinquishment of internalized objects. In less developed societies, the counterpart of the internalized object is the ancestral image. This is a subject that is worthy of continuing study.

In our society, adolescents who leave home demonstrate considerable variation in their affective responses to this change. A similar range of variation occurs for ending analytic treatment, for which typical feelings include, conflictually, joyous anticipation, anxiety about the future, and, for some, a period of mourning. A 16-year-old boy expressed his feelings in this way: "Leaving this treatment [is] not like dying, because you [can] see the person again, but it [is] like having someone close die, because you [are] really on your own" (Schmukler, 1990, p. 473). If we consider responses to final separation—death—in various societies, we find degrees of prescribed responses, from joyful interaction to mourning, which Freud perceived as part of a healing process (Furman, 1990). The Balinese, for instance, joyously celebrate the deceased's moving on to join his ancestors, and the Wari of Brazil have cannibalistic rituals in which the dead are roasted and consumed by specific members of the community. Thus we uncover a breadth of material that can illuminate our understanding of identification, incorporation, and impulses and defenses at every level of development. Specifically, here, we can learn about fantasies that address final disengagement, the ultimate aim of a well-conducted termination phase in an analysis.

What is the intrapsychic response to such endings? The renunciation of infantile wishes typically involves some measure of disappointment. While aspects of internalized objects are relinquished, that which remains intact undergoes a series of transformations (a subject addressed by Weiss in chapter 12 in this volume) and may appear in a myriad of disguises during a lifetime. Images of such transformations are suggested by Ariel's song in The Tempest:

> Full fathom five they father lies,
>   Of his bones are coral made,
> Those are pearls that were his eyes.
>   Nothing of him that doth fade
> But doth suffer a sea change
> Into something rich and strange.
>   Act I, sc. ii, 1. 397–402

Poetry, mythology, and fairy tales are natural cultural elaborations of issues of separation and loss that can enhance our examination of therapeutic endings, can enrich our grasp of associative productions, and can expand our analytic function. A well-balanced synthesis of clinical, theoretical, and interdisciplinary studies can ultimately provide us with a broader perspective to grasp the intricate and crucial questions raised in this volume.

It is hoped that this volume will contribute to our understanding of the psychoanalysis of children and adults, that it will demonstrate the value of a careful study of analytic process at termination for those who practice psychoanalytic psychotherapy, and that it will be helpful for those who study the processes of grief, mourning and creative forms of healing.

References

Abend, S. (1988), Unconscious fantasies and issues of termination. In: *Fantasy, Myth, and Reality*, ed. H. Blum, Y. Kramer, A.K. Richards & A.D. Richards. New Haven, CT: International Universities Press, pp. 149–165.

Abrams, S. (1978), Termination in child analysis. In: *Child Analysis and Therapy*, ed. J. Glenn. New York: Aronson, pp. 451–469.

Arlow, J. (1987), Perspectives on Freud's "Analysis terminable and interminable" after fifty years. *International Psychoanalytic Association Educational Monographs*, No. 1, pp. 73–88.

Arlow, J. & Brenner, C. (1969), The psychoanalytic situation. In: *Psychoanalysis in the Americas*, ed. R. Litman. New York: International Universities Press, pp. 23–55.

Burgner, M. (1988), Analytic work with adolescents—terminable or interminable. *Internat. J. Psycho-Anal.*, 69:179–218.

Eissler, K.R. (1958), Notes on problems of technique in the psychoanalytic treatment of adolescents. *The Psychoanalytic Study of the Child*, 13:223–254. New York: International Universities Press.

Firestein, S.K. (1978), *Termination in Psychoanalysis*. New York: International Universities Press.

Freud, S. (1937), Analysis terminable and interminable. *Standard Edition*, 23:216–253. London: Hogarth Press, 1964.

Furman, R.A. (1990), New perspectives on preparation. In: *Child Analysis*, ed. D. Paris. Cleveland, OH: Cleveland Center for Research in Child Development, pp. 26–41.

Harley, M. (1967), Transference developments in a five-year-old-child. In: *The Child Analyst At Work*, ed. E.R. Geleerd. New York: International Universities Press, pp. 115–141.

Muensterberger, W. (1975), The adolescent in society. In: *The Psychology of Adolescence*, ed. A. Esman. New York: International Universities Press.

Novick, J. (1976), Termination of treatment in adolescence. *The Psychoanalytic Study of the Child*, 31:389–414. New Haven, CT: Yale University Press.

Nunberg, H. (1926), The will to recovery. In: *Practice and Theory of Psychoanalysis*, Vol. 1. New York: International Universities Press, 1948.

Sandler, J, Kennedy, H., & Tyson, R.L. (ed.). (1980), *The Technique of Child Psychoanalysis: Discussions with Anna Freud*. Cambridge, MA: Harvard University Press.

Schmukler, A.G. (1990), Termination in midadolescence. *The Psychoanalytic Study of the Child*, 45:459–474. New Haven, CT: Yale University Press.

Van Dam, H., Heinicke, C.M. & Shane, M. (1975), On termination in child analysis. *The Psychoanalytic Study of the Child*, 30:443–474. New Haven, CT: Yale University Press.

Weiss, S., Fineberg, H., Gelman, R., & Kohrman, R. (1968), Technique of child analysis. *J. Amer. Acad. Child Psychiatry*, 7:639–662.

I

Clinical
Contributions

Early Latency

The chapter by Alan Sugarman describes Sarah, who at six and three-quarters, began a termination phase during the fourth year of her five-times-weekly analysis. A schedule of sessions of decreasing frequency was established, so that each month one weekly session was eliminated. Sarah was told that she could determine the date of the final meeting, provided she gave sufficient notice so that there would be time to talk about her decision.

The rationale for this pattern included Sarah's early traumata over separation and her relatively undeveloped sense of time. Sarah's analysis had involved extensive work with sadomasochistic impulses and separation anxieties. Although the termination phase was characterized by symptom revival and various modes of regressive behavior, Sarah responded rapidly to interpretation and demonstrated evidence of increased synthetic function of the ego, development of defenses typical of latency, and reworking of earlier conflicts and developmental delays. The analysis of Sarah's conflict between her feelings of loyalty to her mother and her loyalty to her analyst enabled Sarah to move from a position of predominantly negative transference. Her symptom of general indecisiveness during the termination process was ameliorated by the analyst's interpretation of it as representing her worry about choosing the time to end treatment. The analyst's verbalizing Sarah's feelings, which she occasionally had difficulty in expressing, permitted her to deal with material that might have otherwise been avoided because of their painful associations.

The reader is also referred to chapter 13, by Novick and Novick, in which the termination of the analysis of a six-year-old boy is presented.

1

Termination of Psychoanalysis with an Early Latency Girl

Alan Sugarman

"I'll miss you, but I'll see you tomorrow."

In describing the termination phase of analysis of a six-year-old girl, I focus on the manifestations and management of clinical phenomena and on such methodological issues as criteria for termination. A more detailed study of the overall case is presented elsewhere (Sugarman, in press).

While taking into account developmental differences and their manifestations in the content and form of the material analyzed, I emphasize the striking structural parallels in the termination process for adults and for children even this young.

The importance of the analyst's more active role in setting a timetable will emerge as one of the technical modifications that are sometimes needed to effect termination for an early latency child. This case demonstrates too the need for the analyst to address the developmental issue of the child's limited capacity to verbalize and the need for the analyst, certainly in Sarah's case, to assist the child in surmounting pronounced separation conflicts.

Sarah

Sarah's masochistic behavior had been addressed in five sessions weekly of psychoanalysis for slightly over three years, beginning when she was three and a half. Sarah was six and three-quarters when we agreed to set her termination date. She had expressed wishes episodically to terminate throughout her years of treatment and these impulses had been analyzed with regard to their defensive and wish-fulfilling functions. After three years of analysis Sarah's wish to terminate seemed less defensive. Symptomatic improvement had occurred steadily throughout the analysis, and for almost two years she had been free of the masochistic provocativeness and tantrums that had precipitated her initial referral for analysis. Furthermore, she seemed solidly entrenched in latency with a developmental momentum auguring well for continued growth after termination. Thus, it seemed reasonable to agree with both Sarah and her mother that she was ready to end treatment.

Sarah's Presenting Complaints and History

A brief description of Sarah's presenting symptoms and their developmental origins will be the background for understanding the nature of the issues she reworked in termination. More complete information can be obtained by reading about her early stage of treatment (Sugarman, in press). Sarah's mother brought her for consultation soon after she turned three. Her parents had separated, Sarah and her mother had relocated to San Diego, and her mother had remarried during the previous year. The cumulative effect of these environmental stresses combined with her equally stressful earlier history to make Sarah more negativistic, moody, and tantrum-prone than is typical of a child her age. Her mother felt exasperated by her inability to please Sarah. Sarah's wishes to be controlled and punished were manifest at the time of the consultation in her requests that her mother "tell me I'm in time-out" or "tell me I did it really, really bad!" The environmental sources of these problems were abundantly clear in Sarah's developmental history, where parental insensitivity and abandonment were severe enough to warrant being called cumulative trauma (Khan, 1963).

Conceiving Sarah was her parents' attempt to save a failing relationship. Not only did the attempt fail, but the same personal conflicts that ultimately led her parents to be unable to remain with each other led them to neglect Sarah during her infancy. For example, they left Sarah with a sitter for over two weeks while they vacationed when Sarah was only three months old. Sarah's lack of manifest reaction to the separation led her mother to feel comfortable about progressively returning to full-time employment over the next several months. This reaction to the infant's anaclitic and narcissistic needs oscillated with excessive gratification of other infantile needs; Sarah was not weaned from the bottle until she was almost three years old and was still sleeping with a diaper when the analysis began.

Sarah's father left the family at the mother's request when Sarah was only 21 months old. A brief reconciliation between the parents failed, and her mother moved out, leaving Sarah with her father between her 26th and 33rd months. The mother then regained custody of Sarah only to move into an apartment where Sarah was not allowed toys because they made a mess. Within a few more months they relocated again and moved in with Sarah's stepfather-to-be. The mother quickly became angry at Sarah's refusal to treat this new man in her life as if he were her father.

Sarah's presenting complaints, coupled with this history, led me to recommend analysis for what appeared to be a nascent masochistic-obsessional character neurosis.

Early and Mid Phases of Sarah's Analysis

From the beginning of the analysis Sarah amply displayed the multiple determinants of her masochistic tendencies. Separation issues were manifested from the beginning after I unexpectedly canceled our third session because of illness. What probably felt like both a repetition of her mother's inconsistency and her fears about my reaction to her aggressive play in the first two sessions led to a shift in Sarah's attitude toward me. She sat on her mother's lap and complained of feeling ill herself, instead of happily accompanying me from the waiting room to the office as she had done previously. Separation themes became a major focus of our play for the first year of the analysis, and they would emerge again at every separation for the second year also. Drive determinants of her masochism were also prominent throughout much of the analysis. Conflicts over rage were evident early in treatment, alternately being expressed in efforts at sadistic control and, more directly, when she would draw her face close to mine and spit or call me a "fuck face" or "asshole." Primal scene exposure was evident in surprisingly frank and repetitive expressions of sexual fantasies. Within the first month of the analysis Sarah requested that I remove my clothes, lie on top of her, and make love.

Defensive elements to her masochism also were exhibited. Projection, externalization, intellectualization, and reaction formation were all prominent, but a triad of related defenses played a particularly important role in Sarah's masochism. *Reversal, identification with the aggressor,* and *turning passive into active* were all exhibited by Sarah in her desperate attempts to maintain control of her emotions and her interpersonal world. Being the passive victim was turned into being the sadistic tormentor in an effort to feel actively in control of an otherwise traumatizing maternal neglect and/or sadism. My role in her many enactments was almost inevitably that of the passive, helpless child in these derivatives of the unconscious beating fantasies characteristic of masochistic children (Novick and Novick, 1987). Identification with the aggressor contributed to the harsh, punitive superego evident in Sarah's repetitive accusation during these enactments that I was "bad," "dumb," or despicable. Externalization of her superego was a particularly salient contributor to her masochism. Gradually, we realized Sarah's need to provoke criticism and punishment in order to avoid her anxiety about losing her mother's love.

Working through these conflicts and components of her masochism allowed development to resume, and oedipal aggression toward Sarah's mother became evident after two years of analysis. At home Sarah expressed her anger directly and complained that her mother was the worst possible. Continued primal scene exposure, which included seeing a videotape depicting fellatio, led to Sarah's stimulated discussions with her peers about ladies sucking on men's penises and about her older stepbrother's penis and buttocks. Competition with her mother for her stepfather's attention began; Sarah repeatedly accused her mother of trying to make her ugly or insisting that she go to brush her teeth so that Mrs. T could have the stepfather for herself. During one session I interpreted her oedipal competition through a displaced enactment. I said that the kitty (Sarah) was angry and wanted the doggy (the stepfather) to love her more than he loved the kitty's mommy. Sarah agreed with this interpretation, and the intensity of her oedipal behavior at home subsided gradually as we worked through variations on this intervention.

But anxiety over these impulses became manifest as themes of guilt and punishment emerged at home and in sessions. A new symptom appeared in which Sarah worried that her parents would run out of money because they spent so much on her. In one enactment I was to be punished by having my clothes removed. Then I was killed and my "girlfriend"—Sarah—came to grieve: This echoed my bemoaning, based on Sarah's earlier play that week about being deprived of lovemaking, that we would no longer be able to make love because I had been punished and killed. Sarah, in the role of my girlfriend, agreed that she was sad that we would no longer be able to make love.

Somatic complaints escalated during this phase of the analysis and prompted Sarah's pediatrician to request an upper GI series, which proved negative. I interpreted her problems in swallowing and her headaches as resulting from her problems thinking about (and swallowing) her sadness, guilt, or anger. One such interpretation led Sarah to attempt to provoke me by knocking over a desk chair. I said that she was trying to get me to punish her so that she did not have to feel guilty. Sarah responded that I should have people make love in my office. Then she began to rip the clothes from two dolls so that they could have intercourse. In this way she graphically linked her guilt to oedipal dynamics.

Oedipal conflicts began to be displaced to competition at school: Sarah experienced difficulty learning to read and handle numbers despite her superior intelligence. She repetitively played at being the sadistic teacher who always criticized Timmy (me) for failing to do things correctly. In one session the police were summoned because I had been so bad. Then my girlfriend spurned me in order to make love to Jonathan. Furthermore, my parents said they were leaving me because I was so mean. Finally, I was killed.

Guilt over aggression became more direct in our sessions as Sarah ordered her mother not to tell me about her accusations that her mother was bad. I said that she must worry that her mother would not love her for having such a feeling. Sarah responded that such a feeling was "mean." I said that maybe she was afraid I would not love her either. Sarah responded by asking her mother, whom she had not allowed to leave the office that particular day, why she had hit Sarah as a baby. Then Sarah was reluctant to allow her mother to leave the office. Screen memories about being beaten by her mother characterized the midphase of the analysis and helped to assuage Sarah's guilt over her oedipal aggression toward her mother.

Finally, after three years of analysis Sarah's conflicts seemed sufficiently worked through to consider termination (van Dam et al., 1975). Her defenses and affects were more balanced and flexible. She was happy much of the time and could comfortably complain to her mother when she was not getting sufficient attention. No masochistic need to provoke her mother's attacks remained evident, and Sarah's ego was far more integrated. Her school inhibitions had resolved as she worked through her oedipal conflicts, and she was progressing well. Latency defenses of repression were being deployed. Sarah, whose enactments in play had always been so affectively charged, began to color, read, and play at banal and neutral themes. Modulated use of reaction formation and intellectualization was occurring. Sarah could talk about interactions and events without being overly intellectual but also without intense affect. Neatness in her play was now the rule rather than the exception. Progressive forces were in ascendance over regressive ones. At home and in our sessions she focused primarily on developmentally appropriate themes such as peer relations, school, and athletics. She handled separations well and easily went on overnights with friends. Drive development was clearly on track with oedipal themes in ascendance over preoedipal ones in her play at home and in sessions, and Sarah was moving into latency with a marked reduction of drive derivatives in our sessions. No longer were sessions characterized by rage or manifest sexual themes. Her self-esteem was considerably improved although she remained preoccupied with her physical attractiveness. This preoccupation was also an identification with her mother's vanity, and therefore seemed, in part, to be a manifestation of her oedipal resolution. Peer relations were vastly improved, and Sarah was one of the most popular children in her class. She was able to traverse the cliques that were prominent at her prestigious private school and to have friends in rival groups without unduly provoking either rejection or competition.

Anxiety about her positive transference still occurred, so Sarah was more hostile toward me than affectionate. We had analyzed her oedipal anxieties, loyalty conflicts, and fears of abandonment as determinants of her negative transference, but I thought that we needed the opportunity to analyze her fears of abandonment once more as they were mobilized in the termination phase to finally resolve her fear of her positive feelings toward me. Thus, in agreement with Sarah's mother, whose alliance remained positive but reactive to her own conflicts, I felt that Sarah was approaching a terminal phase in treatment.

Sarah's Termination Phase

The Decision to Terminate

Sarah herself raised the question as we drew close to the third anniversary of the analysis. Our exploration of her question led her to express the wish to terminate and to acknowledge that her worries had disappeared and that our sessions interfered with other activities she wished to pursue. Sarah denied any ambivalence at this time despite my query. Consequently, I agreed with her that she seemed ready, and we negotiated a schedule of gradually reducing the frequency of sessions by deleting one session per week each month during the next six months, with Sarah exercising complete control of the frequency of sessions during the last month of the analysis. I encouraged a prolonged termination phase because Sarah's separation conflicts had been so prominent that I wanted to ensure ample time for working through, but her counterphobic tendencies also made me concerned that she might decide to terminate "tomorrow" if allowed to make the decision herself. I tried to allow her some feeling of choice by allowing her to decide the frequency of sessions after we had started meeting once a week and to choose our last session, provided that notice was given at least one session in advance.

We planned to terminate in the middle of July. Sarah's anxiety about the termination was manifested quickly and strikingly. After concluding this negotiation Sarah asked to go to the bathroom in order to clean the pierced earring holes in her earlobes so that they would not get infected. I reminded her of previous insights about her somatizing and said that worrying about her body was often a displacement from worrying about feelings. (Past work on her somatizing led me to make this general interpretation rather than pursue the content about dirty holes. More content-oriented interpretations had been less effective in illuminating her somatic preoccupations.) I went on to say that perhaps she was worried over the prospect of not seeing me. Sarah replied that she did not care about seeing me—in fact, she did not even like me. I interpreted this defense and said that not liking me allowed her not to miss me. Her counterphobic defenses escalated as she exclaimed, "I can stop whenever I want and I can walk out and stop now." I struggled to avoid being drawn into the sadomasochistic transference–countertransference interactions that had characterized an early portion of the analysis. Instead, I replied that even though the big-girl part of Sarah now felt ready to stop the analysis, the little-girl part of her remembered how unhappy and unsafe she felt when she was not the boss of saying goodbye—at those times that her mommy had left, her daddy had left, or when she had been left crying in the crib for what seemed like forever. Now she wanted to feel safe and to be the boss of when she stopped with me. Sarah put her hands over her ears in her attempt to deny the anxiety engendered by this interpretation. The session ended with her dragging out part of a box from my office to the waiting room, trying, as she had in the past, to take home things of mine in order to cope with her separation anxiety.

At the next session Sarah and her mother were discussing termination in the waiting room when I came for her. Sarah's mother was saying that she hoped Sarah could terminate the analysis before starting first grade but that she could not promise it. My own countertransference anxiety about Sarah's termination led me to ask Sarah if she had forgotten that we had decided the termination date yesterday. To my surprise, she replied that we had not discussed the issue. At that point her mother asked for the details that we had arranged; unfortunately, I summarized them instead of waiting to explore the issue with Sarah in private. Sarah burst into tears that continued even after her mother accompanied her into my office. Sarah continued to insist tearfully, ''That's not right!'' After Mrs. T returned to the waiting room, I tried to sympathize with Sarah and said that stopping the analysis was so scary that it was hard to think about and to understand. Sarah began to insist again that she could stop whenever she wanted. I pointed out how this insisting was similar to when she had been little and had tried to boss her mommy so that she could be the boss of her feelings about being away from her mommy. I said that I thought she was trying to boss me in order to be the boss of her worried feelings about saying good-bye to me. This interpretation enabled Sarah to become calm and to grasp the planned reductions in frequency. Then she asked how many days there would be between sessions when we reduced to four sessions per week. She checked the calendar so as to figure out exactly when this reduction in frequency would begin. Needless to say, I began to wonder if Sarah's dramatic reaction to the idea of terminating indicated that she was not ready for it, and I paid close attention in the weeks that followed.

The First Month of the Termination Phase

Soon Sarah began to calculate the precise number of days until we would stop seeing each other. Simultaneously, she reenacted both in her play and in the transference the sadomasochistic conflicts that had characterized the early and midphases of treatment. Thus, she became the cruel, critical teacher, and I was the ''dumb,'' inept student who was humiliated, abused, and punished. Such issues expanded to our relationship as she began to kick over furniture and to create gigantic messes in the office while trying to provoke me by insisting that I had to clean up her mess. I pointed out that she was trying to make me angry and that sometimes people start fights so that they do not have to miss the person they are leaving. She told me to shut up and called me a ''dummy.'' Sarah wanted to play hide-and-seek, a game she had used during the first 18 months of the analysis to bring her separation anxieties into our sessions. I told Sarah that sometimes people liked this game because of feelings they had. Before I could expand this interpretation, striking negation appeared as Sarah emphasized that it was *not* because she was hiding her feelings. Accepting her defense, I said that some people like the game because it feels so good to be found and to be together again after being left. The game was played repeatedly throughout that session while Sarah demonstrated her ambivalence by hiding in the same place each time, after telling me that she was hiding somewhere different. Thus, her wish to be found and her need to deny such a wish with its implications of conflict over emerging independence were both apparent.

The transferential nature of her separation anxieties and their relationship to her early experiences with her mother became clearer, since Sarah began to have trouble saying good-bye to her mother before entering my office at the beginning of sessions. For example, she began one typical session by running in and hiding behind my chair. Sarah seemed to be reenacting the separation conflicts that were evident early in the analysis. But just as I began to lament the legion of feelings about being left that she had taught me, Sarah ran out to her mother at the elevator in order to give her one more good-bye kiss. Then she returned and announced that she wanted to play hide-and-seek. I pointed out that we had been playing that game more often recently, just as she seemed to be having more trouble saying good-bye to her mother in the last several sessions. Then I added that I thought the little-girl part of her feared that her mother would not come back. An instant and reflexive denial followed. Soon I was able to add that part of her worried if she would ever see me again once treatment ended.

Similar themes were evident at home as well. Sarah began to ask her mother about the times her mother had left her when she was a baby. Problems around going to bed began, and Sarah would object and cry when she was left alone with a sitter for the evening. Still, her overall mood remained predominantly happy, her academic performance continued to improve, and Sarah seemed able to maintain an oedipal engagement, manifested in her continued preoccupation with her new "boyfriend" at school and whether he would find her pretty. The latter seemed an identification with her mother's preoccupation with appearing attractive to men and was an expression of Sarah's continued working through of oedipal conflicts.

Separation conflicts continued to be expressed in sessions through various kinds of hiding play, but anal issues around messing and sadomasochistic insistence that I clean her messes or suffer her verbal attacks began to occupy a more prominent place. In part, Sarah's provocations around messing were an externalization of her superego and the guilt she felt over her wishes to steal something of mine in order to help her cope with the impending loss of our relationship. Sarah tried to take items from the office without my knowing, as she had done during the midphase of the analysis. But her messing also seemed to be an effort to cope with the conflicts over messing that had always made her an unusually tidy child. Consequently, I began to reconstruct that she was remembering how it felt when she was little and lived with her mother in a place where she could not make any kind of mess, even while playing. I said that Sarah must have wished that she could make a mess and have her mommy allow it. Sarah instantly denied that such events had ever happened or that she had ever had such messy feelings. Nonetheless, she asked her mother about this stage of life when she was at home.

The Second Month of the Termination Phase

Taking things from my office in order to cope with separation continued, and I continued to link these actions directly to termination. My interpretations seemed indicated both by the prominence of Sarah's symptoms and her age-typical cognitive limitations with respect to time sense. For example, she greeted me in the waiting room at the beginning of one session by asking what had taken me so long. I asked if she had worried that I had forgotten her. Sarah persisted with her question of why I was late (she had, in fact, arrived early) but refused to speculate about my reasons. Instead, she tried to sneak some checkers into her backpack after she entered the office. This time I interpreted her wish to take something of mine in order to help her with her feelings about my absences, particularly the impending one wherein we would stop seeing each other. She responded by putting the checkers back and moving to hide-and-seek play in a manner that seemed a behavioral confirmation of this interpretation. Sarah then began to stuff my pants pockets with toys and told me not to look at them until she left. I interpreted that this behavior was to ensure that I would be reminded of her in her absence. Within days Sarah needed to clarify again when we would reduce the frequency of sessions. I pointed out her unusual difficulty in remembering the schedule and wondered if she felt worried about it. Sarah denied anxiety and rubbed her crayon into my carpet. Once again, in making such marks she was leaving me something permanent by which to remember her, but she also seemed to be expressing her anger at me for allowing the separations, as well as demonstrating the relationship between her separation anxieties and the sadomasochistic provocativeness that had received much analytic scrutiny during the midphase of the analysis. I continued to make interpretations along these various lines.

This revived sadomasochism began to crop up at home: Sarah's mother had to set limits on her hostile, controlling behavior at a slumber party. It also became more intense in the analysis: during one session Sarah became impatient with my difficulty grasping one of her anecdotes and complained, "Don't you listen?" She then slowly and carefully enunciated every syllable as though I were quite unable to understand her. At the end she contemptuously asked, "Got it?"

Sarah's provocations escalated. During one session she began to swing a toy phone by its cord so wildly near both our heads that I had to set a limit; I interpreted her need to see if I would still be the boss of these wild feelings. In another session Sarah continued to knock books from my shelf, shower the office with torn Kleenex, and slam the shutter doors on the closet even after I asked that she desist. Finally, I insisted that she stop and held the doors shut. An enraged Sarah marched out to her grandfather in the waiting room. I followed and reminded her that she used to behave in this angry, defiant way when she first started to see me. Then I interpreted that she was doing so again because she was worried about who would help her with her angry feelings when we stopped seeing each other. Sarah replied that she would not return to my office. I interpreted that she felt she had to control me by leaving in order to control her anger. Using the technique of avoiding a direct power struggle, which had been so essential early in the analysis, I explained that I would wait in my office and reminded her grandfather that he would have to get her to return. I saw, ruefully, that my angry delegation of responsibility for returning her to the office was a demonstration of Sarah's continuing ability to draw me into sadomasochistic enactments.

Her grandfather was able to persuade Sarah to return although she refused to talk about why she had left or how she felt about my telling her grandfather to return her. Instead, she talked about her mother, and I interpreted the displacement onto me of her anger at her mother for being away on a business trip at this time. I explained that this was why she had been so angry with me at the beginning of the session. Sarah's reaction was striking: she began to cry while desperately insisting that she was not angry with her mother. Her use of the negative transference to split her ambivalence toward her mother was clear: I was the bad, depriving object so that her mother could remain the good, loving one. Sarah's provocativeness escalated, and she called me a "butt face" while slamming the wall with a toy. I suggested that she wanted to make me angry in order to avoid feeling angry herself; that way she did not have to feel bad for her angry feelings. Sarah regained her composure as the session drew to a close. But at the next session she claimed that her mother had threatened to take her to another "worry doctor" if I were not nice. I said that she seemed worried that she had made me so mad the day before that I wanted to get rid of her and so she wanted to be the boss and get rid of me first. Sarah seemed to confirm this interpretation by pretending to call the other "worry doctor." She then acknowledged that she enjoyed making me mad.

The Third Month of the Termination Phase

Symptoms precipitated by the return of some of Sarah's sadomasochistic and separation conflicts reemerged during the third month of the termination phase; for example, her midphase fear of going to the bathroom alone surfaced again. This symptom was foreshadowed in our play during one session as Sarah climbed the bookcase and told me to pretend that I was a shark. Then she threw Kleenex into which she had blown her nose and told me to pretend it was "poop" while I ate it. In another session shortly thereafter, she hinted at having a worry but complained that I made her worries last longer when she told them to me. I acknowledged that when I put them into words they seemed to last longer to her. Then Sarah admitted that she did have a worry and that she would rather tell it to her mother than to me. This time I replied that this option must feel nice because Sarah would have her mother to help her with her worries even after she stopped seeing me. Interpretation of this defense allowed Sarah to tell me that she feared that a shark would come up behind her in the bathroom. After telling me more details, she asked me to make her a "dot-to-dot" picture. I made one of a shark. Sarah criticized the way that I had drawn the teeth and insisted that I draw another one in which she drew the teeth. In this way she tried to turn her passive fear into active mastery. When Sarah wondered why I had drawn a shark, I explained that I had drawn a picture since words seemed to make her so worried. She exclaimed, "Good idea!" and wondered if she should hang the picture in the bathroom to help make her "shark worries" disappear.

Such reemergence of symptoms corresponded with Sarah's more open acknowledgment of her anxieties about termination. Early in this third month of the termination phase she became anxious about when we would reduce the frequency again. My pointing it out on a calendar led her to exclaim, "And after that it will be one time!" Then she asked if she would see me anymore after we no longer met even one time a week. At this point I stressed that this decision was up to her. Sarah responded by asking if she could return with worries that she developed after termination, get rid of them, and leave again without having to engage in a prolonged analytic process. I emphasized, "Of course you can." Sarah relaxed visibly at this point. Efforts to explore her anxiety met resistance and a refusal to discuss the issue, perhaps because I had reassured her before exploring her question.

Within a few sessions Sarah announced that she had gotten rid of her shark worry. (I learned later from Sarah's mother that this was not so). Sarah went on to explain that she had figured out that seeing how the movie *Jaws* was made when she toured Universal Studios had caused the fear. Then she talked about the movie *Beetlejuice* and how disgusting it was.

Soon I reminded Sarah that we would reduce our frequency to three sessions beginning the following week. She demonstrated dramatically the relationship between her shark fear and separation anxieties by immediately adopting a scary voice and demanding to know what I thought. I adopted the complementary role that she had taught me in such play and quavered and said that I was scared. Sarah bellowed that she was a monster while I again emphasized my fear. At that point the monster "changed" into a great white shark. In turn, I announced my fear of the shark's teeth, which Sarah had elaborated in a previous session. Sarah responded, "I'm somebody who eats people!" Then the shark demanded my first-born child. I asked what the shark would do to it and was punished for my audacious questioning by being turned into a snake. Sarah then began to play a hiding game. At the end of the session she brought her mother into the office from the waiting room to clarify the new schedule and which days we would meet. Thus, Sarah's phobic fear seemed a reaction to her aggressive feelings about termination.

The Fourth Month of the Termination Phase

During the fourth month Sarah employed counterphobic mechanisms to deal with her fears about terminating. In one session, for example, she tried to destroy my desk blotter and told me to get a new one. Sarah seemed to be trying to master the passive experience of, and fears about, impending change by actively causing change to occur. Similarly, she began to anticipate the end of our sessions and to count off the remaining seconds: "One Mississippi, two Mississippi," and so on. But the anxiety that she was attempting to master proved disruptive: she made numerous mistakes in counting despite her precocious mathematical abilities. Similar conflicts over the termination appeared at home as she alternated between cheering at the thought of ending treatment and asking eagerly if she would see Doctor Sugarman that day.

Sarah's phobic anxieties about sharks continued, and Sarah told her mother that she now feared that the shark was in the middle of her bedroom floor at night. Finally, I was able to interpret to Sarah that she was afraid of the part of herself that wanted to gobble me up and carry me with her when we no longer saw each other. Sarah confirmed the interpretation by asking whether or not we would meet the following day. She also told her mother that she wanted to pretend that her mother was Doctor Sugarman and talk to her about her worries after we terminated. Her shark fear subsided soon after but was quickly replaced by a fear of being kidnapped. As she had done with her shark worry, Sarah requested to be allowed to work on this worry with her mother. I agreed while interpreting again her wish to ensure that she have someone to help her with her worries once we terminated. Her immediate request to take home from my office the pencils that I kept for her confirmed Sarah's anxiety about being apart from me. As her kidnapper fears evolved at home and in our sessions, it became apparent that they too were a reaction to her wish to devour me as mother in order to avoid feeling apart and worried that she would be left alone. I finally interpreted that Sarah herself was the kidnapper and wanted to kidnap both her mother and me, just as she had earlier wanted to gobble us up as a shark. Sarah retorted, "That's a dumb idea! I'm worried somebody will kidnap me." Further work on her guilt for her aggressive and competitive wishes led to the disappearance of both of these fears by the end of the month.

Her predominantly negative transference began to shift as we worked through her need to split her ambivalence toward her mother, her loyalty conflicts about caring about me, and her need to be angry with me in order to avoid the pain of losing another adult for whom she cared deeply. Signs of greater comfort with her positive feelings toward me emerged both at home and in our sessions. Thus, she told her "boyfriend" that she had been in my building lots of times as they were eating frozen yogurt at the stand next door. Sarah then asked her mother if she could bring him up to my office and introduce me to him. In a session about the same time, she leafed through a book on my shelf and asked about the pictures of pioneering analysts in it. Finally, Sarah pointed to one and said, "She's so ugly. I would never want her for my worry doctor. I'm glad I've got you."

The Fifth Month of the Termination Phase

The fifth month was heralded by Sarah's asking when we would reduce our frequency again. She wanted only an answer and refused to discuss her feelings about reducing the frequency. She then hid a book and told me that I would have to look for it all day if I could not find it. I replied that hiding it would ensure that I would then be thinking of her all day as I looked for it. More hide-and-seek play followed. I finally reconstructed that the anticipation of not seeing me any longer was bringing back the feelings that she had as a little girl when she feared that her mommy might never come back. For the first time Sarah openly acknowledged such a fear with her response that she *no longer* worried about that. An additional response to my interpretation was Sarah's asking at each session, for nearly a month, for me to remind her of what we had done most recently. I would comment that it was harder to remember now that we met less frequently, but my attempts to interpret her concerns about either of us forgetting the other after termination were ignored.

Soon a new symptom appeared when this formerly obstinate child became strikingly and suddenly indecisive at home. Sarah began to insist that her mother make all the choices. Decisions such as clothing purchases, picking a Father's Day card, and choosing a restaurant were all deferred to her mother as Sarah anticipated the need to choose when to reduce her frequency of analytic sessions to once and then "no times" a week. Finally, I interpreted that her worries about choosing at home were due to her worries about choosing how often she would see me and, finally, when to stop the analysis. Sarah retorted that I was wrong and that she would make the decision about reducing our frequency further when she went home that day. She then wanted me to choose which colors she should use in a picture she was coloring; I pointed out that she was worried again about making the wrong choice.

At the conclusion of the fifth month, we came to the session in which Sarah could choose whether to continue twice-weekly sessions or reduce the frequency of sessions to once a week. She asked what I wanted her to decide. The prominent work on her guilt over aggressive impulses that had also occupied this month led me to interpret her fear that I would regard her as bad if she chose to see me less frequently, because it was completely her choice for the first time. Sarah stated that she sometimes did not like to come to see me, but she was unable to elaborate what she disliked about it. More work on her sadomasochistic conflicts followed as she asked me if I hated anybody in my office suite. Sarah then said that she hated some kids in her class at school; she wondered if I had ever tried to kill somebody. Sarah questioned whether I thought that she was strong enough to kill somebody. I said that I did know that kids her age often felt like killing somebody and then felt bad about themselves for having such feelings. Such an interpretation, expressed in general terms, allowed Sarah to admit that she often kicked her puppy when it nipped at her and then she felt bad. During our next session she played at being a judge and sentencing me, the criminal, because I "stole a TV from the President" and "shot him in the head." This series of themes indicated both Sarah's guilt for what she viewed as the aggressive act of separating and also her need to suffer and to be punished in order to reestablish the bond with me that she anticipated losing.

The Sixth Month of the Termination Phase

Sarah's indecisiveness in the previous month had resolved after interpretation of its relation to her anxiety about choosing to terminate. But it reappeared briefly when it came to the session in which she would decide if the next one would be our last. Again Sarah asked what I wanted her to do. I said that she wondered if I wanted her to stop seeing me or not. "Right!" was Sarah's retort. I went on to say that perhaps Sarah was wondering if I cared about and loved her. If that were the case, she might worry that I did not if I said that I wanted her to stop. Sarah emphasized that she did not want me to love her, but she balked at leaving the session, prolonging her leave-taking by coloring. She then returned from the waiting room in order to clarify that she did want to stop following the next session, one week hence.

Sarah's Last Session

Sarah began the session by coloring and did not mention that it would be our last time. Therefore, I mentioned it. Sarah responded that she was glad to be stopping and wondered if I also felt that way. I said that I had two feelings: I was glad for her because she had worked hard to understand and get rid of her worries, but I was also sad because I would miss her. Using her typical denial of unpleasant affects Sarah said that she would not miss me. I responded that she must be glad because I remembered how pained she used to feel when she missed her daddy. She said that she still did miss him but would be seeing him soon. Sarah then requested that I tell her the funny things she used to do in our sessions. I reminded her of some of her earlier play. Then she remembered that she used to blame the pen for doing things and that I had believed her. She soon said, "It's doing it again," and marked my rug with the red pen. I interpreted that Sarah wanted to leave something in the office for me to remember her because she was worried that I would forget her when we stopped seeing each other. At that point Sarah began to order me around and to criticize my coloring while I remembered out loud how she used to do this when I first saw her. Soon she started to color pictures to take with her, and she requested more time when I gave her the usual five-minute warning before the end of a session. I said that I understood that she wanted more time because it was hard to say good-bye to me. After delaying for a few extra minutes Sarah requested to take home one of the toys that I had always reserved for her. I agreed to this wish, but Sarah wanted me to choose the toy. I said that I would not do so, that I thought she was still worried whether she had made the correct choice about no longer seeing me. I reminded her that she could always change her mind about coming back to see me. Sarah responded that she would come back tomorrow. I reminded her that she was leaving town the next day but said that she could see me when she returned if she wished. Sarah agreed happily to this. She discussed the matter with her mother in the waiting room in my presence. Sarah decided to wait and make an appointment when she returned from her trip to see her father. However, she never did so. When I telephoned, her mother informed me that Sarah had reconsidered the matter and said that she would see me again "in a while." At last follow-up Sarah was doing well.

Technical Issues

Sarah's termination phase raises a number of issues about termination with an early latency child. One is the setting of the termination date. As in adult analysis one can debate the value of having one party or the other set the date. In agreement with Greenson (1965) I chose to make the decision a mutual one. Once Sarah seemed ready to terminate, I decided to acknowledge her request while exploring her feelings about terminating and how we might approach that goal. But I was clearly the more active of the two in setting a specific date. Like Novick (1982), I failed to see the value of being completely passive on this point. My suggesting a process of gradual reductions in frequency and a target period for the actual termination is more in keeping with the positions of Glover (1955), Rangell (1966), and Brenner (1976), all of whom state the traditional rationales for this departure from neutrality.

But there is an additional factor unique to early latency children— their undeveloped sense of time, which affects both their subjective experience and their conceptualization. An hour—let alone a period of months—can seem like an eternity. Thus, it seems unreasonable to give these children as much responsibility for the actual setting of a date as one gives to adults. In Sarah's case, I chose a period of a few weeks during which she could choose which of the sessions would be our last as long as we had at least one session to prepare for the last one. I hoped that such a technique would allow her some sense of control and yet would also take into account the limitations of her time sense. Although I tried also to place the final session in a period that would stand on its own, as suggested by Novick (1982), and not come as the start of an otherwise planned prolonged recess (Firestein, 1978), my plans went awry. Sarah's mother provided an example of the complexities of dealing with parents when treating children. Her change of plan caused the family vacation to coincide with the prearranged termination date and interfered with Sarah's freedom to adjust that date under the terms we had agreed on.

Another technical departure from the analysis of adults, or even older children, was my decision to taper off sessions. Such a tactic is at odds with what usually is recommended for adult patients (Lipton, 1961; Kramer, 1967; Firestein, 1978). I adopted this approach for several reasons. First was the degree to which separation conflicts associated with external cumulative trauma had been a factor in Sarah's protomasochism (Sugarman, in press), which made me think that Sarah would need the advantage of a method that both weaned her and yet provided her with numerous real but shorter separations around which we could work. Children this age so easily use avoidance as a defense that presenting them with a graded series of concrete losses can be helpful in working through the final loss. Indeed, Sarah's dramatic responses to each reduction in frequency highlights the value of having given her an opportunity to work through her separation conflicts in this fashion. Another factor in the decision to taper off sessions is the tendency of children of this age to react to the impending loss of the analyst with other immature defenses (van Dam et al., 1975). The pain and pressure of the impending loss of the analyst is so vivid at this age that tapering the frequency is helpful in attenuating the resistance to final working through of the transference that can occur in such cases (Kohrman, 1969).

The final factor justifying this approach is the analyst's function as a developmental object with children of this age (van Dam et al., 1975). Accordingly, I looked for every opportunity to put Sarah's feelings about termination into words. Other issues continued to be analyzed also, but I think that termination material demonstrates how important it is for the analyst to repeatedly verbalize the child's feelings about the impending loss. The immature state of the ego and the relative problem of attaching words to abstract concepts and to emotions necessitate greater activity by the analyst. Sarah's need to deny or minimize the impact of this loss, despite her behavioral and symptomatic communication of its pain, highlights how difficult it was for her.

Despite these issues that are unique to early latency children, Sarah's termination phase was also remarkably similar to such stages in adult psychoanalysis (Firestein, 1978; Novick, 1982). She showed, for example, the dramatic symptomatic flare-up that characterizes many adult terminations (Glover, 1955; Miller, 1965; Kubie, 1968; Hurn, 1971). Clearly, my interpretation of Sarah's rekindled shark phobia and her new kidnapper phobia reflects my agreement with Ekstein that her symptoms were a "final adaptive active mastery which is the dress rehearsal for future adaptive behavior" (1965, p. 62). Thus, I interpreted Sarah's phobias as a reaction to her separation anxieties and a defensive attempt to ward off her wishes to incorporate me as mother and keep me with her always. In doing so, I concur with Novick (1982) that the patient struggles more to give up the analyst as a transference object than as a real object. In fact, I thought it was Sarah's wish to make me the omnipotent, idealized mother that promoted the loyalty conflicts that, in part, caused her to deny the positive transference.

I do not believe that such new symptoms and reemergence of previous ones indicate failure (Kubie, 1968) or insufficient working through (Miller, 1965). Sarah's symptoms during the termination phase always responded to interpretation very quickly. Even more important was Sarah's ability to maintain her developmental momentum as these symptomatic flare-ups occurred. She remained in the oedipal stage of development at home while consolidating her identification with her mother. Her self-esteem continued to be resilient and her academic performance excellent. Even during the most conflictual periods she had no problems with separations that occurred outside her home or treatment sessions. Thus, I believe the symptoms noted were due to the revival of her separation anxieties, stimulated by termination, and to her effort to once more rework and master those anxieties.

Finally, Sarah showed the common feature of again reworking conflicts previously worked through. (Some work was done on primal scene material but was omitted here for reasons of space and emphasis.) Similarly, her sadomasochistic issues were again revived and worked through. Such work focused on superego determinants, object relational ones, and drive factors. Again, Sarah used the termination phase to master these conflicts; they did not seem to indicate insufficient working through. In fact, they were far less intense than when they had first appeared and were analyzed during the early and midphases of the treatment.

In summary, the termination phase of a latency-age child has been presented in detail in order to allow for an appreciation of its phenomenology. Although certain technical features of terminating in a child of this age are unique to this developmental stage, the material suggests that the termination phase resembles, more than it differs from, the termination phase with adults. Sarah's material makes amply clear that this phase of treatment is at least as important for consolidating the gains of analysis for young children as it is for adults and that studies of the termination phase of analysis of early latency children can be as fruitful as research on this phase of adult analyses.

References

Brenner, C. (1976), *Psychoanalytic Technique and Psychic Conflict*. New York: International Universities Press.

Firestein, S. K. (1978), *Termination in Psychoanalysis*. New York: International Universities Press.

Ekstein, R. (1965), Working through and termination. *J. Amer. Psychoanal. Assn.*, 13:57–78.

Glover, E. (1955), *The Technique of Psychoanalysis*. New York: International Universities Press.

Greenson, R. R. (1965), The problem of working through. In: *Drives, Affects, and Behavior*, Vol. 2, ed. M. Schur. New York: International Universities Press, pp. 272–314.

Hurn, H. T. (1971), Toward a paradigm of the terminal phase: The current status of the terminal phase. *J. Amer. Psychoanal. Assn.*, 19:332–348.

Khan, M. (1963), The concept of cumulative trauma. *The Psychoanalytic Study of the Child*, 18:286–306. New York: International Universities Press.

Kohrman, R. (1969), Panel report: Problem of termination in child analysis. *J. Amer. Psychoanal. Assn.*, 17:191–205.

Kramer, C. (1967), Maxwell Gitelson: Analytic aphorisms. *Psychoanal. Quart.*, 36:260–270.

Kubie, L. S. (1968), Unsolved problems in the resolution of the transference. *Psychoanal. Quart.*, 37:331–352.

Lipton, S. (1961), The last hour. *J. Amer. Psychoanal. Assn.*, 9:325–330.

Miller, I. (1965), On the return of symptoms in the terminal phase of psychoanalysis. *Internat. J. Psycho-Anal.*, 45:487–501.

Novick, J. (1982), Termination: Themes and issues. *Psychoanal. Inq.*, 2:329–365.

Novick, K. K. & Novick, J. (1987), The essence of masochism. *The Psychoanalytic Study of the Child*, 42:353–384. New Haven, CT: Yale University Press.

Rangell, L. (1966), An overview of the ending of an analysis. In: *Psychoanalysis in the Americas*, ed. R. E. Litman. New York: International Universities Press, pp. 141–173.

Sugarman, A. (in press), Developmental antecedents of masochism: Vignettes from the analysis of a three-year-old girl. *Internat. J. Psycho-Anal.*

van Dam, H., Heinicke, C. M. & Shane, M. (1975), On termination in child analysis. *The Psychoanalytic Study of the Child*, 30:443–474. New Haven, CT: Yale University Press.

Midlatency

As Calvin Haber describes him, Stanley began to talk of "endings" after four years of an analysis in which his gender-identity symptom was reorganized. Interpretations and reconstructions were made in the context of Stanley's rich, productive enactments in play; and although he rejected or denied many of the interventions offered, he clearly processed the material and the effects of interventions were patent in subsequent sessions. After some negotiation about a date for ending treatment, and an initially joyous reaction, Stanley responded to the setting of a specific time as if he had been presented with a threat: the castration anxiety that had been so prominent earlier in treatment reemerged. In spite of renewed anxiety, his masculine self-representation remained stable, and vulnerability to narcissistic injury replaced the earlier cross-gender defense. As Stanley's negative oedipal conflicts were analyzed within the transference, he developed a comfortable relationship with his father. Age-appropriate developmental conflicts emerged as early struggles were worked through. Stanley's remembering his presenting symptoms and contrasting them with his current level of function, and his ambivalent feelings about leaving his analyst were prominent at the time that his treatment ended. Haber's follow-up material is included.

In chapter 3, Remi Gonzalez discusses Paul, who at nine had been in analysis for nearly three years. His five-month termination phase began with his expressing ambivalence over separating from his analyst and his longing to be remembered. At that time, his parents were in the midst of divorce proceedings.

Paul's aggressive, destructive behavior at the onset of treatment had found targets in those around him, while simultaneously he was plagued by obsessive fears, sleep disturbances, and learning difficulties. When the destructive impulses emerged within the transference during the termination phase, they responded at once to interpretation. As the analysis drew to a close, Paul was able to verbalize his love for his analyst and acknowledge the analyst's maternal role in his feelings and fantasies. Paul worked through his intense fears of abandonment within the transference and was relieved of the defensive aggressive stance which had led earlier to his social isolation.

Both Stanley and Paul denied much of what was presented in the form of interventions, yet the material was apprehended, comprehended, processed, and this was reflected in their subsequent play enactments and direct interchanges with the analyst. The significance of this necessary defense cannot be underestimated, since it can induce countertransference feelings of withdrawal and boredom, and otherwise rich clinical material may be cast to oblivion. The denial of interpretations in mid-latency represents, in part, reaction-formation. Additionally, the latency child wants to exhibit mastery, the interpretation may induce a sense of loss, and dismissing this perceived intrusion serves a protective function, for the moment.

In chapter 15, Paulina Kernberg describes the termination phase of an eight-year-old, James, whose experience with ending analysis provides useful comparative material.

2

The Reorganization of a Cross-Gender Symptom

Calvin H. Haber

*"Well, I did a lot of writing, playing, and a
lot of screwing and unscrewing, remember?"*

The focus of this chapter is the fate of the gender symptom in a
latency-age boy as well as the development and conflict in the
termination phase of his analysis (Haber, 1989, in press), which
occurred in the fifth year of treatment, at age eight. Material from a
follow-up is included; the last visit took place when the boy was 11
years 10 months of age.

Course of the Analysis

Stanley was brought for evaluation at three years nine months
because of his persistent desire to cross-dress and play with dolls
and carriages. Stanley's parents first observed this behavior when
Stanley was two and a half. Some time later Stanley became
indignant when a friend accused him of being a girl because he
played Cinderella. This accusation, and Stanley's reaction to it,
precipitated the referral.

Stanley suffered from chronic ear problems, which persisted
through the time of evaluation. Allergic in origin, they required
injections, which involved forcible restraint by his mother, grandmother, and pediatrician, from the time Stanley was six months old.
At 21 months toilet training failed; at about the same time, Stanley
was weaned from the bottle. A second toilet training attempt failed
during a period in which Stanley showed fear and withdrawal

which seemed to be related to the fact that his uncle wore a cast following a motorcycle accident. A few months later Stanley reacted in a similar way when his grandfather, who lived in the house, was required to wear a postsurgical bandage over an eye. At two and a half Stanley demonstrated a recurrence of fear and withdrawal when his uncle had another operation. Nevertheless, toilet training was successfully completed at this time; upright urination occurred shortly thereafter. Stanley was removed from the parental bedroom to his own room four months prior to the initial consultation.

Stanley's parents and maternal grandparents resided in a single-family home. His mother was the dominant force and was prone to fierce temper tantrums. She acknowledged feeling isolated in her family of origin; she had two brothers, one older and one younger. During childhood she had wished for a younger sister and confessed that she would have preferred a daughter to Stanley. Father, a quiet man, immersed himself in home improvement activities during his free time. He played little or no overt role in Stanley's life and appeared intimidated by his wife's personality and temper.

The grandmother was an active, vital working woman in her early sixties who was supportive of her daughter. Grandfather died of cardiac problems when Stanley was three. His health began to deteriorate when Stanley was two and a half, and this caused a disruption in their close relationship. Stanley showed profound changes when his grandfather exhibited gradually failing health and died: he became silent and lost interest in play, and he became alienated from the Church because "God didn't allow [him] to visit or phone Grandfather in heaven."

Stanley's separation problem became apparent when he was enrolled in nursery school. A wish for relief from his acute anxiety promoted his eagerness to meet me; the consultation, when Stanley was three years nine months, coincided with his visit to nursery school.

Stanley was a tall, blond, unsmiling child who insisted that his mother be present during sessions for the first months of the analysis. He ignored me. When I said he might be afraid because he thought I was like the doctors who took care of his grandfather, Stanley abruptly left the consultation room with an anguished scream.

Initially, Stanley's play centered on a series of famous, powerful heroines, including Princess Diana and Wonder Woman. This was followed by scenes in which a woman was rescued by a man and thus protected from a monster. Another theme was one of moving and relocating to a different home.

Stanley enacted a scene of oral genital sex in doll play. When he repeatedly referred to me as ugly or an idiot and chased me, in play, into the cold, I complained that he didn't like me because I am a man and perhaps he would prefer a lady analyst.

Stanley's parents reported that while he was in nursery school, he was unable to socialize. At home he exhibited temper tantrums and tended to be obstinate and cranky. During sessions he intentionally spilled water, became angry with me, and left the room. I interpreted his efforts to overturn furniture by referring to his anger and lonely feelings when he was forced to leave his parents' bedroom.

During the first year of treatment Stanley reacted in an analytic session to his parents' first vacation away from him by playing a game in which I was to sit silent and alone in an apartment. I connected my loneliness with how he must have felt when his parents were on vacation. His demeaning view of me I interpreted as a response to my being male: if Stanley didn't want to be alone, he pretended to be a girl, and this was enacted during his analytic hours. During one such session he said my office was a girl's office and I could leave. My name became "Ugly." He presented a scene in which the boy doll died and he was left with a Barbie doll. I interpreted his feeling that boys seemed to be dying all the time. He recalled the boy doll from death. The death was connected to his ultimate fear of losing his mother. Moving from a passive to an active defense, he assumed a female role and took loving care of the doll. Temper tantrums seemed to be a partial identification with his mother, whose temper outbursts he had experienced since early childhood. His mother reported to me that she had had such attacks particularly during Stanley's first years, when he had to go to the pediatrician or when her brother had a motorcycle accident. At such times she felt severe stress. Stanley seemed to be using identification with the aggressor and denial of gender difference to allay his fear of separation and loss.

His rapprochement phase, including weaning and toilet training, had been complicated by his uncle's motorcycle accident (and recuperation) and his mother's reaction to it. Stanley repeated some of his reactions to these events in a session during which he spilled water, directed anger toward me, and left me in the consultation room alone.

Stanley's solution to his dilemma seemed to be in identifying with his sister, who was favored by mother. He admired her cheerleader outfit and her baton. He admired and mimicked her music, favorite color, and clothing. I interpreted his wish to be his mother's favorite and added that he had loved his grandfather and was so sad that grandfather had become sick and died. Stanley felt contemptuous of his older brother, who vociferously interfered with and criticized Stanley's cross-gender tendencies. (Yet, during baths, Stanley proudly declared to his mother how large his penis was.)

A superficial paper cut sustained in a session led to my learning that Stanley had a Band-Aid phobia, which began with the uncle's motorcycle injury when Stanley was two and a half. I interpreted the link between his fear of injuries to himself and his uncle's accident, and the Band-Aid phobia disappeared.

Stanley refused to deal with an anticipated tonsillectomy until I suggested that we write a book about it. He expressed his fantasy by drawing a "pretend girl" who didn't like sickness or medicine. Subsequent "books" revealed fantasies in which he appears as a girl, as well as fantasies about his genitals, gender differences, and details of internal genital structures.

During the first half of the analysis we analyzed derivatives of cross-gender symptoms that were understood as defenses against a fear of death and the danger of losing mother. Other issues in the analysis included Stanley's use of denial of gender in fantasy, identification with the aggressor, and shifting from passivity to activity to defend against his fear of his mother when he went to the doctor for injections. He accepted my suggestion that he played at being a girl because he wanted a special relationship with his mother. He appeared to have a fantasy that injuries and death occurred only to males and so it was safer to be a girl.

Oral-phase derivatives emerged in the analysis when Stanley ordered me to eat and drink immediately or else he would take meals away from me. He understood my interpretation that he thought the person who was in charge of food was the most powerful. Anal phase derivatives were observed in the spilling and messing following an angry tirade and exit from the consultation room. He used gender denial, reversal, and identification with the aggressor to punish the analyst instead of being punished himself for losing bowel and urine control, and he pretended to be a powerful superheroine.

The analysis of Stanley's play with dolls revealed that he had probably observed his uncle and future aunt make love when they were his babysitters. On the basis of my observations of Stanley's doll play, I suggested to him that he may have felt uncertain about who was on top and who was on the bottom and who was the boy and who was the girl. He responded by enacting a scene in which he was a millionairess who had several husbands who promptly died.

When I interpreted that he felt "boys died all over the place like his grandfather and grandfather's brother" but he never knew a girl who died, he replied, "I don't want to have a fifth husband." He didn't allow the fourth husband to die and made loud, passionate love to him.

Stanley revealed his masturbatory fantasies after he stopped pretending to be a girl outside of sessions. He imagined scenes in which beautiful women were desired by men. At my suggestion, I played a reporter and he a TV star. During the interview, he said that he had switch fantasies. Ordinarily, he would not share this information with me because it was too embarrassing, but under the circumstances of the interview he did so with hesitation. He revealed that he imagined kissing men if he liked them. He preferred tall, dark, and handsome men. Stanley imagined that, as a girl, he was "pretty, 3'3", gentle, and reasonable." Sexual excitement appeared to accompany his fantasies. In reply to a question he acknowledged that his penis became hard when he was in the company of men who didn't wear a shirt.

During the fourth year a theme emerged in Stanley's fantasy play in which men died but women who were in danger were saved by a fearless man. After further analysis Stanley began to talk about his fears of dying. Oedipal themes of males who were in combat with each other and sustained physical injuries also became prominent. He ended the year by playing at being a girl who was in love with a strong, handsome boy. I suggested that he wanted to steal strength from such a boy. His wish to hide his masculine strivings out of fear of dying or being injured was interpreted many times from various vantage points.

During some sessions Stanley was the teacher and I was told to take the part of the student. I was assigned the role of the student who wanted to be perfect for fear that the teacher would become wild, scream, and break things, as Stanley's mother had done in the past. In the play I stated that I was afraid of being a boy lest I be hurt and die; Stanley offered me solace and told me that he would help me with my worries.

During the fourth year, when cross-gender switching was less frequent, male fantasies emerged within three themes. In fantasies with a medical theme Stanley was a male doctor (when he felt secure); at other times he was a nurse. A second theme involved a detective who rescued a wealthy woman to whom he made love. The last theme involved a rich architect who consorted with royalty and presidents.

The Termination Phase

Child analysis is a tripartite arrangement (Abrams, 1978) among parents, patient, and analyst. At termination it is useful if all parties are in agreement, yet this is sometimes difficult to achieve. Stanley, at eight, expressed interest in termination by asking about "endings," at the conclusion of a session. Thus, he defended against his anxiety over stopping treatment by communicating his interest at the end of a session. Two months later he again mentioned "endings," this time at the start of a session, and added that perhaps he could finish by the end of the year. This was followed by Stanley's playing the role of a science teacher who had left his school the preceding year. When the doorbell at my office rang unexpectedly, the session was interrupted, and I answered the door. Stanley attempted to lock me out of the consultation room. I interpreted his behavior as a wish to lock himself in and me out at a time when he was concerned about endings. This led to further work on his fears of life without his analyst.

In the following session Stanley took the part of a teacher who forced his students to work by threatening to cancel their play time. In play, an earthquake struck and Stanley was transformed into a student who had a teacher who flung computers at him. He sought haven in a bomb shelter and developed an attack of vertigo. The thought of stopping treatment seemed to have precipitated this internal upheaval. I offered a genetic reconstructive interpretation that paralleled the play and said that he must be afraid of the teacher now as he was afraid of his mother when she threw dishes and left the house. (It was when his mother had outbursts of temper that Stanley had first enacted being a girl.) Stanley disagreed with my comment and denied its relevance by commenting that his parents were strangled to death by California snakes. Referring to Stanley's talk about endings at that time, I said that during the last couple of days he seemed to feel that dangers were coming and I wondered if he feared that I might die. He said that he wished I would die. "But it wouldn't happen," he reassured himself. This transference attitude seemed to be the current version of an earlier transference in which abandonment and castration were reenacted when he threw dishes, spilled water, and left me in the waiting room. However, in the earlier instance the transference was accompanied by cross-gender fantasies and behavior. Stanley's thinking about termination precipitated a yet unanalyzed aspect of the transference. During the earlier transference I had interpreted his fear that he or his mother would die and linked it to his identifying with her by the defensive use of cross-gender behavior and denying in fantasy his masculine strivings. In this instance, after an interval in which Stanley twirled rapidly on the ottoman, appearing preoccupied, I said, "Sometimes a boy gets a boner and then it gets soft and then the boy worries his penis is almost disappearing." Stanley made a comment about the date, confirming my suspicion that he was thinking of the time, and denied worrying about "those things" (his penis falling off).

Stanley's parents reported during the Christmas vacation that he was doing well at home, in school, and socially. I indicated that termination might be worthy of consideration and that we had made significant progress in Stanley's analysis. I emphasized that it would be best if I were to discuss this matter directly with Stanley. The parents and I had a good working relationship, and they agreed to this suggestion. During the last session of the year, in a nostalgic mood, Stanley reviewed various drawings and writings he had done since starting analysis. He observed that a girl he had drawn when he was five years old had bags under her eyes—it was a portrait of himself as a girl. I commented that he was looking into his past. He answered, "I was a baby when I wrote the hospital book," implying that matters were different now. He was remembering and working through conflicts, activities for which an ample termination phase provides an opportunity. Stanley was signaling that he felt he had changed since the start of the analysis, and he appeared to be expressing an opinion concerning his readiness to end.

Stanley began the first session of the new year by observing that I had a new calendar. His next thought was in the form of a question. "Could this be my last day?" he asked as he gazed at the calendar. I asked if we could talk about it. After Stanley asked what I thought, I told him that if this were the last day, we would have little time to talk about his feelings about the ending. He said, "Okay, then let's make it February." I said that February was when I had a vacation that could take time away from our scheduled meetings. He looked at the calendar and wondered about stopping about the time of Easter vacation. He chose April as a time to stop, and I pointed to April 30 on the calendar as one possibility. He looked at it and said that was fine, that "April 30th is only a short way off," and he appeared satisfied. "Let's make that up," he said, and then went on to describe his feelings: "It seems like the Army when you get discharged." The importance of the date, which was four months hence, gave impetus to the next fantasy play. After examining several pages of his drawings, from age five, he said, "If you're having trouble with your sexual life, you can tell people to come to Dr. Stanley." Stanley thought he ought to get a medal on April 30th and walked out into the waiting room. He jubilantly told his mother about the date, and she replied, "Great!" Returning to the playroom Stanley stopped to look at a picture he had drawn three years earlier. It depicted a very tall nurse. He said it was disgusting and closed the book. Reaction formation, a typical latency defense, had become prominent.

When the hypothetical end of treatment became an actual calendar date, Stanley's ego responded as if he had been presented with a threat. Mounting aggression was manifested in subsequent sessions by generals, wars, and the most violent act—the assassination of presidents. Negative oedipal themes provided a vehicle for Stanley's struggles with aggression. Sometimes Stanley pretended to be the analyst. Anxiety and aggression became prominent, and in his play he transformed himself into a robber killer to defend against his own death. While I was robbed, he was to take the active position and steal my attaché case (phallus).

As a latency-age child who was in his fifth year of analysis, Stanley was ready to listen to interpretations that link aggression to the fear of being alone in the posttermination period. I asked, "Do you think you're playing a powerful man because you think someone has to die, and does that frighten you?" He said he wasn't going to die. However, his intense pressure to purchase one of my puppet monkeys from me with money from his "piggy bank" betrayed fears of his existence after the ending of treatment. I interpreted that he might feel he needed something of mine to keep after he leaves.

Stanley had been very attached to a soft blanket that he gradually gave up as he entered latency; at the same time, he began to play with the furry monkey in my toy cabinet. He had shown no interest in the monkey for more than a year, but the impact of termination revived this separation issue and his interest in the monkey. When I interpreted his interest, I reminded him of his blanket as well as his fears of leaving me.

Themes in Stanley's play of body integrity, phallic pride, and vulnerability in relation to separation and termination were expressed in fantasies of internal genitals and associated with preoedipal issues that coincided with his shifting identification from his mother (Greenson, 1968; Kestenberg, 1975; Mahler, Pine, and Bergman, 1975) to his father.

A countertransference issue at this point emerged when I considered postponing the date so that we could deal with this material. My recognition of my own feelings and my understanding of their various sources permitted me to proceed with termination at the pace set by Stanley.

The effect of analysis of the earlier intrapsychic conflicts and the consequences of interpretation could be seen in the terminal phase of Stanley's analysis, when there was a reorganization of the earlier compromise formation under the impact of developmental progression. For Stanley, a pre-latency-age child at the start of treatment, the cross-gender symptom was manifested by a need to play superheroines. Now, the positive oedipal compromise formation seemed to be manifested by a replacement of the superwoman with a superman. A sequence of play included the following scenario: The doctor–murderer Stanley, a male version of the TV sleuth Angela Lansbury, was threatened with death from a fire in a building that had only one exit, which led to a terrace that would cause death by freezing. A shoot-out occurred and Stanley again stole my attaché case. Then I became the sleuth that Stanley seemed to want to discover that he had a desire to kill father and get mother. The next day Stanley played a succession of powerful men: a movie director, an oil tycoon, the President, and the richest man in the world.

Stanley was saying, in effect, that with my super-phallus he might be able to leave as an intact boy. His sense of masculinity was not sufficiently consolidated for him to wish to be an "ordinary" male like his father, grandfather, and uncle, who must all have appeared weak to him. This theme crystallized even more clearly when I interpreted his castration anxiety and said, "You still have a worry that if you become a strong, powerful boy, there's a danger that your penis will be taken." Confirming my interpretation, Stanley talked of a movie about alligators living in the sewers and then coming out. I replied that a person can worry that an alligator can bite a penis off. He agreed and jumped on my desk.

During the pre-latency period, Stanley had shared his bedtime masturbatory thoughts with me. In a session in the termination phase he talked about his bedtime ritual. When I asked him what his night thoughts were before he fell asleep, he avoided the question and created a fantasy during the session. In the fantasy he was a writer and his father was the detective who investigated the period in which dinosaurs invaded the planet Earth. Doors and windows slammed open and shut, with sparks flying. "Spitballs" shot around and touched a telephone, which precipitated an earthquake. This implied, I thought, that following termination of the analysis Stanley might join forces with his father and rely on father and father's phallus to protect him from his mother's aggression. His identification with his father and men seemed to persist in the face of termination anxiety with a positive oedipal theme. The dinosaurs could invade and penetrate Mother Earth and cause a quaking orgasm.

The impact of termination permits deeper internal conflicts to emerge and to be interpreted. Maintaining the same frequency of sessions each week until the final week provided Stanley with the opportunity he needed to deal with his conflicts, transference issues, and fantasies about ending treatment. A termination phase of adequate duration can give the analyst an opportunity to follow those aspects of personality change that led to the determination that the time was appropriate for setting a termination date. It also offers an opportunity for continuing further work with issues that require further resolution. Two months prior to termination Stanley's parents reported that he became impatient, particularly at school, if he were unable to grasp a concept immediately. This impatience was related to his vulnerability to narcissistic injury, revived somewhat during our work on issues of termination, and to his experience with multiple illnesses during infancy. Into the matrix of narcissistic vulnerability was woven a series of psychic traumas involving his dying grandfather, his accident-prone uncle, and his emotionally distant father. These experiences appeared to lead to the development of low self-esteem, a collapsing sense of masculinity, and meager self-confidence. Acquiring a sense of boyhood seemed to stimulate in Stanley a need to be perfect. The cross-gender symptom appeared early in the analysis and seemed to be replaced by narcissistic vulnerability, providing a new outcome. In one instance, Stanley recited a report to his teacher; when the class laughed, he left the classroom in tears. Stanley was upset because he thought the teacher had laughed at him. In this instance, the phallic aggressive woman was present in the form of the teacher and he defended against the narcissistic injuries by leaving the classroom. Stanley sobbed during this session and related how "mean" his mother was that she forced him to return to school. During subsequent sessions he became tearful as he reluctantly related the incident. I linked his feelings of humiliation in response to the female teacher to similar feelings from his mother's bursts of yelling and cursing. He replied that his mother yelled and used to hit when it was unnecessary. Now, he said, "she gets in a bad mood but doesn't hit." We worked through earlier issues and linked Stanley's reaction to his mother's anger and withdrawal of approval to his feelings of insult and humiliation in the classroom situation. This was obviously an area that required further working through and the termination phase provided the opportunity for this.

In a later session Stanley played a game in which he made a phone call to the police and reported a tornado. He told them that everything was "A-OK." The former cross-gender compromise did not emerge.

At one point during one phase of play, Stanley threw keys in the air, caught them, and said, "I can hypnotize someone." He attempted to hypnotize me and seemed somewhat disappointed that I had not fallen into a real trance, only a pretend one. I responded, "You'd like to keep me under your spell and that would make you feel very powerful because sometimes you don't feel so strong and you're under the control of someone else. This way, you turn it around and make me feel like the helpless one and you're the one in power." He agreed. The use of reversal and turning passivity into activity defended against the anxiety in his trial at masculine identity. Reworking of his gains and consolidation of his identity were taking place during this phase and were evidenced by the shifting contents of Stanley's personal drawer in the playroom. It now contained two pistols and a telephone. Gone were the Barbie dolls, pots, pans, and necklaces. A powerful man, who was at times a thief, had emerged. This was yet another reorganization of the gender symptom. The powerful male burglar was a compromise formation of conflicted self-representations that defended against fears of abandonment and body damage.

Stanley seemed to be more conforming. The female representation in play did not share equally with the male self-representation, as it had earlier in the analysis. A female imago more typical for a latency-age boy was present; it differed from the pre-latency period when the strong Wonder Woman capably apprehended male wrong-doers.

With further work the gender conflict evolved into one between a gentler woman and a powerful but "bad" man. Both affected the image of the omniscient mother, but "she" represented intellect and "he" was characterized by violence. Stanley had a nightmare in which he was awakened by his sister, who uses "half [his] closet space because [he] has so few clothes." In his associations, his masculine self-representation had yielded to his female self-representation, since to be masculine leads to a conflict succinctly abbreviated by an impoverished male versus a wealthy female.

As a prelatency child, Stanley had avoided his father and had shown a disdain for him, an attitude that, at termination, was replaced with an eagerness to be with his father. A relaxed relationship developed between them, which led to Stanley's developing an interest in life insurance (a defense against the death wish) and asking his father questions, such as the amount of his current policies. Earlier, Stanley had shown no interest in his father, yet he now asked if he could join his father in going to work. Drive neutralization and sublimation seemed to accelerate, and death wishes were deflected into increasing curiosity and intellectual functioning. Narcissistic derivatives of the oedipal complex re-emerged. A cross-gender compromise did not develop, and a masculine gender position, albeit tenuous, was maintained. His relationship with his father was one that Stanley would need for a stable masculine identification following termination. He then would have a satisfactory male figure to incorporate as he progressed into adolescence, when he might consolidate a sense of masculinity and heterosexual orientation.

Stanley obviously wanted a farewell celebration: in play he made a number of calls to various florists, explaining that we were going to have a big party. He told each florist that he had an infinite number of dollars. He defensively had to leave me with a powerful money phallus. His grandiosity expanded to include fantasies of General MacArthur and Governor Rockefeller. This appeared to be a reorganization of the superheroine cross-gender symptom. The party turned out to be a fake—a costume party. This was analogous to his earliest play as Wonder Woman. In the version during the terminal phase, a girl gate-crasher was forced to leave, suggesting that his former self-representation no longer had its earlier significance. As she left, however, which symbolized his leaving the analytic situation, Mr. Death ran in. In a soft voice I wondered aloud if he were afraid. He replied that he was not and immediately enacted a scene of major warfare. Stanley was busy trying to get rid of Mr. Death, a reference to his own termination anxiety. It took a tremendous effort for him to heave Mr. Death out; that finally occurred when a security guard (the analyst) employed a "hypermodern disintegration gun." At this point the question of his returning to visit the analyst after treatment ended appeared in a fascinating manner. Stanley asked what "homonyms" were. He offered the example of *desert*, "to be left alone," and *dessert*, "food served at the end of a meal." I replied that he might feel that I was deserting him on the final day of our meeting together. He disagreed and said deserting to him meant that people were *leaving one another* and *he* might come back to see me once in a while. In the next session he defended against anxiety by trying to imagine life without me. He talked about the year 2012 when the planet Earth would run out of room and people would live in space. This population, whom he referred to as "infinity people," would not have to worry about endings.

An example of how Stanley's working through an earlier conflict led to a version of intrapsychic conflict that was more relevant to his current latency phase follows: Stanley screamed at me to end this talk about being hurt by the teacher, and almost knocked over the furniture. He then said, "Don't be mad at me." He repeated this particular comment, "Don't be mad at me," to two teachers, and it appeared to be inappropriate to the classroom situation. (He had not done anything for which the teachers might be mad at him, but obviously he felt he had.) "Don't be mad" seemed to be, at one level, a defense against the phallic aggressive mother that appeared in the transference. It also could be viewed as a harsh superego attitude that seemed to appear at this particular time but had not been evident earlier, since the pre-latency superego had not developed adequately.

I offered an interpretation, linking his fears of my being angry with him to his fear of his mother. Stanley agreed and in his fantasy play his defenses shifted. He moved from a passive to an active stance and identified with the aggressor when he said that he wanted to be the teacher and I would be the student. We observe here another reorganization of the gender symptom: earlier in treatment Stanley would have regressed to become a superheroine, but in this instance the transformation that took place was not one of cross-gender. Instead, there was a reversal, and he wanted me to be the student. I offered what, technically, might be referred to as a "role reversal interpretation." Stanley became critical of me, yelled, cursed, and threw me out of the classroom. I (as the student) told him that he hurt, disapproved of, and treated me badly. Then I said, "I remember when my mother used to yell, curse, and throw dishes and leave the house in anger. I was afraid she would kill me." He yelled at me for another period of time. Finally, from a superego stance, I said to Stanley, "It's so hard for me because I want to be a good boy. I want to be a smart boy, and this teacher doesn't let me feel that way, just like my mother." This particular facet of his narcissistic conflict and harsh superego attitude seemed to require attention.

Masturbatory conflict was prominent in our talk of ending treatment. Stanley told a story about two "hoola girls" who were "doing it" with an old man. This comment was Stanley's first overt reference to sexuality. He revealed a secret when I asked him if he watched the Playboy channel. He told a story about adoption, which he explained as "when a family gives you away." I replied, "Sometimes a child thinks his family will give him away if they discover he watches the Playboy channel and touches his penis." Somewhat later I mentioned to him that this leads a child to want to be perfect in school and to worry that the teacher might criticize him. He didn't disagree, and revealed the circumstances that led to his watching the channel at his friend's house, since his parents have theirs locked.

The next week, exciting play revolved around a volcano blowing up with lava pouring out. After admitting he had seen an X-rated film on television, Stanley spoke of his fear of being discovered as he looked at a *Playboy* magazine. During the volcanic play, everyone died. I connected the death with the X-rated film and the excitement of observing people having sex. He listened quietly. After a few subsequent interventions I suggested that he might be afraid that his volcano would erupt at night. Stanley responded to this comment by enacting a scene in which people thought he was a mad killer and he was imprisoned. He didn't disagree when I said that he worries when he touches his penis and thinks his mother will discover it and think he's a madman. World destruction fantasies emerged. He reluctantly related the nightmare of the preceding night after having reassured himself that his mother couldn't hear and I wouldn't tell her. It was about the world and capital cities being attacked by a small country. Stanley awakened at the moment that guards chased him into the water, where he swam for 25 years and ate only shark meat. At that point his mother had come into his room because he was crying. She thought he was upset because he was returning to school after the winter vacation. His fear that his mother would learn about his masturbation was represented in his associations to the nightmare: Stanley feared that if his mother learned of his secretive activities, he would be banished, and the fear was elaborated into a world destruction fantasy.

Verification of my tentative assumptions about the castrating woman occurred when Stanley began the next session in the waiting room by asking his mother for his pistol. In his play the good G.I. Joe and the evil Cobra interacted; Cobra was beaten in the presence of a woman. This suggested a fantasy in which Stanley acquired the phallus from the woman and succeeded in the end. However, the woman still had the capacity to make him feel vulnerable to humiliation.

The forbidden topic of masturbation and the overt sexuality of *Playboy* and films that portrayed explicit sexual behavior was an aspect of Stanley's early- to mid-latency development. However, he seemed more willing to share his secrets and accept interpretations during the termination phase.

The sexual theme was followed by a story that revealed increasing castration anxiety. In the story a married woman fell into an alligator pit. Her son arranged the funeral. I said, "You're worried that father and son can argue, which leads to thoughts of dying and may have to do with thoughts you have when you touch your penis." He denied worrying about his father. During the next session he switched the waiting room lights on and off. Since they were controlled by a switch in the consultation room, he appeared to want to annoy his mother, who was waiting for him. When I said he worried that his mother would be angry if she discovered his secrets and might even take what he owned, he smiled and replied, "She'll reach into my pants and rip it off." In this instance, we can observe an identification with the analytic work and a progression in the capacity for self-observation and interpretation.

During the termination phase negative oedipal issues reemerged and were reinterpreted and worked through. In one game Stanley used my initialed desk paperweight as a magical object that gave him many powers, including the capacity to leave earth to travel the "forest of feeling which is somewhere in space." I offered an interpretation: "Maybe you want to have my magic paperweight to protect you from having your penis cut off, especially if you feel you are banished from here when you leave." He asked me for my magnifying glass and became a sleuth, a role that represented power to him.

Three weeks before our final meeting Stanley played a game in which he was a rich doctor who gave a patient a physical examination. Then he told a story: "One day I was sitting in front of my big [musical] organ with all my patients. I played the organ with my hands and then my feet." I said he was proud of his organ and liked playing with it but was afraid "you know who" would find out. He changed the game and helped a man with a heart attack. In each case he seemed to deepen his awareness of the relationship between his masturbation, his castration anxiety, and his fears of the phallic woman. The sequence of his turning to the man seemed to help him to sustain and stabilize his male self-representation. The reorganized gender symptom remained gender-appropriate.

As he helped the heart attack victim, I asked if the man were dying because his mother had discovered him. He said, "Maybe," thus demonstrating his continuing fear of his mother's power over him. Progression in development was suggested during the next session, in which Stanley pretended to be a busy doctor who had won a Nobel Prize and was honored by an audience with the President. He agreed when I said he's not afraid to be a bigger doctor than I. The cross-gender symptom was transformed from a super-heroine to a superscientist, an identification with the analyst but one that still required super powers. Stanley no longer felt that he needed the Wonder Woman's lasso, as he had earlier in the analysis, but he did look for sources of magic power, such as a paperweight to help him hold onto his gender-appropriate stance as he left the safety of the analytic situation.

The transference theme that repeated itself was the wish to rob, or acquire in some way, aspects of the analyst to carry him safely through the perils of being alone. The repetitiveness seemed to enhance further progression of gender development without the cross-gender defense. In one play sequence Stanley took the role of a man who supervised women and tossed utensils. This was a latency version of a pre-latency experience in which his mother had yelled, thrown utensils, and left the house. I said, "Instead of being afraid that you play with your penis, you change things around and place yourself in charge and no girl bothers you." He then dueled with a woman called "Joan Collins." A wild fracas ensued, and in the midst of it he stood on a chair, looked at my diploma for a few quiet seconds, and proclaimed, "Zeus, the God, the only God, gave me the power to command Joan Collins' death." This fantasy had two components. At that time gender development had progressed to the point that Stanley was capable of utilizing the man to enhance his growing sense of masculine identity. Also, we might view the death of Joan Collins as a shift from the pre-latency self-representation, in which masculinity and femininity are equal to one in which the male position is more prominent.

Two weeks prior to termination, Stanley gave some clues concerning his wish to be like, or be, his sister. This was a significant pre-latency position. He noted that a pair of glasses looked like his sister's and placed them back in the drawer. Then he picked up a pair of high-tech glasses and said he wanted to have something of mine when he leaves. The pre-latency cross-gender fantasy surfaced briefly and was replaced by a male gender identification. It seemed that Stanley needed my glasses to defend against the reemergence of the sister/female representation that was so well entrenched during the first half of the analysis. He seemed to reluctantly relinquish his wish to be his mother's favorite child—his sister.

Oedipal rivalry and castration anxiety re-emerged when he rolled up three papers, taped them, and called them diplomas. I said they looked like three penises. He said that he would be good and France is free. He shot a prince, his father, or his best friend. He left to go to the bathroom to blow his nose and returned, pulling up his zipper. I said thoughts about wanting to shoot his dad got him upset so he wanted to be sure that everything was okay down there. It appears that Stanley was using this vignette to reveal his anxious feelings and associated fantasies about the future after the end of treatment. Preconsciously, he played out his fears and allowed me the chance to deal with his anxiety of having an appropriate gender identity.

Stanley began his final session with a request for an appointment three or four months hence. I told him that I would be available and that he could ask his mother or father to make an appointment for him. Robbers then appeared in his fantasy play, and I said it seemed as if he felt that I was being stolen from him. Memories from age three emerged. Stanley's earliest male identification was his grandfather, who lived with Stanley's family. The grandfather died after several months, and shortly thereafter the family dog, "Happy," died. At the time, Stanley defended against this loss by saying that Happy and grandfather would keep each other company in heaven. This was linked in associations to his present dog, Muffin, who was small compared to his large old dog, Happy. I reminded him that when Happy died he thought his grandfather would have company. I then said, "You told me that you loved and missed your Popup." He replied, "I know and I loved Happy too. He was a big dog. Muffin is a small dog. Muffin is fun too." He appeared to be anticipating my departure from his life. The loss, the sadness, was rekindled, as was the mastery. Stanley invented a game, a contemporary version of one of his earliest at age four. He turned over the furniture and played tornado. The "twister" could injure him so he protected himself. Another person was trapped. Themes of losing an organ and an object appeared. I said, "When you were a little boy, Grandfather and Happy died and it was like a tornado that overturned furniture and your life at that time."

Then Stanley related a fantasy: he awoke in 1864 as a rich Abe Lincoln. Nostalgically, he mentioned that this was the last time he would see this room. He recalled that he had first met me at age three or four and that he had wanted to be a girl. On the evening following our final meeting a family celebration was to take place. Stanley said good-bye to my sculptures of Helios and Freud. He reminisced and said, "Well, I did a lot of writing, playing, and a lot of screwing and unscrewing. Remember?" He was referring to the period when his masculinity was budding in the form of a tentative identification with his father and he used my screwdriver to loosen and tighten screws in the office furniture. He talked of school and his early wish to be a girl; "But not anymore," he said. When we parted he seemed to be aware that although he felt a sadness in leaving and saying good-bye, there was also joy in being able to anticipate a promising future. Stanley asked to see me after termination. I was curious to learn if developmental progression would proceed unencumbered. An unexpected event was his mother's separation reaction to his ending treatment. She was eager to have the security of knowing that I would be there for Stanley if need be (Glenn, Sabot, and Bernstein, 1978). She wanted to know if we could arrange appointments now for the future. I suggested that we talk from time to time on the telephone, leaving it open whether I would see Stanley.

Follow-Up

Stanley requested an appointment to see me four months after the analysis ended. When he arrived he checked the drawer in which his play materials had been stored, and he observed minor changes in the office. He blushed as he reviewed a book that he had written at about age five, prior to his hospitalization for a tonsillectomy. He spoke of his current activities and seemed to have a sense of self-confidence in coming and going on his own initiative. I saw Stanley again at age 10; he was rather quiet and reflective on that occasion and again made a "customs inspection" of my office. Stanley moved from passivity to activity when he felt anxious, and there was no trace of cross-gender defense. At 11 years 6 months Stanley asked his mother to make an appointment with me. Apparently, a problem had arisen in school when he left the building without permission. The principal sent him to the school psychologist. He explained the circumstances of his leaving the building, and she asked to see him again. He politely refused and told her he had his own analyst, whom he once saw four times a week, and would prefer a visit with him. The psychologist did not believe him and subsequently checked with his mother, who confirmed Stanley's statement. He came to the office and related the problem with a sense of confidence and poise. (He appeared to be as comfortable in the office as he had been during his analysis.) He related that he had been part of a five-person team that had worked on an art project. One of the members, Tom, purposely spilled paint on the project in anger because he had splattered paint on his shirt. Stanley was furious that the efforts of the team were in vain and that Tom's behavior might cause them to receive a poor grade. He said it was unfair and told the teacher what occurred. Tom turned out to be a tough youngster with friends who threatened Stanley. Stanley was afraid and so he abruptly decided to leave school at noontime. He thought that to stay would place him in danger of not only fighting Tom, with whom he might be able to hold his own, but also his cronies. By the time of the appointment the threatened problem had receded owing to the intervention of the teacher, and he was now on speaking terms with Tom.

During that session I learned that Stanley went with a girl, Christina, who left him during Christmas and began to spend time with Tom. I asked Stanley if he thought that might be one of the reasons he was mad at Tom, aside from Tom's ruining the project. He didn't disagree. Then he spoke about people in his classes. He noticed the children in school didn't seem to stay friends. "They're on and off." He talked about a child who was teased, so I asked him if that ever happened to him. He said that sometimes the kids call him "brain." Turning to another interest, Stanley said his class was involved in one-act plays. He was assigned the lead, which led him to think that he might be interested in the theater.

At age 12 years 3 months, Stanley's mother reported that there were some indications of what girls meant to him. He seemed to be developing an active interest in girls during the past two months and spoke of pretty girls. On one occasion he commented that a girl was "growing boobs" and that another had great legs.

Stanley's mother reported that he has an amnesia for the analysis prior to the second grade. He told the school psychologist, as he told me when he was 11, that his problem had been a bad temper, and he recalled turning over a school desk in anger during the second grade. At 11 Stanley's areas of interest were numerous, and he had many avocations and belonged to many school clubs. One of them was the literary club, and his mother reported that he was busy writing a book but had not shared the contents with the family. His career plans vacillated, as might be expected during this phase of development. At that time, Stanley said he was interested in being an architect, a prominent fantasy during the terminal phase of his treatment. I met with Stanley for the last time three years, three months after termination, when he was 11 years 10 months. At that time he appeared slightly overweight. He mentioned spontaneously that he had four best friends and talked a little bit about each. He belonged to several clubs but decided to drop the science club because he disliked the teacher. He did not plan to go to camp that summer but wanted to go to work with his father instead. He likes a girl called Sally, he said, although he used to like Katy. Sally said she liked him. Generally, he explained, he doesn't like girls from Sally's neighborhood because they appear to be snobs. He mentioned some favorite TV programs, including "Murphy Brown," told me some gossip about the sexual activities of teachers, and admitted that he doesn't like gym and avoids it when he can. He proudly announced that he now has a color TV in his room. He'd like to be an actor, he said, and is currently a lead player in a school production. He'd like to be a Clark Gable who could do everything and be "cool."

Discussion

Gender development and the fate of the cross-gender symptom were discernible in the terminal phase of Stanley's analysis. In the reorganization of the compromise formation, the superheroine became a superhero. In Stanley's fantasies only a man whom he considered powerful (a president, general, or millionaire) could withstand the aggressive, phallic woman, who at times evoked images of abandonment and castration. During the terminal phase the analyst was the powerful man whom Stanley feared losing. Stanley's identification was patent in his enactment of scenes in which he was a doctor who dealt with sexual problems. Stanley's lingering doubts about maintaining his gains were expressed in his wanting an object that belonged to his analyst to take with him—a medal, a toy monkey, or an attaché case. This fearfulness appeared to reflect the incompleteness of his male self-representation. He seemed to feel that he had to depend on another man in order to stabilize his masculine representation. Legitimacy and a sense of confidence in his newfound sense of masculinity were not yet secure. For Stanley, the termination phase presented an opportunity to define and revise aspects of the transference neurosis. Stanley's asking to purchase my stuffed monkey appeared to be an attempt to individuate and separate from his female object world (mother, grandmother, sister). He wanted to leave with something of mine that he did not have to steal—a transitional object. At the same time, his interest in his father and brother was heightened. The brother's interest in World War II and soldiers was a link to Stanley's failed identification with the grandfather who had died when he was 3. Stanley's real relationship with his father began during the analysis.

Analytic material suggested two interacting lines of development—female gender identification and separation–individuation—with the progression of the former being most sensitive to the progression of the latter. Stanley started analysis during an acute state of separation anxiety, when he began nursery school. During termination a recrudescence of this stage occurred in the transference. At issue was his fear of loss, which could be defended against either by a reidentification with mother or an advance in separation from mother. He was desperate and attempted to purchase a displaced transference object (a furry toy monkey) from me.

Stealing a phallus (attaché case) and associating my gender with my profession represented for Stanley a break in the female gender identification and coincided with the simultaneous availability of father, brother, and uncle. Stanley's bedtime masturbatory fantasies suggested an alliance with his father during the dinosaur invasion of planet Earth. Stanley moved from intensely disliking his brother to becoming interested in him and emulating him. Following work in which the analyst represented the brother in the transference, Stanley's brother seemed to provide the means for a reidentification with the grandfather, whom Stanley barely remembered during mid-latency. Although the role of the analyst would become increasingly less prominent and ultimately fade, both brother and father were available to provide Stanley with the figures he needed for continuing male identification.

Progressive gender development appears to be an undulating variable in a child's life. Stability of the masculine representation of the self may be vulnerable and dependent on the stabilization and parity of the female and male self-representations, as well as on the quality and resolution of the conflicts with the representations of the female object world. In Stanley's case aggressive scenes of death and desertion were very much in evidence during the termination phase, and Stanley offered a solution: he might have to return to visit me after termination. This was a natural request for Stanley, who had used the analyst as a figure for identification, and he reasonably imagined that he might require the analyst's presence in the future.

Stanley eagerly came to follow-up sessions. He requested one session when he was in an oedipal rivalry with a boy who had an interest in the same girl. A posttermination compromise formation occurred. He remained gender-stable but defended against his fears of rivalry by making an appointment to discuss his concerns. Thus, he attempted to rejoin forces with the fantasied male superdoctor who respected his right to have a phallus and a growing sense of masculinity. Stanley indicated the direction of his sexual drives in his interest in the female body. Nevertheless, the future of Stanley's gender sense, which is the flourishing, personal experience of feeling masculine throughout life, is still prone to the vicissitudes of adolescent developmental conflict. Disidentifying from female imagos and identification with males can advance and stabilize only after episodes of conflict, gender progression, regression, and resolution that will be confronted again during adolescence.

References

Abrams, S. (1978), Termination in child analysis. In: *Child Analysis and Therapy*, ed. J. Glenn. New York: Aronson, pp. 451–469.

Glenn, J., Sabot, L.M. & Bernstein, I. (1978), The role of the parents in child analysis. In: *Child Analysis and Therapy*, ed. J. Glenn. New York: Aronson, pp. 421–423.

Greenson, R.R. (1968), Dis-identifying from mother: Its special importance for the boy. *Internat. J. Psycho-Anal.*, 49:370–374.

Haber, C. (1989), A three-year, nine-month-old boy with a gender identity disorder. *Assn. Child Psychoanal. Newsltr.*,   :19–20.

_____ (in press), The psychoanalytic treatment of a preschool boy with a gender identity disorder. *J. Amer. Psychoanal. Assn.*

Kestenberg, J. (1975), *Children and Parents*. New York: Aronson.

Mahler, M., Pine, F. & Bergman, A. (1975), *The Psychological Birth of the Human Infant*. New York: Basic Books.

3

Termination in a Midlatency Boy

Remigio G. Gonzalez

"I'll write my name in the cement."

An evaluation of a child's readiness to end treatment that is determined by a multiple-aspect view (Van Dam, Heinicke, and Shane, 1975, p. 445) using Anna Freud's (1962, p. 151) developmental profile is, I have found, most useful in that attention is focused on all areas of functioning. This was the approach used in evaluating the patient in the case that follows as well as in determining his readiness to terminate therapy.

Background

Paul entered analysis when he was six years two months old, and his treatment ended 3⅓ years later when he was nine and a half. He had been in a once-a-week treatment for a year prior to his being referred for analysis. Paul's parents, who were both in therapy, were concerned about his long-standing history of hostility, aggression, and destructive behavior, manifested earlier by biting and later by hitting. The aggressive, disruptive behavior first appeared when Paul went to nursery school at about the time of the birth of his younger brother. After some concerted effort both at home and in school, his aggressive behavior diminished. At three Paul had speech therapy because of problems with articulation. He related well to the therapist, who was firm but empathic. This therapy lasted until the summer of his fourth birthday when Paul became negativistic and demanding of the teacher's attention and reencountered difficulties with other children because of his wish to be in control. Also, he would become enraged when his demands were not met immediately. The teacher, feeling frustrated and powerless in dealing with him, suggested psychological evaluation.

Psychological testing revealed superior intellectual endowment but poor impulse and emotional control as well as a "definite developmental lag." Paul's explanation for his physical attacks was that he had two brains and the one that controlled his muscles was not working. Just before he came to analysis and while in weekly psychotherapy, he reverted to episodes of baby talk, was preoccupied with wars and weapons, and feared that his mother would die while he was on vacation with his father. These fears and regressive behaviors occurred after his parents separated and were seriously considering divorce. Further psychological testing at five years seven months revealed Paul's verbal intelligence quotient to be in the very superior range while his performance level was at the lower end of average. Paul's parents were dissatisfied with his progress in treatment, and his therapist agreed that once-a-week sessions were inadequate.

In addition to his aggressive behavior, especially toward his brother, against whom he launched constant verbal and physical attacks, Paul was preoccupied with wars and weapons, was unable to learn, and had sleep disturbances. He had obsessive fears that he was a failure and incapable of competing with his peers (because he "couldn't even catch a ball"), that he would be injured, and that his parents would die. He had nightmares in which he was being attacked by monsters and was in danger of being killed because of his "badness." In waking life his fantasies were quite active and manifested similar concerns. Paul also lied but insisted that he was just making up stories, thus denying the importance of his actions.

History

Paul was born five years after his parents' marriage and was described as a wanted child. His brother was born when Paul was two and a half. Both parents were in their early 30s and both were in treatment in their attempt to better understand themselves, save their marriage, and learn how best to cope with Paul's behavior. With much guilt they admitted that discipline had been inconsistent; Paul's father, especially, believed that inconsistency had contributed greatly to his son's problems. Paul's mother felt more competent and was capable of performing her duties but seemed lacking in warmth; she would rely on intellectual explanations while engaging in acceptable contact such as holding and kissing the children, but with limited affect.

Paul, who weighed eight pounds at birth, suffered from respiratory distress syndrome and was placed in an incubator for his first 36 hours. There were no subsequent problems in infancy. A tonsillectomy and adenoidectomy were done when Paul was three because of repeated bouts of upper respiratory infections and otitis media.

Paul was breast-fed until four months, when he was switched to the bottle. No feeding problems were reported. Weaning took place uneventfully at about 12 months. Toilet training was not a problem, according to his mother, although there were some accidents when his brother was born. This was the time when Paul became obstinate, angry, and aggressive. The parents recognized, in retrospect, that there had been significant sibling rivalry.

Paul's mother tended to minimize his problems, emphasizing his verbal skills at an early age as well as his ability with numbers. She seemed to attach little importance to his earlier articulation problems but was concerned about his reverting to baby talk just prior to his entering analytic treatment. At the same time, both parents noted that despite his aggressive, demanding behavior Paul could be affectionate and likable, especially with his mother.

Paul's father was a caring person who experienced a great deal of anxiety about his own adequacy; he was concerned about being an appropriate role model for his sons. He was very supportive of his son's therapy, although he was in constant search of a magical solution because of his own conflicts.

Paul became a vegetarian at four, at the height of his aggressive behavior and his repeated monster dreams, because he could not bear the idea of animals being killed and eaten. His phallic strivings were evident, and his erotic interests became apparent by his giggling at the sight of pictures of nude women and his constant search for magazines with explicitly sexual pictures. He was also interested in entering his parents' bed. Just before his analysis began, Paul would try to enter the bathroom or bedroom while his mother dressed. He was fascinated by breasts. His mother discouraged him, explaining why it was not proper, but at the same time she was pleased by his interest. This seductiveness was both stimulating and confusing to Paul. His mother was afraid of his experiencing her as rejecting because of her own personal experiences and because of separations from her husband in the past.

Assessment

The significant environmental influences evident at the beginning of Paul's analysis included the birth of his brother when he was two and a half, a tonsillectomy and adenoidectomy at age three, an atmosphere of seductiveness and a lack of deeply felt positive emotion albeit from well-intentioned parents, parental conflicts in the marriage resulting in several separations, and the parents' need for Paul to fulfill some of their real or imagined inadequacies, that is, their need for Paul to be a superintellect.

In my developmental assessment of his libidinal strivings, Paul was in the phallic-oedipal phase, with clear indications of regressive moves to both oral and anal-sadistic levels. His vegetarianism, for instance, represented a defense against regressive cannibalistic and sadistic fantasies. His ritualistic counting and messiness pointed to behavior characteristic of the anal phase. There was also evidence of defensive ego regression secondary to extreme castration anxiety: his baby talk. At the same time, his self appeared to be fairly well cathected although he needed frequent reassurance and lacked self-esteem and, consequently, a firm sense of well-being. Paul engaged in a great deal of aggressive behavior, both verbal and physical, and this aggression was directed at the object world, not at the self.

The Analysis

At first Paul exhibited no major resistances to coming to his sessions. He readily separated from his mother. He was initially anxious, however. He would want to know how much time was left in the session, and he would try to bargain with me about the frequency of the sessions because they interfered with his favorite television programs. He also reminded me that his previous therapist saw him once a week, and he thought I should do likewise. Typically, Paul was neatly dressed and brought his own toys, reminding me that *his* were better than *mine*—while mine were better than those of his previous doctor. He was very curious about all things related to me and concerned about the potential danger I represented.

After a brief initial period of careful, passive scrutiny, Paul's aggressive play took prominence, and he engaged in battle games and car-crashes. He enacted struggles in which the Japanese and German armies fought the American army, and he orchestrated card games in which he would have to cheat in order to win. Occasionally, he would give me some cards to keep me happy and interested. When I commented on his representing the Japanese or the German (bully, bad guy) and his wish to win, he would sometimes stop and tell me that this was not true; at other times he remained silent. Paul dealt with his anxiety and fear about my anticipated retaliation by assuring me (and himself) that he liked my beard better than his father's. Although there was evidence of much sadism in his play, castration was his principal concern. On one occasion he told me to set up the armies. When I wondered why he was ordering me around, he became furious and destroyed them, telling me that he had better soldiers and better guns. Other games followed, accompanied by fantastic stories. When I said that they sounded to me like dreams, he answered angrily, "Do I have to interrupt my card playing to tell you about my dreams?" This was followed immediately by his telling me a fantasy of "crawling monsters that can get all over you." I wondered what they did when they crawled like that, and he said with extreme anxiety, "They bite off your wiener because it itched" and made a masturbatory gesture, adding that a friend of his had a habit of scratching his penis. As his castration anxiety and his masturbatory guilt were interpreted, he became pensive and said he had no such concerns. But he soon acknowledged after some thinking, "You are right."

This was the culmination of prior episodes of play in which much castration anxiety was exhibited but during which I had refrained from explicit interpretation, feeling that such intervention was not timely. Soon after the episode just described, Paul's anxiety noticeably decreased and his frequent trips to the bathroom during the session practically ceased.

Up to this point Paul had not been interested in doing anything with pencil and paper and his mother was reporting that his work in school was sporadic. He had difficulty concentrating and caused frequent class disruptions, so that his teacher questioned his ability to continue in her class. In addition to avoiding his work, he bullied smaller children. The teacher wondered if he should be placed on medication in order to control his "hyperactivity," aggressivity, and apparent inability to concentrate. After six months of analysis, Paul's classroom behavior improved, and his parents indicated that he was easier to manage at home. His father thought he was friendlier, and they began to go places together. I felt that this represented an example of symptom relief secondary to a decrease in castration anxiety and that further structural change was required for defensive equilibrium to be maintained.

With his anxiety level lowered, Paul was able to draw and write and took much pleasure in these activities. The drawings involved air battles in which the Red Baron was playing havoc with enemy planes and anti-aircraft guns. In other drawings there were battle scenes between Japanese, German, and American armies. Paul gave me the opportunity to participate in his games, but in the end I was usually the loser. It was clear that in the transference I represented the ambivalently feared father figure whom he tried to please. Paul contrasted me with his father, and he would remind me of all the things he liked about me.

Soon Paul's constant physical activity diminished, and he no longer threw objects—which sometimes barely missed me—about the playroom. He wished only to play cards and checkers and did not care to tell me what he was thinking. He wanted to feel that he was in complete control. In trying to understand this change I realized that the stalemate, at least in part, was due to my wish to avoid the turmoil that had characterized the previous months of treatment. Paul's restful, quiet behavior was ego-syntonic with my desire for a respite from the earlier high level of aggression and conflict.

Once I examined this material and became more active in dealing with the resistance by avoiding accommodating to Paul's requests for me to engage in games in which I was forced to remain passive, the conflict reappeared. Paul was preoccupied with being defensively protective of his parents and of his analyst in the transference, for he was about to move to a new house and a new school; Paul did not wish to move and feared that his rage would become uncontrollable. For the first time he was able to connect his anger with his feelings. He cried in anger, expressed sadness, and wanted to sit very close to me. We were then able to explore his feelings concerning separation, abandonment, his parents' separation, and his sense of guilt. He was able to experience much sadness and deal with it appropriately. As Paul's defensiveness diminished, his ability to experience genuine feelings enabled him to feel less conflict and have a happier summer, camping with his father and being able to make significant friendships for the first time. His mother was especially pleased that he was now invited to spend the night at friends' houses, and these visits were reciprocated. This was quite a contrast, she thought, to the time when no mother in the neighborhood would allow her children to come to their house. She also reported a further decrease in Paul's aggressive games and in his overt expression of sibling rivalry.

To the surprise of his parents, Paul adjusted well to the new school although he experienced considerable anxiety at first. He was able to make friends but felt inadequate academically. He would bring books to his sessions and was ashamed that he could not write to his satisfaction. When I pointed out the similarities between his feelings during analytic sessions and his feelings at school, Paul disagreed, saying that what he learned in his sessions was about what bothered him in his head. Then he mentioned that he did not want to agree with everything I said, as he did with his mother and his teacher.

When his dog died, Paul became quite angry and displaced much of his frustration for his feelings of impotence onto his father for having failed to take the dog to the veterinarian early enough to save his life. This loss, among other things, served to revive his feelings about his grandmother's death, which occurred early in the analysis, and his parents' separation, and it helped in focusing on his treatment and my function in it.

Why did he come to see me? He felt that it was because of his use of foul language and because he was bad. At that time Paul was not yet able to connect the multiple losses with his rage and his aggressive behavior. The relationship between various events in his life, his feelings, and his behavior were gently interpreted. He was attentive and pensive but did not comment. This issue was explored over several sessions, utilizing his anger and concern about his dog as the point of departure. He could understand that the dog was sick, but he could not understand his dying. He was particularly disturbed by a sense of helplessness and frustration and by his resulting anger. Paul was also able to talk about his fears and his feelings of helplessness. He said, "I am just a little boy; I can't do everything." This was, in part, a response to the fantasy that he could and should "fix everything."

With continued interpretations of Paul's aggression within the transference, he became friendlier and more considerate, saying that he did not wish to get completely well because if he did, he would have to leave me and he did not want to do that. There was also a change in the nature of his games; he was now concerned with rules and cheating, thus showing the emergence of the superego striving more typical of a mid-latency boy. When he lost a tooth during one of his sessions and became quite concerned about it, we had another opportunity to deal with his castration anxiety, which, in this instance, occurred without the defensive helpless rage and aggressivity that had characterized his earlier responses.

After a year and a half of analysis, it was clear that the main transference was one in which I represented a nurturing aspect of mother. His father was trying hard to fulfill the paternal role but was still having many problems in feeling adequate to the task. His mother was now much more emotionally available and capable of setting limits without inducing in Paul a sense of rejection. It was obvious that the nature of Paul's object relations was also changing and that there was a beginning fusion of libidinal and aggressive drives as well as the emergence of sublimatory activity. Paul was also capable of differentiating between the analyst as transference object and real objects, and he could think of himself as a boy with some degree of independence. His ego function demonstrated a fair degree of integration. Although his ability to learn was still below his potential, he felt more competent and his teacher was pleased with his progress.

Paul had by now been in analysis for two years and was gradually better able to understand how his mind functioned so that at times he would say, "I know what it means; you don't have to tell me." He was also much more aware of his feelings toward me, and he understood his displacement of feelings from me to his parents. While his parents were on a short vacation trip, he willingly, though not happily, stayed with his grandparents. He said he was angry with them and with most of his family, and knowing that I was going to be away for a week soon after their return, he said that he was unhappy with me for also leaving him. This marked a specific shift in behavior in which Paul demonstrated verbalization instead of acting out; in the past he had been unable to show open displeasure with me, fearing retaliation.

Paul was aware that in the past, and obviously to a degree in the present, he experienced ambivalent feelings toward both his parents and me and feared being punished or abandoned as a result. His ambivalence was clear on one occasion when he was kissing my tie while quite unconsciously stepping on my toes. At other times he would embrace me affectionately as he came into the session while laughingly telling me how he would like to shoot me. When I pointed out the discrepancy, Paul claimed that he was just joking. At other times he would draw people carrying knives, guns, and other weapons. Once he drew his father holding a pocket knife, which he said would not be very dangerous; he wondered if I had a gun. On an earlier occasion, he tried to kick me in the genitals and threatened to cut off my penis. After multiple repetitions of this theme and my interpretations of their meaning he would teasingly laugh, saying that he knew what his behavior was all about. I said that he was making light of it but that I thought he was having some serious thoughts about hurting and getting hurt and that he had to laugh about it because it was too scary. While he was aware of the accuracy of what I said (I learned later), he became furious and, using some foul language, let me know that he thought I was crazy; then he began to pick up some small toy cars that I thought he might use as missiles, but he restrained himself. (Earlier in the analysis he would not only throw them but would angrily step on them in an effort to destroy them.) After a while he dropped the cars and said that he did have angry thoughts but did not want to hurt anybody, especially me.

After 2⅓ years of analysis Paul was most pleased with his sessions and was making drawings of his family, his friends, and me; these were real attempts to capture the likeness of the persons rather than the grotesque unrecognizable figures of the past. Earlier, for instance, during a period of drawing birds he drew a mother figure that looked like one of Picasso's productions of the middle twenties when, following the failure of his marriage to Olga, his women figures were depicted with distorted sawlike mouths and unrecognizable heads and bodies. One of Paul's drawings depicted a woman with glasses and large breasts who he initially insisted was just a girl; eventually, we came to understand that she was a mother. Since these mother figures at first had large umbilici, they provided an opportunity to explore Paul's castration anxiety in relation to the phallic mother. He said with much anxiety and laughter that these were girls before they lost their penises. I suspected that the large breasts represented powerful penises, but my allusion to such a possibility met with his denial of such a connection. Paul liked breasts because they were "beautiful." He was also continuing to bring books with stories that he could now read by himself, wanting to know what I thought about them. He was willing to share his fantasies and his stories, so we were able to deal with his drive derivatives. For a long time there was a fantasy about an invincible Japanese general who could always beat the Americans due to his ability, knowledge, and cleverness, as well as his superior strength. As the analysis progressed the general's endowments (as well as those of his father and his analyst) became less fantastic and his feats were more realistic. Something similar happened to the battles between Japanese, Germans, and Americans.

For months Paul brought a sack of "precious stones" to the sessions. He was involved in the collection of objects, and these stones were among his favorite possessions.

Paul was now able to use fantasy actively and to employ symbols in order to discharge, control, and manage his drives. Paul's progress in resolving his neurotic fixations and conflicts could be seen not only in the process of working them through in the transference, which led to the diminution of symptoms, but also in indications of his ability to resume progressive development. It was clear that Paul had moved fully into latency. He had become increasingly objective about his relationship to his primary objects, was able to establish friendships within his peer group, and could relate to his teachers less as parents whom he needed to both please and fear.

Paul's parents were pleased with his progress although they were not insisting on termination, since they wished to feel certain that his gains were permanent. I was not aware of whether his parents were speaking of termination in his presence, but Paul himself was thinking of an approaching end, since he no longer felt "sick." "I can figure things out now," he said. At one level he was happy because he would have more time for other activities, but he also wished to keep me; maybe he could "come back once in a while," he suggested, spontaneously voicing his concern about no longer having his sessions. He was now relaxed and able to freely talk about what was in his "brain" without fear of retaliation or embarrassment. Paul's gains in his general level of functioning and evidence of structural change gave me the impression that, although he was not completely free of neurotic conflict, he was developmentally on track. My concern was his potential for continued progressive development once the analysis ended.

In our work together Paul continued to deal with his feelings and behavior at school, where he now felt part of the group but was still very competitive with other children, particularly older boys. At home Paul still got into arguments with his brother, whom he characterized as a "pest," and was punished periodically for verbally abusing him. He reported a dream in which he had gone on vacation and did not think about me at all, so that on his return he forgot to come back. He had been consciously thinking about going on his summer vacation and was quite excited about it. When I suggested that perhaps he was thinking that soon we would not see each other, he became quite sad and wondered if other children would take his belongings if he left anything in my office. Several hours later he said that he was not ready to stop because he had gotten into a fight at school with a "mean big guy" who kicked him and made him cry. Paul thought he was lucky that he did not get hurt. Again we explored his anxiety and sadness about terminating. This was followed by his having an argument with his father about the vacation; Paul was not sure he wanted to go where they had previously planned to go. It was an "okay argument," he said; he was not scared to death, because his father was now reasonable. We talked about my speaking with his parents about stopping his therapy. He agreed that we should tell them, but he wanted to do it first.

Termination Phase

It was agreed that termination would take place after the vacation so that we would have five months left to work. I spoke about the idea of stopping, and Paul said his parents had talked with him about it. He was not sure he wanted to end his therapy although, he said, it would be fun to be like other boys, who did not have to interrupt their play to go to the doctor. He wanted to know if he could stay longer if he had problems. I wondered if he were concerned that I would be unhappy with him for wishing to stop and would therefore forget him. He said he would not forget me and would keep in touch. Then he added, "I tell you what; I'll write my name in the cement up front. I did that once by the bus stop and it's still there." Paul was concerned about the stability of his family, since his parents were living apart and were in the process of getting a divorce. Analysis had provided not only a place to explore his feelings but also a safe haven. He rejected the idea that he was worried when I alluded to his concern about family stability but soon admitted that "it was a little worrisome." He proceeded to talk about the home situation as much to reassure himself as to convince me that there was no peril.

Paul's school performance, although not superior, except in subjects that especially interested him, was acceptable and there was no question that he would be promoted. He was now talking about friends, including girls, and wishing he could have a girlfriend; he and a good friend were sometimes spending nights at each other's house. Paul wondered how it would be when he did not have to come anymore. His friend didn't understand why he came anyway, Paul reported, but then "he didn't know about (his) troubles of long ago." All of this was said with much sadness as he sat on the playroom floor facing me.

Paul's parents reported that he was coping well at school and seemed to enjoy his friends. His father felt that it was now possible to reason with Paul while his mother felt that he now behaved in an age-appropriate manner. She summarized it by saying that he was "generally more loving."

Paul now wondered if I would give him a present when he stopped. He had been angry, he admitted, at my not having done so on various occasions in the past. He reminded me, as he had done before, that his previous therapists had always given him presents. Paul became quite angry when I wondered why he wanted one. He said, "Oh no, not again," in disgust. "We've talked about that before. I just *like* presents; you *could* give me one." He still needed to imagine that I was very rich and powerful, perhaps even more so than his father, and my not giving him a present was still incomprehensible to him. I said that perhaps he wanted to be reassured that I liked him and would not forget him. He "knew" that I would not forget him, he replied. He was visibly angry and would not address the issue further. However, in the next hour he asked if he could take some of his drawings home. He had been in the habit of leaving most of them in my office, some as "presents" for me and the rest for safekeeping. Further exploration made it clear to Paul that, at least in part, his wish for a present and his taking the drawings home had to do with his need to have something of mine in order to feel secure and loved. "It would be like having something to share," he said.

Neutrality and abstinence puzzled Paul but, at the same time, once an analytic process was established and under the guidance of his observing ego, he was pleased that I did not make decisions for him. He was able to verbalize both his murderous rage and his warm feelings for me. The therapeutic alliance was good despite his threats that he was not coming back because I was mean and did not understand.

Termination was now being discussed by both patient and analyst. When Paul returned from vacation, he said he had thought about me and wondered if I would recognize him when I saw him again. I said that perhaps he was worried about my forgetting him. Paul became pensive and denied such worries but then admitted his fear that I would become more interested in my other patients. It was obvious that the separation during the vacation had resulted in the resurgence of considerable anxiety. My attempt at helping him deal with the impending separation was only partially successful. Paul's aggressive behavior, both verbal and physical, recurred. He reverted to using foul language while throwing toys about the playroom, some coming close to hitting me. He would break and smash things by "accident" so that on more than one occasion I had to gently restrain him as I interpreted his anger and rage, relating them to his fears of rejection and abandonment.

Paul's reaction to my interventions during these outbursts of aggressive behavior was different from those occurring earlier in the analysis. Now he responded by altering his behavior, frequently he was able to calm down within a brief period of time, either talking about his thoughts or playing quietly.

With three months left until the ending date Paul came in one day and, although quite calm, reported having had some difficulties with his father; they had had a fight because he had been mean to his brother, and his father had punished him. This was reassuring to him because his father was now able to set limits and enforce rules. Paul had not physically abused his brother, as he had frequently done in the past, but he had refused to share his belongings and had called him demeaning names. He added that he understood he had done the wrong thing and had later apologized to both his father and brother and they were no longer angry with him. To my surprise he proceeded to recapitulate the work of the analysis in terms of his past behavior. He said, "I am pretty happy now, but I remember when I used to bite when I was three and Dr. L (his first therapist) couldn't stand me. I used to be all mixed up." Then he recalled how he used to stir anger in his father by talking about the Nazis and the Japanese, especially when he said that General Nacamura was so powerful and could make mincemeat of the American army. Then he spoke about his fights. Now he was not "confused;" he was "not sick anymore."

This was followed by his telling me more about his vacation; he was obviously experiencing separation concerns. And then he said, "I passed to the fourth grade, and I am a little worried about it." I wondered if he was also worried about how he was going to manage when he no longer came to his sessions. He agreed but went back to the comforting thought that he could come back if necessary. Since the termination date was set he had had several episodes of confrontational behavior at home and some encounters with his friends, but his overall behavior remained manageable.

Paul's confrontational behavior in the sessions of the termination phase was well controlled. Throwing things about would seldom occur now, but he would try to cheat me "a little" when he played cards, especially when he had difficulty in sharing his feelings with me. Once, after losing a card game, he angrily threw the cards to the floor and threatened to beat me up. When I related his anger to issues of termination and control, he said I was an "ass" and that I was "no doctor." I was the kind of doctor who always said that things meant the opposite. "I bet," he said, "if I say carrot, you say tomato"; he then demanded to know if I liked him. He said he wanted to be bad so he would have to continue to come and wondered if I wanted to get rid of him. Following this he asked, "Did anybody ever try to beat you up?" I said that he was unhappy about the fact that soon we would stop seeing each other. He simply said, "I really didn't mean to lose control." The session was about to end, and Paul proceeded to put his shoes on; he said, "See you Monday" as he was leaving.

In the next session Paul told me he loved me and was not sure he wanted to get well because it meant having to leave me and he did not wish to do that. Later in the same hour he spoke of his troubles with his mother, who, he said, was being very strict and unreasonable. I felt that the anger had been displaced onto me and tried to clarify the issue with him. Paul claimed that neither his mother nor I loved him. Toward the end of the session he addressed me as "Mother" and, realizing what he had said, quickly added, laughing, "I didn't say that." Before I could comment he said that he knew what it meant.

In the next few hours there was a recurrence of Paul's concerns about being abandoned by family and friends—and, I added, his analyst. Paul said he had the "worries," but he knew that it would not happen, that I would not abandon him or forget him.

One month before the termination date we missed two sessions because of my being away from the office. When I told Paul about my having to be away, he said sadly, "Okay" and on my return did not comment on my absence. During the following session, however, he said he had "forgotten" to tell me about having gotten very angry, during my absence, at his father because he refused to buy him a toy. He said he had thrown a tantrum, and his father had punished him. When I said that perhaps his anger at his father had to do with his being angry at me for missing our sessions, he did not deny it.

During the last week of treatment Paul was quite sad, and although he was not openly verbalizing his thoughts, it was obvious that he was thinking about leaving. He came to the last hour feeling quite happy but also anxious and talked about coming by to check on me. When the time was up Paul insisted on shaking hands, but it was clear that he was conflicted and did not know whether to shake hands or hug me.

Follow-up

Paul's parents arranged for a follow-up visit nine months later, not because of any signs of regression or lack of proper progression but, rather, because they were planning to send Paul away to camp and were concerned about his ability to cope. He had had a successful school year and appeared to be progressing satisfactorily in spite of the fact that the parents had divorced in the meantime. His capacity to form and maintain relationships had continued to improve; in relating to me he was able to express genuine warmth and caring. He expressed some concern about going away to camp but at the same time was anticipating having "a great time."

Paul said that he wanted to see me but did not want to "come to a session." He would have preferred to just see me somewhere else because he "felt OK"; coming to my office brought back memories that were both "sad and happy." The sad ones, Paul said, had to do with his "problems," which made him "feel terrible," the good ones were about some "fun times" in the sessions when his "problems were already better." He had resisted coming for the follow-up visit but apparently had not been very forceful because he did not want to hurt his parents. He wondered if I knew that they were now divorced. I said that perhaps he also felt hurt. He agreed but added that now there was less friction, and that was good. He went on to explain how the custody arrangements worked. They appeared to be quite flexible and he was relatively happy with them although the wish that his parents reunite was still present.

Paul did not express any immediate need to return for further sessions but made it clear that he wanted to preserve the option of coming for another visit should it become necessary to use it. The emphasis seemed to be on his needs and not his parents.

Paul's parents experienced considerable anxiety and ambivalence upon termination of Paul's analysis. The anxiety had to do in part with their guilt about their contribution to his illness as well as with their ambivalent feelings toward me. The father, in particular, felt very competitive with me but was unable to express it openly. He dealt with his conflict by being compliant and cooperative throughout the analysis, and while I hinted at this being a fact on several occasions, and suggested that he explore his feelings in his own treatment, but he remained resistant. I felt that his insistence that I see Paul before he went to camp was still part of this unresolved conflict and difficulty in separating from me and assuming his appropriate role as Paul's father. Paul's mother was less concerned about Paul's ability to function, and although she was not openly opposed to the follow-up session, she did not think it was essential. She was much further in her own analysis than before and felt more competent in her mother role. Both parents, however, were concerned about their children's adjustment and coping capabilities in view of their divorce and were still experiencing a significant degree of guilt about their past inability to function as "adequate parents." It was obvious that they had perceived me as a parent to them, with the resulting ambivalent feelings, and were having some difficulty working through their own separation from me despite the fact that they had their own therapists and presumably had been working on the problem. Following the termination of Paul's treatment I felt much freer to confront his parents openly about their own needs and difficulties in coping with their anxieties and guilt concerning Paul's well-being, about their need to separate from me, and about their competency as parents.

Conclusion

Paul was well into mid-latency when the work of termination began. He was involved with his friends, feeling more self-sufficient both socially and academically, and was experiencing a modicum of success in sports. Parental and analyst omnipotence had diminished in his eyes, and he could now relate to his teachers and coaches, as well as other adults, with a certain degree of equanimity, trust, and satisfaction. Reliance on fantasy was also less prominent, and his ability to perceive and accept reality was improved. This degree of ego integration and phase-appropriate functioning facilitated the work of termination. As is the case in most analyses, the topic of termination arose from time to time during Paul's treatment. Initially, the analyst deals with the topic as both a defense and as content (van Dam, Heinicke, and Shane, 1975, p. 469); later, it has to be faced by both patient and analyst as a reality issue. The patient, as a result of analytic work, gradually demonstrates a capacity to cope and function well in his life situations, and both analyst and patient realize that the end of treatment is in sight.

Paul had shown that he was able to cope adequately with his parents' separation, a change of schools, his grandmother's death, his dog's death, and the analyst's vacations, and he began to talk about what it would be like when he no longer had to come to his sessions, indicating his awareness that there would be a stopping point.

Symptom abatement in the developing child is not a reliable indicator of structural change or cure. Paul's symptoms had diminished in intensity after the first six months of treatment, and within a year and a half he appeared to be coping well; yet the underlying internalized conflicts were, for the most part, still present. He was responding primarily to the "real" relationship with the analyst and to his attentive, reliable, predictable presence and secondarily to the analyst's interpretations. As Paul engaged in the analysis, interpretation gained in importance and became the principal tool promoting internal change.

The assessment of the state of the treatment and the decision to end the analysis is a difficult one. Questions that arise include the following: Has the patient gained enough insight? Has there been sufficient working through? Have new adaptations evolved? What is the state of the transference? Additionally, the analyst has to deal with his countertransference resistance to termination, for the patient, as was the case with Paul, is by then healthier and sometimes more engaging.

In Paul's case the general principles outlined in Anna Freud's (1962) developmental profile (p. 151) were used in the initial evaluation as well as in the determination of the appropriate time to terminate. When Paul entered analysis he was chronologically in early latency; however, his behavior and presenting symptomatology manifested oedipal characteristics, with regressive forays into preoedipal anal-sadistic behaviors. He was suffering from overwhelming castration anxiety, augmented by fears of retaliation from dangerous "musclemen." His aggressive behavior was, in great measure, in response to his fear of annihilation as well as a reaction to his passivity. As these conflicts were worked through in the analysis and the oedipal and preoedipal issues were resolved sufficiently, Paul was able to move into early latency. As he gained mastery of his feelings, he could depict his thought processes in his drawings, form friendships, and gain some insight into his erotic interests in the sexually explicit pictures in magazines.

Earlier, Paul had needed to divide the world into "good" and "bad," and he had identified with the "bad guys." This critical state of his superego resulted in a frail intrapsychic balance, making Paul very sensitive to any type of interpretation, which he perceived as criticism. The result was a continuation of open aggression in the sessions that initially was physical and later became principally verbal. As his reality testing improved, a gradual equilibrium began to emerge between ego, id, and superego; latency had begun. Paul's perception of me began to change from critical adult to a helping, understanding person, and although he was initially suspicious and ambivalent about my helpfulness, he gradually accepted it. His communication with his parents also changed so that he no longer covered his ears when they spoke to him (or when I, the parental imago, made an interpretation). His aggressive outbursts both at home and in school disappeared. In the analytic sessions he was now able to express his thoughts rather than having to act them out, thus keeping his aggression under control; additionally, he was able to express affection appropriately. He also realized that his aggression, in part, was linked to his feelings of helplessness, which resulted in fantasies that only the possession of great power could save him.

Paul's work in school improved, and the increase in ego integration was clearly demonstrated in his ability to form friendships and participate with enjoyment in organized games both in the sessions and in his daily life. Another significant change during this period was his shift in identification. He now favored the "good guys," and the "bad" Japanese general disappeared.

Viewing this case more specifically from the vantage point of Anna Freud's developmental profile, Paul's most disturbing symptom, as far as his parents and his teachers were concerned, was his impulsive aggressive behavior. With regard to libidinal distribution, it was clear that Paul's self-regard and self-esteem had improved considerably: he liked himself and no longer needed to be the "bad guy." He derived much narcissistic gratification from his achievements and new object relations. He could read and write stories and took great pleasure in drawing people rather than battle scenes. He felt he was an important member of his baseball team and enjoyed the game, forming a warm relationship with the coaches. He also had other friends and acquaintances and considered himself part of the group, yet his self-regard was not unduly dependent on these object relations; he could deal with the occasional rejection without fragmentation.

Paul's aggression had been directed at the object world; his brother, other students, his parents, his teachers, and his analyst. Although he viewed himself as bad, his punitive superego did not dictate either accidental or purposeful self-injury. Instead, the aggression was directed toward those whom he perceived as his rejecters and persecutors. As the analysis progressed, the physical attacks came under control, with verbal aggression becoming the means of discharge. Still later, during the terminal phase, Paul's impulse control and aggression, both physical and verbal, came within appropriate range for his phase of development. He still experienced sibling rivalry, but this appeared to be developmentally appropriate.

Evaluation of Paul's object relations revealed a close relationship with his mother, his grandparents, and his teachers. He experienced some arousal of erotic feelings toward his mother, but since she had become conscious of her seductiveness and changed accordingly, Paul was able to experience the closeness with her with far less threat. The rivalry with his father decreased, and now he viewed him for the most part as a person genuinely interested in his well-being. There was a dramatic change in Paul's capacity to form and maintain friendships. His relationship with his younger brother became protective at times; he would play the role of the big brother, was far less physically and verbally aggressive toward him, and could now apologize for causing him pain and unhappiness. Paul was also able to openly express affection and concern for me. He said, "I am embarrassed about wanting to kill you a long time ago; I was stupid." When I wondered what was going on in his mind he said that he liked me a lot and wished he could have understood it "a long time ago."

There was still some anger and conflict about the fact that his parents did not reunite. When Paul came back for a follow-up session, at his parents' request, I was concerned about his having accepted somewhat passively their decision to call me for an appointment for him but encouraged by his indicating that the next one, if one should be needed, would be the result of his initiative and decision. Despite considerable work on his longings within a strong transference and a good termination, Paul still needed to be reassured that the analyst would be available. This need for reassurance of my availability was also true of the parents, especially the father.

His defense organization upon termination was balanced, (Abrams, 1978, p. 463) though Paul still needed to depend on his parents, to an extent, to control his aggression toward his brother. The "hyperactivity" manifested early in the analysis was well under control also, and his defensive regression to preoedipal, anal-sadistic, and oral levels had long since been worked through. Generally, his defenses were well in place and he could now be spontaneous and enjoy a sense of accomplishment.

While it is not uncommon for symptoms to return during the termination phase, this did not occur with Paul to a significant degree, perhaps because sufficient working through had taken place. Still, his initial responses to the idea of ending the analysis were, at least in part, related to his fear of abandonment rather than to an age-appropriate desire for greater independence. Paul's preoccupation with being left, reviving his original concerns about his parents' separation as well as other losses he had suffered, was dealt with by interpretation within the transference. The loss of the real object as well as the transference object was not easy for Paul. He reported thinking and daydreaming about me; in his thoughts he wished to continue to attribute to me great powers. At the same time he said he "knew" that it was not true. He felt sure I would not forget him because he recalled that I always remembered things he had reported or said during his sessions; he comforted himself with the thought that he could come back if necessary. I suspect that thinking that he could come back played into his not being more resistant to his parents' wish for a follow-up session for him several months later.

Paul's termination phase took five months; I felt that the aims of the analysis had, in general, been achieved and that it was reasonable to expect that he would continue in the path of normal development.

References

Abrams, S. (1978), Termination in child analysis. In: *Child Analysis and Therapy,* ed. J. Glenn. New York: Aronson, pp. 451–469.

Freud, A. (1962), Assessment of childhood disturbances. *The Psychoanalytic Study of the Child,* 17:149–158. New York: International Universities Press.

Van Dam, H., Heinicke, L. M. & Shane, M. (1975), On termination in child analysis. *The Psychoanalytic Study of the Child,* 30:443–471. New Haven, CT: Yale University Press.

Late Latency

Paul Brinich's chapter is about John, a 12-year-old boy. John had completed two years of analysis when his mother insisted that his five-times-weekly sessions be reduced to twice weekly, ostensibly because of reality commitments in a new school. By that time, John was substantially relieved of his initial symptoms, which had included migraine headaches, inability to perform to capacity at school, and intense competition with his older brother. Themes of competition and aggression, oedipal rivalry, concerns about his mother's psychiatric illness, and issues about time were analyzed within the transference as John related jokes, dreams, and fantasies in his play with clay figures. Conflict over his aggressive (and loving) feelings toward his mother was still problematic.

One phase of John's termination was initated by decreasing the frequency of sessions, at a time of increased resistance, yet continuing analytic work. The final phase began when his analyst told John that he would be leaving the country several months hence.

John's initial shock in response to this news was followed by his asking for specific details of his analyst's departure, and he decided at once that he would not seek treatment with another analyst at that time. John had gained considerable strength during his treatment and was able to tolerate his mother's fury over the analyst's leaving. He was also able to continue to work analytically with material of the termination phase. During this period, his headaches reoccurred but responded to interpretation. An involuntary eye twitch followed the same course.

For interesting comparative clinical material, the reader is referred to the case vignette of Erica in chapter 13, by Novick and Novick.

4

Echoes of a Family Secret

Paul M. Brinich

The boy whom I shall call John L. began his psychoanalytic treatment when he was ten years old. He was suffering from migraines, underachievement in school, difficulty in making friends, an unusually strong rivalry with his older brother, and a very demanding relationship with his mother.

The consultant diagnostician who recommended an analysis noted signs of permanent regressions that were impoverishing John's personality. It was his impression that early narcissistic injuries were acting as traumata, carrying their aftereffects into John's latency phase development. The diagnostician was particularly worried that John's timidity, his "belittled younger brother" role in his family, and his "loner" role outside the family would become solidified, with a subsequent constriction of his social relations and continued academic underachievement. The diagnostician also thought that John was at risk for an adolescent depression. Psychoanalysis was recommended in order to help John resolve his internal conflicts and help free him from the ongoing, tense, and conflict-laden relationship with his anxious, hostile, and fragile mother.

John came to treatment five times each week for two years; his mother then reduced the frequency of John's sessions to twice each

I wish to acknowledge the helpful guidance of Mrs. Maria Berger of the Hampstead Child-Therapy Clinic (now the Anna Freud Centre), London, in my treatment of John.

week for the last nine months of treatment. John still had some active, significant internal conflicts at the time his treatment ended, particularly regarding aggressive impulses (and, less visibly, loving impulses) toward his mother. However, his symptomatic picture had improved quite markedly: his migraines were absent, he had gained entrance to a competitive school and was doing well there, and he had become captain of an athletic team at school. His inhibitions regarding aggressive competition with his brother had remitted, and he had become a feisty adversary, one who was not easily beaten and who often won out over the older boy. John was still struggling with important difficulties in his relationship with his mother, but in *most* areas of his life he was doing remarkably well.

Termination did not come "naturally": the specifics of its timing were forced by my decision to move from England. Yet John's treatment appeared to have gotten him back on the developmental track. (I shall leave it to the reader to imagine how the termination described here might have been different had it not been imposed on John, that is, had we been able to make termination a mutual decision and a mutual process rather than a decision imposed by the analyst on the patient.)

General Considerations Regarding Termination

Other authors in this volume, as well as Ablon (1988), Abrams (1978), Bergmann (1988), Erlich (1988), A. Freud (1970), Limentani (1982), Novick (1976, 1982, 1988, 1991), Shane and Shane (1984), Shopper (1989), and van Dam, Heinicke, and Shane (1975), have extensively described and clarified many of the issues involved in the termination of psychoanalytic treatment with children. Nonetheless, and at the risk of bringing coals to Newcastle, I would like to preface the description of my work with my patient John with some general comments about termination.

My own touchstone regarding termination is a familiar one: Has the child managed to get back onto the main track of development from the intrapsychic detour or crash that prefaced his treatment? This is a *relative* judgment, one that must take into account the internal dimensions of drive development, cognition, object relations, and overall integration of the personality, as well as the external dimensions of age-appropriate adaptive functioning (progress in school, peer relationships, and so on). This criterion does not suggest or demand that a child be free from symptoms or conflicts in order for termination to be appropriate. It examines the *balance* of forces in the child, asking (much as Anna Freud, 1965, does in her Developmental Profile) whether or not the progressive forces of development outweigh the regressive forces. This judgment is not always easy to make; and in the case of children like John, who might fairly be characterized as "at risk," it is particularly hard to peer into the future.

A comparison springs to mind from my work with adoptive families, for I have been asked many times: "When is the right time to tell a child that he is adopted?" My reply, developed over the years, is that there is no right time to tell a child he is adopted but there are many wrong times. It is wrong to tell a child that he is adopted when he is already struggling with major internal or external difficulties. It is wrong to tell a child that he is adopted in the heat of anger, that is, as an attack. "Telling" needs to be accompanied by a commitment on the part of loving parents to see their child through the difficulties encountered in digesting some unpalatable news.

Similarly, I would argue that there is no clearly right time to terminate a child's analysis though there are many wrong times. It would be wrong to terminate an analysis while important portions of a child's personality remain frozen in defensive regressions. It would be wrong to terminate an analysis when it is clear that external developmental threats to a tenuous adaptive balance are likely to overwhelm a child. It would be wrong to terminate an analysis out of the analyst's need to prove some point to the child or to his parents.

Termination must involve genuine sensitivity to the range of losses and gains implied by such a "graduation" (to use Bergmann's phrase), with its related moves toward greater maturity and independence. The decision to terminate treatment does not mean that all bridges have been crossed; indeed, the termination process is itself an important bridge. But it does reflect a judgment that the road ahead is *relatively* open and that the analysand/graduate has sufficient resources at hand to make the trip both successful and pleasurable.

Given life's vagaries and the increasing length of child analytic treatment (reflecting both the widening scope of analysis and the increasing ambition of analysts), it is not surprising that few terminations are ideal. The present case is certainly not an ideal; it is, however, real.

John's History

John is the youngest of three children (a girl followed by two boys) born to Mr. and Mrs. L, a middle-class couple living in the south of England. The family had many stresses, not the least of which were Mrs. L's own psychiatric difficulties. These had been obvious in her teens but they became painfully obvious in the years following her own mother's suicide (which occurred a few weeks after Mrs. L gave birth to her second child, Peter). Mrs. L managed, with difficulty, to keep going at that time; she reported to the diagnostician that she had "avoided breaking down by the skin of my teeth." Two years later she gave birth to her third child, John. However, when her mother-in-law, to whom she had become quite close, died, Mrs. L could no longer manage, and she was admitted to hospital for treatment of an illness that was characterized as manic–depressive and/or schizophrenic in character.

John had just turned two years of age when his mother was hospitalized; Mrs. L remained in hospital for 11 weeks. Her oldest child, Patience, was six years old at the time; she was said to have a "very close" relationship with John at the time, but she was sent off "on holiday" some distance away and lived with friends for the duration of her mother's hospitalization. Peter (4 years old), John, and Mr. L moved in with Mrs. L's father and his new wife (i.e., the boys' maternal step-grandmother).

The step-grandmother decided to take this opportunity to begin John's toilet training and, according to Mrs. L, did so quite rigidly. The step-grandmother also insisted that John begin to eat meat; up to this time Mrs. L had kept John a vegetarian "because it's healthier." Mrs. L reported that during this three-month stay with his grand-parents John cried every morning when his father left for work; when he came to visit mother in the hospital, he was terribly fat, "as though he had been consoling himself with food." John shied away from his mother on these visits.

Mrs. L reported that when she returned home, she found John "a disturbed two-year-old who was a complete baby with all the spirit knocked out of him, fearful and clinging, and that's how he's been ever since." She decided that this was partly to do with the sudden toilet training and therefore put John back in diapers. Mr. L, however, insisted that John continue to eat meat; this marked the beginning of a severe battle over feeding. When John was five years old his parents finally conceded; John remained a vegetarian.

At the time Mrs. L brought John to treatment she believed and insisted that he did not know the reason for her hospitalization.

Further, she did not want the matter discussed; although the hospitalization had occurred eight years earlier, she still felt very vulnerable. She described how, during the year following her breakdown, she had felt unable to give John any stimulation or companionship: "I don't think I had much time for John because I had Peter and also I had a very demanding daughter. I couldn't do much at all to compensate him."

John's experience of his father during his first few years was mixed. While his father was the one familiar adult available to him throughout Mrs. L's hospitalization, John felt his father to be miserly and cut off from him: during the course of his treatment John told me, "My father wouldn't notice if I was painted blue!"

Despite all of this unhappiness John maintained a kind of resilience that was picked up by the psychologist who tested him during the diagnostic evaluation. She described him as a "wiry-looking, rather small, fair-haired boy" who showed "very good perseverance in the face of difficulty." (John achieved a Verbal IQ of 139 on the Wechsler Intelligence Scale for Children [WISC]; his WISC Performance IQ was, however, only 106. He appeared to have special difficulty with the competitive aspects of the timed performance tasks.) When I first met him I found John to be an attractive boy, quite short for his age, with an engaging smile and a very shy manner.

Treatment

When we began his analysis John dealt with his initial anxiety by sticking closely to the familiar: he used clay to make some soccer players. At the same time he questioned whether I had to take Latin in my first school. He also wanted to know about my "character" and how I had voted in a recent election. And he was intensely preoccupied with time.

Three themes that persisted throughout John's treatment were already visible. One had to do with aggression and competition; John repeatedly used his clay figures, as well as reports on the successes and failures of his favorite sports teams, to express this theme. A second theme had to do with John's early memories of his mother's "strange" behavior; his interest in my "character" turned out to be (amongst other things) an expression of his worries about his unpredictable mother. The third theme, John's intense concern about time, appeared to be a residue from the periods when he felt deprived of his mother's time and attention.

Theme 1: Aggression and Competition

When I replied to John's questions about my character, my voting record, and my exposure to Latin with queries about why these things were important to him he quickly became angry with me. A clay model football came sailing toward me rather than toward the goal. When I commented on this he denied it and built a wall between the two of us to stop the ball.

Fortunately, however, we were able to discover how other important questions lay behind his question about how I had voted: John wondered if I had voted as his parents had, how long I would be in England, and where my true loyalties lay. Once we had these concerns out in the open he told me three "jokes," which were analyzed and reanalyzed throughout his treatment:

(1) A: Mummy, Mummy, I don't like Daddy!
   B: Shut up and eat your dinner!

(2) A: Mummy, Mummy, why is Daddy staggering up the drive?
   B: Shut up and get more bullets!

(3) A: Mummy, Mummy, why are you sprinkling salt and pepper on me?
   B: Shut up and get back in the oven!

John wondered why these jokes were "funny"; the first was about "eating Daddy." What was so funny about that? He added that he himself was a vegetarian. I simply remarked that jokes were sometimes a way of talking about forbidden thoughts or feelings.

Some weeks later John made a clay bust that he designated as "St. Alban, the first English martyr." He explained that St. Alban had been beheaded; he demonstrated this with a ruler, then pretended to cut up and eat the head while watching to see how I would respond. I recalled for us both that John's older brother, Peter, attended a school named after St. Alban.

John began bringing material regarding his aggressive and competitive impulses in more verbal ways. He told me endless stories about his favorite soccer team, especially about their matches with Peter's and his father's favorite teams. Not only did the stories contain, in displacement, John's rivalry with his father and brother but they also expressed his fear of abandonment (a player was "secretly up for sale"), of injury (his team suffered four broken legs in one season), and of loss of control (a player was fined for "late nights and heavy drinking").

As we moved into the analysis of John's competitive and aggressive wishes toward his father and brother, John told me that Mr. L had just gotten a new company car; the man who had it before Mr. L had died suddenly of a heart attack. Part of John's aggression toward his father was fed by his feeling that his father never noticed or approved of John's accomplishments. He fantasized that he would do "the impossible" and that the newspaper headline would be "Boy Does Impossible!" His father, reading the article, would say, "John L, John L . . . that name rings a bell."

Just before our first summer break (i.e., ten months after the start of his analysis) John spoke of a boy's wish to "overthrow the king" and about how dangerous such a wish could be—it could lead to "execution." For John the danger was dual; his fear of aggression was intimately linked with a fear of loss of control, of acting "strange."

John returned from the summer break to begin his second year of analysis with a tale about a couple on a television show who had won the "husband and wife of the year" award because of their polite behavior toward each other. In private, however, they were extremely sarcastic and nasty toward each other. John recalled a line from a popular song: "I knew that snake was not my dear old dad." He began to tell me about his migraines and about being a vegetarian.

I suggested to John that when he was little, he had wanted to get rid of some people by eating them up; those same angry feelings, locked up inside, led to migraines. In response John insisted that he was a vegetarian; that meant that you didn't eat living things.

During the weeks after the summer break, John's brother, Peter, was preparing for his religious confirmation. Despite a good deal of work around issues of envy and competition John missed his analytic sessions the entire week during which his brother was confirmed. He was "ill" in bed, his condition causing a serious disruption of his mother's elaborate plans for the celebrations surrounding Peter's ceremony. When he returned to treatment John thought of accidents that might befall Peter: an 80-year-old woman might play darts and accidentally hit Peter. When I said that was his wish, John replied, "Better she should do it; no one can blame me then."

With the death wish toward Peter out in the open it was only another week before John recalled an incident in which his father had been on a tall ladder outside the family home. Mr. L had tapped on a window, scaring John and Peter inside, and John had thought of pushing his father off the ladder onto the ground. He then told me of a television program in which a man, the earl of a castle, had a cigarette lighter that looked like a pistol on his table; he also had a *real* pistol there. The earl's son came in, picked up the pistol, and tried to light his cigarette. The shot killed his father and the son inherited the castle.

Oedipal aspects of John's death wish toward his father emerged in displacement on to his brother: Peter claimed to be the "best man" in table tennis, but John thought he could beat his brother. John added that that phrase was sometimes used in weddings. When I asked who then would be the bridegroom, John said, "It couldn't be me!" "And the bride?" I asked. "My mum?" he replied. John missed the next two sessions with an "intestinal flu." Oedipal rivalry also appeared in the transference; John became intensely jealous of the patient I saw in the session before his, a boy who was two years older than John (i.e., the same age interval as that between John and Peter).

The sudden, unexpected death from meningitis of a 15-year-old cousin frightened John; he linked this both to his migraines and to the sudden death from a heart attack of the dead cousin's father three years earlier. John's worries about the effect of his aggression on his father and siblings were so strong that he found it necessary to repeat to me the "rules" of the clinic: "I can't destroy the room, I can't hurt you—and I guess the other one was I can't hurt myself."

John told me how he could beat Peter in dart games called "301" but always lost when they played "Killer." The time seemed ripe for linking John's fears of competition with (1) his wish to do better than his father and brother, (2) his fear of destroying them, and (3) his fear of their retaliation. John responded by telling me about the book *Jaws*; it was about a man-eating shark. I recalled his joke about eating father.

The link between John's fear of competition and his death wishes bore dramatic fruit that very weekend. John returned on Monday to tell me about a soccer match; he had done "rather well." In fact, he had scored eight goals, four of them with Peter as goalkeeper. Peter had, in desperation, "rugby-tackled" John on the third and fourth goals. John had been awarded penalty shots by the referee (Mr. L) and had then scored easily.

John described a dream: He and Peter both ran for a new table tennis paddle, but John got there first. The paddle was new, large, and covered with foam rather than with plain rubber; that is, it was the best, a professional paddle. I interpreted John's wish for a new, large penis, adding that he seemed to feel that if he had larger equipment he'd be in charge. John told me that he had managed to beat his father three games to nothing in table tennis the previous weekend. This material emerged a matter of weeks before John took the school entrance exams that he had failed the previous year. This time around he was able to face them with less conflict about doing well, and he gained admittance.

John's aggression began to change its focus. In the fifteenth month of treatment he told me about an essay he had written in school entitled "I Thought It Was a Good Excuse":

> Wakened by my sadistic mother, I told her I had a sore throat, a headache, and a stiff neck; I couldn't go to school. Breakfast is waiting, she said, completely ignoring my remarks. She had prepared a horrible breakfast and gave me a foul lunch, something that the dog would not eat. As I left the house that morning I looked back and saw my mother smiling brightly and waving. I threw the lunch away on the way to school; the old bag would never know.

John played with his parents' names, changing his father's from "Gordon" to "Gorgon"; that made his mother into "Medussa . . . if you looked at her you turned to stone." He told me, "If you can get rid of the two Gorgons, my dad and Peter, you can have Medussa all to yourself." I noted John's mixture of fear and desire.

Psychoanalytic treatment allowed John's aggressive impulses to find a way out of the shell he had built up around them. At the beginning of treatment they were expressed through the clay figures and jokes; they later moved to competition between soccer clubs. Analysis of death wishes toward his brother and his father was accompanied by fears of retaliation. The analysis (and remission) of John's migraines was followed by oedipal strivings; after these were analyzed I began to hear about the effects of the analysis on John's performance in the "outside" world. He did better in school, he competed successfully against his brother in sports, and he passed the exam that he had failed a year earlier.

Theme 2: Memories of Mother's "Strange" Behavior

In the seventh week of his analysis John told me of an incident he and his family had witnessed in a "pub" in France: a woman in the pub was drunk and people were laughing at her. This memory elicited an uncanny feeling in both John and me; it was affectively overloaded and John's description of it was punctuated by anxious laughter. Some weeks later John talked about Anne Boleyn; she had "lost her head." John volunteered that this could mean "going mad."

Later John told me of a woman who seemed "crazy"; she kept changing her name and she neglected her children. He made a series of sarcastic remarks about the clinic receptionist's poor memory for names; she didn't seem to be qualified for the job. John went on to wonder about his mother's qualifications for her profession. The following week he brought in the essay "I Thought It Was a Good Excuse" (presented earlier in this chapter) and then told me, for the first time, that his maternal grandmother had killed herself.

John then began worrying about me and my reactions to critical things he might say about me. He thought I might "fall backwards off my chair and die" if he really spoke out. He told a joke about a woman who, while away on holiday, phoned her husband to see how the family cat was. Her husband told her that the cat was dead. The woman berated her husband for being so blunt; she suggested that he could have told her one day that the cat was stuck on the roof, the next day that it had fallen and been hurt, and the third day that it had died. The man apologized and said he'd remember that. The woman then asked, "And how is my mother?" "She's stuck on the roof," the husband replied.

John brought up the frightening deaths of his young cousin (from meningitis) and her father (from a heart attack). He noted that people in *that* family didn't like to talk about what had happened. I said that the feelings stayed around and sometimes caused things like migraines. John talked of the shock of hearing about the father's death; I asked how he had heard about his mother's hospitalization. He said he didn't know; he wasn't sure if he had begun to talk yet. "I can ask, if you want me to," he volunteered. The next day John told me that he had asked his mother and she told him that she went into the hospital when he was two and that he wasn't quite talking then. She came back when he was two years three months and he was talking. She had been in the hospital with a "nervous breakdown."

While the secret was out, this was only the beginning of the long process of working through. John told me that when Schubert met Beethoven he had run away, he was so frightened of the questions Beethoven might ask. Interestingly, while tales of "strange women" and of Anne Boleyn (the woman who "lost her head") had appeared repeatedly throughout John's treatment up to this point, they disappeared almost completely once Mrs. L was able to tell John the secret of her "nervous breakdown."

Theme 3: Concern About Time

John was intensely preoccupied with time from the very beginning of his treatment. In his first session he was surprised and disappointed to find that the 50 minutes went by so quickly. The following week John adjusted his watch to coincide with mine, then complained that I had stopped our session 30 seconds early. A few weeks later he expressed a hope that he was the only one I saw. He brought his transistor radio to his sessions to do a time check with Greenwich, then added a second watch, then a third, and even a stopwatch to make sure that he got his full 50 minutes. John suggested that we lengthen his session to 51 minutes to make up for time he believed he had lost in earlier sessions. He thought we should not begin counting the time until *he* said something; that way he could wait silently for the first 30 minutes of a session and thus extend his time.

Mrs. L was also preoccupied with time; she felt she was depriving her older son because of the time she was spending in transporting John to and from his sessions. Clearly, John came by his hypercathexis of time quite honestly and his concern about time certainly brought many of his conflicts to a focus within the transference.

Analytic work revealed that John's preoccupation with time was overdetermined. It contained (1) a memory of a painful early deprivation, (2) an angry accusation related to this deprivation, (3) an attempt to gain control of his mother's love, and (4) a rebellious reaction to his sudden toilet training (i.e., his wish to do things in his own time). He repeatedly experienced my looking at my watch near the end of each session as if I wanted to get rid of him. Thus, it appeared that John felt left behind, lost, neglected, and unloved when his mother disappeared. In addition, he felt responsible for her disappearance and expected retaliation and further rejection because of his own hostile wishes toward his mother.

Preface to Termination

The termination of John's analysis came in two phases. The first phase, which I have called the "preface to termination," was initiated by Mrs. L when she insisted that the frequency of John's treatment be reduced. The second phase was initiated by me when I told John that I would be leaving England and moving back to America.

At the end of the second year of John's analysis Mrs. L announced that John would have to change from five-times-weekly to twice-weekly treatment when he moved from his primary school to grammar school in the autumn. She thought that the new school's academic demands would prohibit daily attendance, and she refused to budge on this matter. In retrospect, it seemed that once John had gained admission to grammar school, Mrs. L felt that her main objective for his treatment had been accomplished.

Mrs. L's attitude about John's treatment wavered, however. She still wanted John to be seen daily during school breaks, but she often canceled one or even two of the five appointments. It seemed that while she did not want him to continue with five-times-weekly treatment, she definitely *did* want him to continue in treatment. Mrs. L appeared to regard John's treatment as a kind of "safety net," not only for John but for Peter and Patience and herself as well.

The reduction in the frequency of John's analytic sessions had a very definite effect on John's attitude toward treatment; he became much more resistant, and he used his familiar defenses (especially denial and reversal of affect) in ways that were quite obvious. In this way John sided with his mother; yet this was not without its problems, for he then worried that she was going "crackers" when she called me to request an extra appointment without mentioning this idea to John first. John asked me if a person could have more than one "nervous breakdown." He noticed that the windows in our treatment room had blocks that prevented them from opening more than six inches; he thought that this was "to prevent children from throwing themselves out the window." When I recalled his maternal grandmother's suicide, John told me that his mother had been far away at the time. I said that John worried about his own mother getting "out of control," and John replied, "you mean that her mother killed herself when she was away . . . mine might do the same?" I confirmed that John worried about such things.

We were able to link some of John's worries about Mrs. L killing herself to John's own angry feelings toward her. John was angry with a receptionist who kept him waiting for me; he decided that her "proper title" was Miss Stupid Old Bag. She reminded him of a cuckoo clock, popping in and out of the door. Of course, cuckoo had another meaning too, and we were back to John's thoughts and feelings when his mother was "mad." While some of these feelings seemed to go back to John's earliest years, others were responses to his mother's current functioning. It was harder for John to talk about these current problems than to talk about the past. John told me that a favorite soccer player had been going back and forth between two teams; he seemed "mentally disturbed; he can't decide which team he wants to play for." John added, spontaneously, that a two-year-old wouldn't know what "mentally disturbed" meant.

Phallic and competitive oedipal thoughts and feelings emerged through John's wish for better table tennis "balls" and "bats." When Guy Fawkes Day (which commemorates the quashing of a rebellion) came, John recalled that it was exactly a year earlier that he had first told me the "joke" about the earl who was killed by his son. Now John's aggression was directed toward me: he remarked that he had never sent anything flying at my *face*, though he had repeatedly shot bits of clay in my direction in the past. He told me Irish jokes, emphasizing that Irishmen were always doing "crazy, stupid" things. He then asked if it was true that many Americans (my nationality) came from Ireland.

Some of John's anger toward me was organized around his jealousy of Robert, an older, taller patient whom I saw in the session before John's. This anger led in two directions: (1) toward John's father, who so often seemed to downplay John's accomplishments and (2) toward Mrs. L and Peter, who often spent time together while John was meeting with me. John thought that Robert looked disheveled and unkempt and wondered how long he had been coming to see me. John added that he (John) "wouldn't be coming to treatment 40 years from now." I agreed but added that John seemed to like the idea that he'd always be able to come and talk and be understood and that he hated the idea that I might spend time with someone else.

John switched to talk of World War II, when the English and Americans were allies. There weren't any "famous" Americans in the war, and it wasn't always certain that the Americans were loyal. I noted that the Christmas holidays were fast approaching (John knew I planned to be away for three weeks).

Over the holiday Mrs. L referred her oldest child, Patience, for evaluation for psychoanalytic treatment. According to John, Patience had not been eating enough and was very thin; he had also told me, earlier in his treatment, of her habit of barricading herself in her room in order to study long hours. She required absolute silence in the house at these times, which John found very oppressive. And, like John, Patience was a strict vegetarian. John seemed relieved that Patience was going to see a diagnostician. (In retrospect I have wondered if Mrs. L was perhaps preparing herself for the termination of John's treatment by getting another child "in line." Mrs. L was aware that she needed help in her own right, but she could not make this kind of commitment. She had seen a therapist regularly for several years after her hospitalization, but that therapist had died unexpectedly and she was not willing to engage in such a relationship again. Instead, she met infrequently but regularly with a senior member of the clinic staff for parent guidance.)

John continued to worry about his mother; he brought a new radio to his session to show to me. It was wrapped in a plastic bag that was imprinted with a warning to keep the bag away from small children. John said, "Well, I don't think I'll keep this away from my mother." I agreed that John couldn't keep all such potentially dangerous things away from his mother, but we certainly could understand the basis of his fears.

John wondered about Patience's visit to the diagnostician. He didn't think two members of the same family would see the same therapist; that would lead to "favoritism." I agreed. John then wondered about my patient Robert; he had not seen him in the waiting room in some time. When John returned after an absence of two sessions (he had had a "virus"), he wondered what I had been up to while he was away. I took this up as a memory of times when he had felt that his mother was spending time with others, when he had felt unloved, abandoned, and angry.

John's comparison of British Marvel comic books with American ones led me to suggest that sometimes he felt he'd rather be with me than with his family, rather like the family dog who was always running off with other people. John laughed and said, "I have the thoughts, she [the dog] actually does it." He then told me he'd be loyal to his soccer team even if they lost ten to nothing. I agreed that his family was very important to him.

Mrs. L began to insist that John come to some sessions on his own; John did not like this at all. He noticed that a figure in a painting on the wall of the treatment room was "missing a head." I said that when his mother didn't give him her time, he felt angry with her and that made him notice the figure without a head. He said, "You mean like Anne Boleyn." I agreed and he pointedly said, "You've never made that connection in the past." I said that it was clear that he worried that *his* anger would make his mother lose her head; he must have felt that *he* had caused her illness. John asked if it were time to stop for the day.

In a subsequent session John told me how he had defeated Peter in soccer. He had *not* gone so far as to "cut his [Peter's] head off with an axe," he assured me. He wished that the desk in the treatment room were larger; if it were we could play a game of table tennis on it. I said he really wanted to show *me* who was boss. It seemed that John was becoming more comfortable with some aspects of his aggression.

Further links between John's aggressive impulses and his mother's illness emerged through "Irish" jokes:

An Irishman saw his doctor on the street. The doctor said, "I haven't seen you in a long time!" The Irishman replied, "No, I've been ill."

I said I thought he could probably translate *that* joke by himself. John replied that we both knew what it was about. I said yes, his mother *had* been away for a long time. John then told a second Irish joke:

> An Irishman goes into a pub and orders 20 bottles of whiskey, 10 bottles of champagne, and cases of chips. The owner looks at him with astonishment and says, "That'll cost a bomb!" The Irishman says, "I left it on the counter."

This reminded John of evidence of "vandalism" he had seen at the clinic; he had wondered if someone had been trying to tear up the linoleum in our room. "I'd prefer to do that myself," he said.

John's anger was linked to his feelings of deprivation. His mother had bought new jeans for John, but Peter got a track suit that cost twice as much. Mrs. L had insisted that John get to the clinic on his own; it was "more convenient." I said it might have been more convenient for her, but I was sure it didn't feel convenient to John, especially when Peter had outscored him by so much in the clothing department. I added that for John one of the most important things about coming to treatment had nothing to do with treatment: when his mother brought him, he got at least one hour of her time, uninterrupted by anyone else in the family. John smiled his agreement. (It seemed at this point that John and his mother were using the treatment as a medium within which to continue their long-standing struggle. John felt deprived and angry while Mrs. L felt guilty, oppressed, and angry; each played a part in the carefully orchestrated movement back and forth.)

Termination

Ever since Mrs. L had decided to reduce the frequency of John's treatment from daily to twice-weekly sessions, I had been wondering when and how John's treatment might end. At first I was concerned that it would end precipitously because of a decision by Mrs. L. But Mrs. L's referral of her daughter to the clinic during the Christmas holidays made me realize, in hindsight at least, that she wanted to maintain a link with the clinic.

At about this time I decided to return to America at the end of the summer. While at first I waited to see if a move toward termination might surface from John's side, I finally felt compelled to tell John about my leaving. I told John that I had some news for him: I would be leaving England at the end of July. "What!" he exclaimed. "Permanently?" John was shocked but went on to inquire precisely how long I would be available. He said he hadn't thought of stopping in the summer. Nonetheless, he volunteered that he didn't want a new therapist, he "didn't want to start a new trail." The news of my departure was very upsetting for Mrs. L. She called me on the phone, her voice rigid with anger; she wanted us to meet to discuss "the situation."

I met once more with John before I met with Mrs. L. John asked me why people have to go to the hospital when they have a "nervous breakdown." I decided to respond in a straightforward way and said that it's usually because other people are worried that they might hurt themselves or someone else. John said he didn't think his mother would hurt other people . . . (his pause indicated that he thought the other half might be true). Then John's right eye began to close involuntarily. (John had often rubbed this eye throughout the course of his treatment, but the mannerism was so smoothly integrated into his movements that I had never noted it consciously before this.] The eye would not stay open, and John finally held it open with the fingers of his right hand. He said he must have something in the eye but he did not report any pain or go to wash the eye out. I interpreted to John that he must have a *feeling* stuck in it that he wanted to say was not true, so he closed the eye. John thought that what I said might be "twenty-five percent true".

John decided that he wanted to be present when I met with his mother (this was our first and only joint meeting). Mrs. L was furious with me; her first question, spat forth, was "How long would you have envisioned John's treatment continuing if you were not leaving?" I said I didn't have any specific time—any number of months or years—in mind. I knew that John had not thought of stopping treatment himself, and thus my departure was unfortunate; but, at the same time, I felt that we had made significant progress.

Mrs. L agreed that John was doing much better. Peter, however, was now "deteriorating"; he could not bear to lose to John. She asked if I had left "topics A or B untreated. And would they be a problem for John later in life?" I said I was satisfied with the work we'd done; but, of course, new phases of life would bring new challenges and John might want some help again in the future. Mrs. L asked John what he thought of that, and he replied that he'd "wait until the time."

I was impressed by John's ability to tolerate his mother's disturbance during our joint session, but it was obvious when next we met that it had not been easy. At first John said he couldn't remember what we had talked about. He then recalled that his mother seemed to think that treatment lasted for a set number of days. I agreed. John said that his father had been out of town when Mrs. L and John and I met; I remarked that we had all left Mr. L quite out of the discussion. John then asked me what I had meant when I said to his mother that "we had made reasonable progress given the time"; he said, "that sounded rather vague." I agreed and said that I thought John still had some very important questions and feelings about his mother—worries that made him feel disloyal—that we might explore.

The remaining three months of treatment were marked by frequent instances of tardiness, cancellations, and rescheduled appointments. John had a brief bout with headaches again; these yielded, however, when I interpreted his comment that "the clinic wasn't exactly a dump" as a reflection of his feeling that I had dumped him.

John noted that we'd been meeting for three years in the same room; it was "almost automatic." He was angry when British Rail canceled the train that was to bring him to one of our sessions; it made it worse knowing that I would not be back in September. He said, "I've been on the train for three years; now you're letting me off at the wrong station." I interpreted that he felt as if he'd been dropped off with no one to look after him.

Matters of loyalty were often in the foreground in John's sessions. He told me that Wimbledon was full of tennis players who would wear the clothes of whichever manufacturer paid the most. The players used the companies, and the companies used the players. Again I compared this situation to his treatment, where he felt both used and user. He felt I was "skiving off" (skipping off) to America, just as his mother skived off from her duties as mother in favor of her profession.

In our penultimate session John said he'd been coming for three years and he knew two things about me: my name and my nationality. He asked where it was I had said I was going (I had said San Francisco). He thought I'd said Philadelphia, "the middle of nowhere." He then wondered how I'd get there—perhaps by swimming? John asked exactly when I'd be leaving England. When I said I'd be in and out of London during August he thought that sounded like someone who was "ready for Shenley [Hospital], right 'round the bend" (this was the local psychiatric facility where Mrs. L had been hospitalized ten years earlier). John asked what kind of work I'd be doing in San Francisco. When I asked for his thoughts, he said I'd probably be doing the same kind of work, "not sweeping the streets.'' I said that was what he felt I deserved under the circumstances.

At our last meeting John noticed a wisp of smoke from a rubbish pile in the garden; he imagined that the clinic might burn down as he left. He asked for my San Francisco address and I gave it to him. He then talked about a soccer player whose club had been offered a lot of money for his contract but they had refused to sell. He felt that America had bought me from England; England should have refused to sell.

John alluded to something "mysterious" that he had noticed his mother doing. I said he'd feel better if she were seeing a therapist and he agreed.

John compared his vegetarianism to that of some peers; he felt he was stricter about it than they since they ate fish and he did not. I said he felt his vegetarianism kept him from taking a bite—"out of Peter,'' he finished. He assured me that he "wouldn't bite his [Peter's] head off.''

In our last moments John recalled how I had shown him the way to the treatment room three years earlier. We had met five times a week for two years, then twice weekly for one. I said he felt cheated by that last year and he agreed. Our time was up. I told him, "Best wishes,'' and he replied, "and you too.'' He said good-bye and left.

Discussion

Themes in the Termination

The three themes that predominated the first two years of John's analysis continued to express themselves during both the "preface to termination'' and the termination phases of his treatment. Each, however, took some new steps forward.

For example, John expressed the first theme—aggression and competition—more clearly and with less obfuscation during the final nine months of treatment than he had earlier. An important advance occurred when we were able to link together the following sequence: (1) John's anger toward mother; (2) mother's strange behavior; (3) no head/missing head/Anne Boleyn; (4) mother's "madness'' (i.e., how she lost her head); (5) John's guilt about mother's illness and its relationship to his anger.

In addition, during these last months of treatment John expressed anger toward me (directly or in displacement through the clinic and other clinic staff) more directly, clearly, and consistently than during the first two years. He seemed less frightened by how I would be affected by his angry thoughts, as well as less concerned about the possibility of angry retaliation by me.

John's ability to tolerate and to make use of his aggressive impulses also affected his progress with the second theme of his treatment: his memories of his mother's strange behavior. Here he was able to ask questions about "nervous breakdowns" and "mental disturbance," get new information, and make use of this information. This was not accomplished without difficulty; John's transient eye tic bore witness to the tension that built up around these topics. But John was able to use the information to gain a new perspective on his mother's behavior, one that seemed to leave John feeling less guilty about his mother's continued fragility.

The third theme of John's treatment—that of deprivation, with a specific focus on time—was also very much a part of the termination. First, John was angered by the fact that his mother began to insist that he get to treatment on his own; he felt this as a (repeated) deprivation. Second, John felt I was running out on him, leaving him "off at the wrong station." He felt conflicting feelings since part of him seemed to want to join my family while another part maintained loyalty to his own.

In addition, it became obvious during this termination that the treatment was itself (1) a gratification of the longing that stood behind John's feelings of deprivation *and* (2) a medium for the expression of the anal demanding/retentive relationship between John and his mother.

Technical Issues in the Termination

John's analysis and its termination highlight a number of technical issues that bear discussion. First, John's treatment and his transportation to and from treatment had great symbolic value for both John and his mother. John was gratified by the fact that he got something that his siblings did not get. He was delighted that the trips to and from the clinic gave him more than an hour alone with his mother each day, and he was quite jealous of that time. This gratification, built as it was upon the longing that underlay John's feelings of deprivation, was a powerful secondary gain associated with John's analysis. Termination implied the loss of this gratification and left John feeling lonely and abandoned again.

When, in the final months of John's treatment, Mrs. L began to bring Peter along for the trip to the clinic, John's attitude toward coming to treatment changed dramatically. Instead of feeling special he now felt excluded. Similar feelings emerged as Mrs. L began to demand more independence of John during the last nine months of treatment. John did not want to make the train trip to the clinic on his own. Thus, a second technical issue in John's treatment had to do with the fact that treatment and its associated travel were, in part, a medium through which John and his mother continued to express their long-standing tug of war/love.

The third technical issue I would like to highlight is the fact that for Mrs. L John's treatment was never just John's treatment. Her intense reaction to the announcement of my planned departure suggests that she had established a strong transference of her own, albeit a silent one, in which my role and that of the clinic extended beyond John's analysis to the safeguarding of the other two children and of Mrs. L herself. In other words, it was not just John's treatment that was ending; Mrs. L felt abandoned in her own right.

In looking back at John's termination I find myself thinking of it as a "forced" graduation, a termination in which, ready or not, the analysand had to move onwards. This kind of situation is not uncommon in daily life, but it is one that we try to avoid in treatment, since it often repeats earlier experiences of having to make do with limited resources. The crucial question here, which I cannot answer, is whether John had gained "enough" from his analysis to continue progressing. Unfortunately, I have no follow-up information about John that might give a clue as to how he negotiated the move into adolescence, with its age-appropriate increases in independence.

A final technical question I would like to raise has to do with countertransference in analyses of training cases. After all, John was not the only one who was terminating; so was I. In addition, John knew, from the first session to the last, that I was an American living abroad. He had raised the question of "loyalty" many times, highlighting the differences between American and English ways. Was he perhaps aware of my decision to leave England before I was? Or at least before I chose to tell him of that decision?

It seems to me that insofar as the analyst remains a foreigner to the analysand, there is a danger that the gains of analysis may also remain foreign—a partly encapsulated collection of affect, thought, and linking interpretations that belongs to the "other" world of the analyst.

Conclusion

It is more than a decade since I last saw John. Reviewing the material from his analysis at this distance has the advantage of hindsight and the disadvantage of the disengagement that comes with distance.

Was John out of the woods, psychologically speaking, at the end of his analysis? I am sure he was not. His conflicts with his mother, his demanding relationship with her, his concerns about her vulnerability to his aggressive impulses—these were all still active to a significant degree. And yet I doubt that further analysis would have carried us much further at the time. There were two areas in which external obstacles prevented us from making much intrapsychic progress. One area had to do with John's aggression toward his mother. I do not think John could have gone much further than he did in this area, given his perception of his mother's *real* vulnerabilities. After all, she *had* "lost her head" in the past and could do so again in the future.

The second area where external limitations made themselves felt was the inverse of the first, that is, John's libidinal impulses toward his mother. I found myself wondering, What becomes of a boy's libidinal strivings if their "natural" object is severely and obviously and frighteningly impaired? This may have been part of what underlay John's concerns about loyalty, especially when he saw his favorite team falling apart and couldn't decide whether to continue his support or not.

Still, on balance, it was my impression at the end of John's analysis that he *was* moving forward in many areas of his life. Academically and socially, he was holding his own and more. More important, his character seemed to be freed of what John would have called the "gormless" (that is, spineless) attitude that concerned the diagnostician who had recommended analytic treatment. His difficulties with "migraines" had shrunk to the size of occasional "headaches." And rather than being easy pickings for his older brother, he was a feisty, resilient competitor who understood and could tolerate the anxiety he experienced when he felt like biting off someone's head.

I wish that I could say that I had identified an "heir" to my role in John's life by the time we terminated, but I had not. There were suggestions that he was looking to his table tennis coach for some encouragement and for an age-appropriate source of ego ideals. But this was still in its early development. I also wish that I could say that John's family environment was reasonably stable and supportive. That, however, would be stretching the truth. His sister, Patience, certainly was symptomatic and Peter probably was, too. Mr. and Mrs. L's marriage was an unhappy one which Mr. L tried to evade by spending long hours away from home. And Mrs. L remained at serious risk of an exacerbation of her ongoing disturbance. So many of the dominoes of John's life were poised quite delicately.

Is this the stuff of a "proper" termination? Not in the world of ideals. I would suggest, however, that it may have been a "good enough" termination (with Winnicott in mind), that is, a termination that left John with enough wind in his sails to carry him on into adolescence and, hopefully, beyond.

References

Ablon, S. L. (1988), Developmental forces and termination in child analysis. *Internat. J. Psycho-Anal.*, 69:97–104.

Abrams, S. (1978), Termination in child analysis. In: *Child Analysis and Therapy*, ed. J. Glenn. New York: Jason Aronson, pp. 451–469.

Bergmann, M. S. (1988), On the fate of the intrapsychic image of the psychoanalyst after termination of the analysis. *The Psychoanalytic Study of the Child*, 43:137–153. New Haven, CT: Yale University Press.

Erlich, H. S. (1988), The terminability of adolescence and psychoanalysis. *The Psychoanalytic Study of the Child*, 43:199–211. New Haven, CT: Yale University Press.

Freud, A. (1965), *Normality and Pathology in Childhood*. New York: International Universities Press.

——— (1970), Problems of termination in child analysis. In: *Problems of Psychoanalytic Training, Diagnosis, and the Technique of Therapy*, ed. A. Freud. New York: International Universities Press, pp. 3–21.

Limentani, A. (1982), On the "unexpected" termination of psychoanalytic therapy. *Psychoanal. Inq.*, 2:419–440.

Novick, J. (1976), Termination of treatment in adolescence. *The Psychoanalytic Study of the Child*, 31:389–414. New Haven, CT: Yale University Press.

——— (1982), Termination: Themes and issues. *Psychoanal. Inq.*, 2:329–365.

——— (1988), Timing of termination. *Internat. J. Psycho-Anal.*, 69:307–318.

Novick, J. (1990), Comments on termination in child, adolescent and adult psychoanalysis. *The Psychoanalytic Study of the Child*, 45:419–436. New Haven, CT: Yale University Press

Shane, M. & Shane, E. (1984), The end phase of analysis: Indicators, functions, and tasks of termination. *J. Amer. Psychoanal. Assn.*, 32:739–772.

Shopper, M. (1989, March), Discussion of Dr. Schmukler's "The Termination of an Adolescent Analytic Case." Presented at annual meeting of the Association for Child Psychoanalysis, Philadelphia.

van Dam, H. H., Heinicke, C. M. & Shane, M. (1975), On termination in child analysis. *The Psychoanalytic Study of the Child*, 30:443–474. New Haven, CT: Yale University Press.

Early Adolescence

The termination phase for two adolescent girls is presented in this section with graphic illustrative clinical material. Mary, discussed by Leon Hoffman, experienced intense castration anxiety that had some relation to early physical difficulties. A prominent issue in her analysis was concealment, a form of detaching from the analyst in an effort to effect object removal. Concealment can disguise longings for intimacy, provide distance by fantasies of provoking frustration in the analyst (serving a sadomasochistic function in this manner), and allow the patient to avoid dealing with intense feelings within the transference.

Mary, whose treatment began at nine, wrestled with wishes to end her treatment for nearly two years, and significant analytic work was accomplished in the face of intense resistance and, ultimately, her early adolescent defensive wish for object removal. The exquisitely sensitive handling of this material by the analyst makes clear the necessary distinctions between those defenses which require interpretation in order for the patient to be restored to an expected path of development and those defenses which must remain intact to permit normal maturation. Mary was engaged in an intense transference struggle, and the analysis of this material resulted in greater accessibility of feelings and an increasingly more effective observing-ego. A clear shift occurred when Mary was able to relinquish her defensive humor and could acknowledge genuine feelings over the impending loss of her analyst.

In chapter 6, Lilo Plaschkes describes Anna's treatment, which also dealt with considerable castration anxiety, precipitated in part by her response to the death of her infant brother when she was three and her fantasy that her parents had adopted a son because they preferred boys. But Anna's stance toward private information took a form that was different from that of Mary (chapter 3). Anna was able to reveal her innermost secrets, sometimes in symbolic, disguised forms, and to explore her guilt over her destructive wishes and fear of object loss.

Anna's initial symptoms, when she was eight years old, included enuresis and unexplained stomach pains. She had few friends and was not able to perform at her intellectual capacity at school.

Anna's feelings at the prospect of ending analysis included conflict over her aggression, ambivalence toward her mother (which emerged graphically within the transference), castration anxiety, for which the immediate precipitating factor was a cast applied to her arm, and her clearly articulated conflict between regressive wishes and longings for success and public acknowledgment.

A prominent thread in the material was Anna's initially gloomy predictions and the more optimistic tone of those which occurred as her guilt diminished and the ending of her treatment approached. A focus on future events may assume defensive functions by displacing intense fantasies within the transference to future representations. Additionally, attention to future events may reveal both early and contemporary conflictual material in innocuous forms; remoteness in time frequently permits exposure of that which may be otherwise inaccessible. Pleasure and interest in future predictions may be developmentally appropriate for the early adolescent; they may reflect progressive development based on ego ideals and identification with the analyst.

Analysis of multiple levels of ambivalent feelings within the transference enabled Anna to achieve a level of function appropriate to her chronological developmental level, and, with the analysis of her longstanding guilt, she was able to permit herself the freedom to enjoy these gains.

The reader will find of interest the vignettes from the analyses of two early adolescent girls presented in chapter 11.

5

Concealment in Early Adolescence

Leon Hoffman

"Ha! You think you did it, but you had nothing to do with it. I did it all myself."

It is well known that in early adolescence resistances to analysis may be marked. These resistances may be in part due to the attempts of the early adolescent to loosen his infantile object ties as he repudiates both his needs for preoedipal protection and comfort and his incestuous oedipal bonds (Harley, 1970, p. 100). Resistances of adolescents may manifest themselves both in a reluctance to enter analysis and in an eagerness to terminate an ongoing analysis prematurely. Statistical studies, although rare, show that untimely terminations of child analyses may not be simply a problem limited to early adolescence. In the Hampstead Clinic in the 1950s of 49 patients terminated during a three-year period, 32 ended treatment prematurely. Of those 32, 5 terminations were as a result of "adolescent revolt" (A. Freud, 1971, p. 9). More recently, Lomonaco and Karush (1990) have reported an unsuccessful termination in 12 of the 24 analyses of latency-age children studied.

Katan (1937) describes the problem in the analysis of the transference of early adolescents as a result of the normal developmental need of the young boy or girl to move away from the incestuous objects to objects in the outside world:

> The entire interpretation of transference is aimed against the process of displacement. What has been projected must be referred back to the central place of origin. . . . In puberty . . . one is confronted with the

entire force of the developmental thrust counteracting the analysis [p. 44].

Thus, the adolescent, in order to keep distant, to remain and strengthen his separateness from the parents, keeps secrets—especially sexual secrets. This secrecy is repeated with the analyst when the analyst comes to represent the incestuous object in the transference.

In the following case vignette I describe a young girl who revealed little about her sexual life. Secretiveness was part of her psychology. This was evident from the beginning of the analysis and was reflected in the manifold communications in which she emphasized her need to be her own person. The secretiveness was intensified dramatically in early adolescence. On one hand, one can compare this situation to that pointed out by Reich (1950, p. 181), who states that analyses of adolescents are incomplete to the extent that secrets are never revealed at the termination of treatment. On the other hand, even though secrecy and concealment can be large obstacles to understanding in an analysis (Spruiell, 1979), one has to take into consideration that adolescents *do* conceal from adults who are connected to the oedipal objects. Moreover, concealment can be an important part of feminine development (Ritvo, 1976). In the following case, despite the limitations due to the concealment, a great deal of analytic work was accomplished.

Case Illustration

Mary was the youngest of four. She had one brother, two years older, and two much older half brothers, whom she did not see often and who were thus romantic heroic figures. When Mary was six, her family immigrated from another country (an English-speaking country) because of the father's business. The half brothers came shortly after to attend college in this country. Mary was seen initially at nine because she had few friends; she spent many hours by herself with her favorite toys: cars and trucks. She was slow academically in a prestigious school, was accident-prone, and had problems with fine-motor coordination, difficulty falling asleep, and many physical complaints. Most significant in her history was a congenital rotation of her leg, which was corrected (without leaving physical sequelae) by a brace worn intermittently until she was four years old. At five, prior to the family's move, she had an appendectomy. She always denied that she had physical problems. She was very attached to her mother, yet fought the idea of having anyone help her do any of her tasks.

In the first session nine-year-old Mary clearly expressed her defense against passivity and helplessness as a dominant analytic theme to be worked through: "If I have a problem I go home, go to my room, think about it, and try to solve it by myself. I don't tell anyone, not even my parents." Mary described two memories: a pain in her abdomen after her appendectomy and stitches on her knee from falling. She said that she used to have trouble running because of her leg but did not have that problem anymore. She drew pictures of people with very prominent legs and stressed how "weird" they looked. Her parents reported that in the past Mary had said to them that she was weird because she had braces.

The analysis began with many months during which Mary avoided engaging in play that involved me and did not offer many spontaneous verbalizations. Her games were usually solitary and her verbalizations limited to brief responses and occasional spontaneous utterances. When I interpreted to her that she was frightened of letting herself get close to me, she engaged in a pattern of seeming more attached and then distancing herself. She began to make many references to her close bond to her mother and in a disguised way made clear that separation problems from her were intensified by the family's move to a new country. I was able to interpret that her reluctance to become attached to me was the result of a loyalty conflict and she feared that she would lose her mother.

Over many months Mary gradually increased her spontaneous communications. Phallic themes and worries of castration became the central focus of the analytic work. We examined their genetic connection to her early impairment as well as to the surgery at five. Mary often expressed restitutive fantasies representing an internal phallus. For example, she drew cartoon characters with phallic protrusions outside or inside the body. She often hid money, books, or other objects inside her bulky coat and demonstrated how to magically extrude the secret objects from the inside: she touched her torso, rubbed her legs and arms, and gyrated. Mary often compared herself to the brother at home and was acutely sensitive to issues of fairness. She vehemently stressed that she always avoided being the one who was cheated. At the same time, in games with me, she usually cheated or arranged situations in which I inevitably lost.

During the analytic work Mary and I understood the genesis of many of her compromise formations, which followed her attempts to master her conflicts about her early impairment. Her interest in athletics, especially soccer and racing, in which she seemed to have a real talent, was a sublimation of these conflicts. She was interested in comparing the speed of world-class runners and wanted to become a racing official—that is, to judge others the way she felt judged, as inferior. These discussions allowed us to analyze an almost imperceptible twitching of her legs that affected her school work by interfering with her concentration. That is, she focused on her legs by vigorously rubbing them or squeezing them tightly in order to stop the twitching.

During a discussion in which she was comparing herself to her brothers and father, Mary's legs began to twitch, first one and then the other. She stopped talking and rubbed them and held them. Then she said that she felt weird and that the weird feeling would go away if she could run fast. Her associations included a car accident and her keen interest in hearing about someone whose leg had been fractured. She nodded in agreement when I contrasted the associations of being hurt to the idea of being able to run fast. We understood the mechanism of mastering the early childhood trauma by turning passive to active and vigorously denying that she was impaired in any way.

Termination

Mary's thoughts of termination first arose as a defense and a desire to escape from an emerging erotized transference. She often teased me in an excited way. At one point, when she was 11, she said: "This is the third year we are meeting. The first year you wore a jacket, last year a sweater, and this year just a shirt." I said that she must wonder whether I'll even wear a shirt next year. She responded, "I don't want to see you next year because I'm bored with you. I think about you too much, even in my sleep." She went on to figure out the number of hours in a day, week, and month and calculated that there was maybe one hour in a day or week when she didn't think about me.

During the end of the second year and throughout the third, the sadomasochistic transference was very intense. We played card games that she called, "I win, you lose." She teased me, saying, "I'm going to drive you crazy, right?"

Mary obsessively wondered whether I was more boring than her father. She either did not respond to me or ignored me, just the way she treated her father. An important line of interpretation was that she attempted to push away her excited feelings and fantasies about me. These interpretations resulted in the elaboration of "beating" fantasies. For example, when she won at cards she became very excited but at other times withheld the winning card to provoke me to win the game and "beat her." She described fights between her parents and her retreat to her room because she was frightened. She understood the parallel to the transference when she withdrew from me after she was excited. She realized that her provocative refusal to talk with me was similar to her attempts to provoke her father to get angry with her. She said, "There's no better way than silence to get a psychiatrist very angry at you."

Often, Mary's excitement was so heightened that she ended the sessions with a large sigh, as if in orgiastic release. Her defense to deal with the excitement was to want to decrease the frequency of the sessions because of her forthcoming schedule. At one point, when she discussed the difficulties attending the sessions, she spoke of her concern about cuts and warts on her feet. I interpreted her need to retreat from the frightening excitement of her treatment sessions because she was afraid that she would be hurt. She had a prototypical response: "You are going to have one of your crazy ideas that because I was talking about my cuts on my feet and mouth yesterday I'm worried about parts of my body being cut off. It's just one of your stupid ideas like that I'm silent on Fridays because I'm going to miss you on the weekend." However, the games that followed were an elaboration of Mary's phallic conflicts. She demonstrated her sense of phallic superiority, reinforcing her denial of her sense, as well as fear, of castration by vigorously hitting a ball with a bat, making and flying pointed airplanes, and demonstrating how she could hyper-extend her little finger, thus "making it longer."

Mary became interested in the news scandals of public figures who had extramarital affairs: "Those guys screw around with ditsy women because the wives are all dogs." She stressed that she was not one of the ditsy women but someone with strength and power, a further confirmation of her fantasy of a secret phallus and denial of castration. In addition, I felt that with this fantasy she communicated not only her view of women as castrated victims but also a denial of her oedipal masochistic wishes in the transference. I interpreted Mary's behavior of repeatedly stressing that she was the powerful one who knew everything and everyone else, including me, was weak and dumb as her defense against feeling weak and helpless; she spoke of her various improvements and the cessation of her tutoring.

Toward the latter part of the third year of analysis, after she turned 12, Mary began to discuss termination in a less pressured way than previously. I felt that it was appropriate to consider termination in view of her marked developmental strides but also that further work needed to be done with regard to the resistance against the strongly defended masochistic transference and her denial of her sense of castration. I said that we could think about, discuss, and work toward termination, but Mary seemed to want to end treatment arbitrarily in order to prove that she, not I, had the power. She said that I told her every year that we could discuss ending treatment but next year was definitely our last. As the summer break approached, themes of injury blended with themes of separation. Again Mary referred to her appendectomy at five, denying anxiety but focusing on the fact that her mother did not stay with her in the hospital. She described in some detail how shortly afterward her family left their native country. She spoke of how much she missed her home yet added, "You act as if those were big traumas but they weren't."

Mary laughed at my "crazy theory" of connecting her feelings of missing me during the summer vacation with thoughts about her early separations. She mocked my inquiries concerning the connection between the current separation and the injuries she suffered, including spraining her ankle: "Yeah, I did it on *purpose*."

I told Mary that one motive for her self-defeating behavior with me and also at school was to get back at me and defeat me (or her teachers). I said that she needed to feel that she was in control and not weak, even if it was at her own expense. She mocked me again: "I must have the beast inside me. You know, the best way to drive people crazy is to sit and look at them and let them babble on."

The next fall (the fourth year) Mary seemed more pubertal. Periodically, we had discussions of termination. She recited her improvements many times, stressing that, of course, she alone was responsible for them. When she received all Bs at the end of the first quarter, she said, "I told you I could do it." Silent sessions where she read alternated with sessions where she described her school activities. She was very proud of her extracurricular accomplishments (we missed a few sessions because of her schedule) and her grades. Whenever the idea of termination came to the surface, I pointed out that on one hand we had done a great deal of work to warrant considering termination but on the other hand she also seemed to be running away from feelings that were uncomfortable.

Old symptoms reemerged as a result of our discussion of termination; Mary attempted to reinvolve her mother in her treatment. She insisted that her mother talk to me about terminating and manipulated her to call me to cancel a couple of appointments rather than calling herself. Mary's mother, noting the improvements, especially Mary's independence, was eager for her daughter to end treatment but agreed that it would be most productive to leave the issue of termination to Mary and me as an opportunity for analytic work.

In the following sessions Mary became more silent, and I spoke to her of her need to try to maintain complete control and to deny the importance of our work. In this context, as Mary denied any need for help, I reminded her of one of her activities early in the analysis when she had trouble doing a task but refused to ask for help. If she needed to get something from the top of a closet she always managed to climb, at times precariously, and retrieve whatever she needed. We discussed her denial of her clumsy walk during early childhood and how she made believe that the braces did not exist. Mary felt intense pride that the braces never inhibited her activity and was gleeful as she remembered climbing to the top of my closet. She said, "You know, I have to do *everything* myself!" She compared her annoyance with me to how she felt about her parents, whom she perceived as intrusive. She said, "I'm stopping in two months. Originally, I said November and my mom said wait and see. I said OK but every time we talked about it, you would say, 'We'll see.' So I've decided, that's it."

A few sessions later Mary said that sports were her highest priority and that she would have to miss a session the following week: "I told you that my schedule would be very difficult." She emphasized that she had told me she was going to do well in school. I said, "Yes, I know things have improved with your work, friends, and sports." She responded, "Ha! You think you did it, but you had nothing to do with it. I did it all myself." I interpreted her reaction in terms of the maternal transference: "You know, Mary, your act to me as if I were like your mom, like when she used to do things for you and talk for you. You react as if I want to take credit for what you've done the way she might have." She perked up and asked, "Are you finished? That is the most BS I have ever heard. It's very creative; maybe you could write a soap opera script."

Over time Mary became more open and talked about her various activities. She said that sports made her feel better so she could do her work more efficiently. She stressed her exhaustion and muscle pains from practices and games. She felt that she had to set the termination date herself because I never would. She said, "You think you crawled into my brain and that's how my work got better. You control me; no, I mean I control you." I pointed out that she was anxious about feeling controlled by me the way she felt controlled by her mother when she was very young. She said that every mother spoke for her young child. When I said that she found it difficult for us to work this out, she said, "I hate that word. It's *you* and *I*, not *we*. I hate the editorial we." She said that she didn't need treatment anymore because her activities were more important and added, "I thought you were full of shit when you spoke about maybe terminating. You thought that we would end in June, but I knew that we would end before that."

In the session before a holiday I asked a factual question about her plans. Mary said that she didn't think that I would care and, besides, telling me about the improvements didn't help her get out of analysis any quicker. When I said that she felt as if I didn't care about her, she responded that she didn't expect me to since she didn't think about me. She added, "Besides, it would be creepy if you thought about me after the session."

We continued to analyze the defensive meaning of Mary's need to control. I said that she wanted to decide on termination herself to prove that she was in control because feeling close to me made her feel weak. Her associations shifted to fights with her father, and it became clear that the struggle in the transference was not only a repetition of the struggle to separate from her mother because of preoedipal conflicts. The struggle in the transference represented a defense against, as well as a gratification of, the sadomasochistic positive oedipal wishes. As we explored the parallel in the transference to the fighting with her father, the pressure to terminate quickly subsided. In fact, I learned that, in reality, Mary's relationship with her father had become markedly calmer.

Mary spent a great deal of time in her analytic sessions reading magazines and not talking to me. At one point she said that she did that because "I know it bugs you."

When Mary told me that she wasn't going to come for a whole month because of exams, I responded that she was attempting to provoke me to force her to come. She responded that at times she felt as if she were in jail when she came to her sessions. During the next few weeks, this claustrophobic fantasy became more elaborate. For example, Mary said that she hated to be in the center of a large group because she felt closed in; she felt anxious and wanted to leave, feeling as if she were not in control. Similarly, when she required help in any situation, she felt that she was not in control and "hated" the feeling of helplessness. When a teacher called on her during class, she "froze" because she had many different thoughts and didn't feel in control. Then, when someone tried to help, she couldn't stand the horrible feeling that accompanied her acceptance of the assistance; she just *had* to do everyting by herself. At the same time, we examined her self-defeating behavior in which she routinely followed a good grade with a poor one. When she did well in school, she didn't show *any* feeling, but inside, she admitted, she felt fantastic.

Mary understood that she had difficulty expressing her feelings because then she felt weak and helpless, just as she did when someone tried to help her. I pointed out that before we set a definite termination date we needed to work on her problem of masking her feelings, not only for me but also for others, that this problem affected her relationships with both men and women. Her immediate response confirmed the accuracy of my formulation that she was defending against her masochistic wishes and her castrated view of women. Dramatically, Mary stood up, looked at me, and accused me of saying something very chauvinistic. (She thought I had said that every woman has difficulty expressing her feelings because she has a problem being a woman.) Then Mary complained about the unfairness of her teachers and of the way women were used in business.

At this point in her therapy Mary began to enjoy "resting" in her sessions and once literally fell asleep when I interpreted her denial of her close feelings for me. She maintained that my interpretations about her denial of feelings were *my* fantasies and that she had just wanted to rest.

During the next few months, until the end of the fourth year, there was an increasing elaboration of the positive oedipal transference with associated primal scene derivatives. Mary read books while I spoke, similar to the pattern of behavior that she had described between her father and her mother. She gave detailed accounts of sexual scenes from magazines, the affairs of public figures, bloody scenes from movies, and the fighting between her parents. When I pointed out her avoidance of direct discussions of sex and menstruation, Mary became silent but demonstrated masturbatory movements with her thighs, which were followed by a vigorous rubbing of her foot—all habits, she said, that she would perform even if "handcuffed."

In September of the fifth year, when Mary was 13, we agreed that we would work for a period of time before considering a definite termination date. We focused on her wish for control and her feeling that she couldn't let someone else help her. She contrasted herself to girls who were very interested in makeup and teasing their hair and who spent all day shopping: she and her friends were more spontaneous, casual, and athletic. I interpreted that since she equated femininity with lack of control and weakness, we never spoke about boys, sex, or menstruation. She agreed that she hated feeling passive. "That's just the way I am. Maybe it's because of the problem I had with my legs when I was younger. But I think it has more to do with the way my parents raised me. Whenever I am in a stubborn fight with my dad, I say to him, 'What do you want, you raised me to be that way; I'm just like you!' "

We saw that Mary very much identified with her father and denied her femininity, not wanting to be like her mother. Several times I interpreted that she could not imagine feeling like a woman and at the same time being active and successful. She said, "I am in utopia. Everything is fine in my life. I have no problems right now and that's why I don't want to tell you my feelings anymore. You have a little devil in your head with spikes that you keep trying to push into me and I won't let you." I said that she sounded as if she were protecting herself from feeling that I was going to attack, maybe even rape, her. In the following sessions she maintained that we were in disagreement. She knew that I was wrong and she was right—that she did not feel as though I were trying to hurt her. She said that she would just sit and listen to me and let me "babble on." One of Mary's significant associations was that I sounded like her father, who lectured to her mother and grandmother, telling them what to do. She said, "I am not like them because I know what is right for me."

In the middle of the fifth year, Mary was generally nondefensive in most of our discussions, which focused mainly on school subjects, her good grades, and her activities. She spoke in detail about her interests and ambitions. She was critical of others as well as herself whenever the highest standards were not met. She stressed her competitiveness, self-critical nature, and anxiety about succeeding; she said that she had been taught that one ought not to focus on one's weakness but on one's strength. She spoke of the subjects in which she excelled as well as those in which she had problems. She said that the problem areas did not bother her because everyone in her family had similar problems. I said that she had always wanted to be like everyone else but often felt different and inadequate. She was concerned about her future; she knew she had to earn money when she got older, she said, because her parents were not going to take care of her forever. She fantasized entering her field of interest but worried because it was "even more competitive than investment banking." She reiterated that she was much improved and stressed that even though she got mainly 80s and 90s on tests, she would always be hard on herself. She said, "Maybe when I get ninety-fives I'll be satisfied; but I don't think I will ever be completely satisfied."

Mary told me that she realized that she was like both her mother and father, always harsh with herself. She discussed her "decision two years ago [when she was in the sixth grade] to stop being lazy." She realized that she had tried before but couldn't change and improve her grades until then. She said that when she overcame this inability and improved her study habits and grades, she had felt that she no longer needed analysis; in the sixth grade (when we began our discussions of termination) she had become freer and felt more responsible for her own decisions. She always hated when people told her what to do; she felt that she had to do things her own way. She had decided, however, that she was not going to be like the youngest of her brothers, who waited too long to "shape up," but like the two older ones, who were admired "heroes" and very successful. She said that she was already thinking about college because she knew that some of these grades went on her college application. She wanted very much to go to the prestigious college that both older brothers had attended. She stressed her improvement, especially the disappearance of her shyness, and stated in many different ways that we had gone as far as we would. She maintained her refusal to discuss sexual issues despite many interpretations of her resistance to the exploration of her sexual feelings.

There was a persistent shifting between Mary's communicating that she had real insight into her phallic competitive conflicts and her resistance to fully and openly discussing the positive oedipal masochistically tinged transference. The positive oedipal transference was demonstrated by the clear pleasure she displayed when she brought in her schoolwork and projects to show and share with me (in contrast, for example, to her verbal denial of missing me during weekends or holidays). This distinction between her affect and her verbalizations in the transference was similar to what she communicated about her relationship with her father. For example, even though she denied any positive feelings about him, she spoke enthusiastically when she described a planned excursion alone with him. However, my attempts to directly discuss these pleasurable feelings, like those in the transference, led to a denial and silence.

It seemed clear that in the transference I represented the incestuous object for Mary and because of the developmentally appropriate need in early adolescence for "object removal" (Katan, 1937), we would not be able to fully analyze her defenses against positive oedipal transference wishes. I told Mary that I agreed with her assessment of her improvement and that even though there were issues that we hadn't worked through it seemed that we should stop at the end of the year. She said that no matter what I said, it would happen anyway. When she missed a session right after this discussion, I said that perhaps the miss indicated an ambivalence about terminating and that she anticipated missing me. She gave one of her usual tirades about not having any feelings about me.

A few weeks later Mary said that I could go on "blabbing" and she would listen. "You need to have two people to have a conversation. That's why I keep coming, because you need me to talk to." I interpreted that she seemed to be treating me the way she treated her parents: she felt that they forced her to be with them for their sake, and she had to deny that she wanted to be with me the way she had to deny that she wanted to be with them. Her silences increased and she spent more and more time reading magazines. I noted the increase in her silences since our finalization of a termination date and wondered if she was angry with me about that. She denied this strenuously and continued her silences.

Mary stopped telling me about her activities and her school work, and I eventually realized that her complete lack of communication was different from what it had been over the last few years and was a reemergence of the old symptomatic pattern at the very beginning of the analysis, when she literally avoided interaction with me for many months. I told her this and for many sessions she repeated that she had nothing more to say. She denied any significance to missing sessions. She said, "You know, Sigmund Freud was the father of this stuff, and he said that a cigar is sometimes a cigar. Anyway, ninety-five percent of the time a cigar is a cigar." She said this with great pleasure and smiled coyly. She often laughingly "predicted" that I was going to comment that she "shut me out."

Another symptom that reappeared during the sessions in the termination phase was Mary's leg twitching. Usually, Mary denied any significance to this symptom. At times she rubbed her legs saying that they were just bothering her. Once she put her legs on top of a table, rubbed them as they twitched slightly, and predicted that I was going to say that she was thinking about the braces she used to wear.

Eventually, Mary began to interact more with me and did not deny that she would miss me, even though she emphasized the projection of her feelings onto me: "You want me to stay with you." When I interpreted this projection, she began to communicate that she would miss me, albeit in a displaced way. We were discussing sports, and her legs twitched. She responded to my query and said that she was thinking about a player on her favorite ball team. She laughed about him because he was old and was not as good as he used to be; she thought that it was funny that he was still trying to play. She thought that this was going to be his last year and that he would certainly become an announcer. She told me, as she rubbed her leg, that she imagined next year's championship game: he would be announcing her team's plays and would fondly reminisce about the team and the people he played with. She stopped talking, smiled, and looked at me, saying: "I know what you are thinking." She said that I was thinking that she was talking about herself, that she would miss me next year. I said that maybe she was thinking the same thing. She said that she didn't say that and that after all these years she knew how I thought. I said that it was very hard for her to say directly that she would miss me. Sometime later, in a somewhat begrudging way, Mary spontaneously said, "I guess this has helped me; maybe I'll miss it a little."

After a silent period she joked that it was a good thing we were terminating because she had run out of things to say. I told her that being silent and feeling that there was nothing more to say was a way of preparing herself for not being with me. She looked at me and became silent. The next day she discussed various news articles dealing with separations: a favorite ballplayer traded to another team, a movie star leaving his girlfriend, and another separating from his wife. She said, laughing, that it was funny that the newspapers ran those stories. I said that for these people the events were difficult and involved a lot of feeling. She stopped, thought, and then remembered that she had to confirm our schedule because she did not remember certain times we had changed. I eventually said that it was hard for her to talk directly about her feelings about leaving me. She said, "I try not to think about that, like I try not to think about missing my parents when I go to camp."

I said that perhaps she denied missing me because it hurt too much to think about it; she looked at me sadly without speaking. She reported a dream in which she was riding a bicycle next to a car and she passed a car accident. The dream reminded her of an accident she had had in the country. She liked to ride her bike a lot during the summer and felt good when she was active. I said that even though she felt good and strong, maybe she was worried about being on her own. I added that it would be as though she were on a bicycle by herself rather than in a car with me and she was worried that she might have problems, like the accident in the country. She then remembered a funny part of the dream: On the bicycle she could almost keep up with the car. Mary talked about the strength of her legs and her skills as a cyclist. I said that there was a part of her that was confident that she would continue to perform well after we stopped. She had further associations involving her phallic power as she stressed how well she did. She agreed with my statement that she wanted to forget about the time when she had problems with her legs.

Mary avoided direct discussions that she would miss me until the last couple of weeks of her analysis, when she started to figure out how long she had been coming and laughingly stressed the extra free time she would have. During the last session she acknowledged that it would feel a little strange not coming to see me after such a long time.

Case Summary

Mary was helped by her analysis to return to an appropriate developmental track. She changed from being a very withdrawn child to one who could interact with adults and peers, and she was significantly more comfortable with herself, no longer thinking of herself as "weird." She was able to separate from her mother as a result of working through many preoedipal conflicts. The analysis of the sadomasochistic transference allowed her to work through to a great extent her sense of damage and castration in being a girl, which had been intensified by her actual physical defect and her operation.

When Mary entered early adolescence, it became clear that the analyst came to represent the incestuous object for her and that we would not be able to fully analyze her defenses against positive oedipal transference wishes because of the developmentally appropriate need for "object removal." These wishes were demonstrated by her pleasurable reactions to interactions with me as well as by her ambivalent expressions as, for example, in the fantasy of "being in utopia."

Two symptoms reappeared in the transference during the termination phase: Mary's extreme silence and withdrawal, which had been the preponderant theme of the opening phase of the analysis, and her leg twitching during her analytic sessions. When we understood that the withdrawal was a reaction to the impending separation and a repetition of the early behavior in the analysis, the symptom disappeared. Usually Mary denied any significance to the leg twitching, but finally her true feelings about separation from the analyst were understood in the context of the reemergence of this symptom.

The analysis and working through within the transference of her castration conflicts enabled Mary to utilize her excellent native endowment and excel in her schoolwork. However, her defenses against passivity were intense, leading to a defense against a complete feminine identification. The discussion about termination, lasting two full years, re-evoked her profound attachment to her mother, which had already been analyzed to a great extent. Furthermore, analyzing the defensive meaning of her desire for a premature termination fostered the emergence of positive oedipal transference material, including primal scene derivatives of the sadomasochistic fantasies. During the last several months of the analysis, after a final termination date had been set, the reemergence of the old symptoms—complete withdrawal from me and twitching of her legs—was analyzed, and Mary acknowledged, in a muted way, that she would miss me.

Discussion

Abrams (1978, pp. 462–463) delineates four key questions to be addressed when assessing whether a child is ready to terminate treatment:

1. "Are the dynamic issues engaged? Have positive and negative oedipal matters been confronted and linked with specific references to the past? Are the preoedipal anlagen delineated?"
2. "Have specific drive-derivatives become manifest?"
3. "What is the direction of the restructuring? . . . Have more appropriate defenses evolved?"
4. "Has the resolution of past conflicts found a more fortunate pathway?"

With regard to the first question, one can compare the situation two years prior to Mary's actual termination, when termination first came to be seriously entertained by the analyst, and the situation at the end of the analysis. At the earlier point the preoedipal conflicts seemed to have been worked through to a sufficiently therapeutic extent, enabling Mary to be more independent and have a greater sense of herself. However, it became clear that additional analytic work needed to be accomplished with respect to the positive oedipal conflicts. After a period of further analytic work on Mary's positive oedipal conflicts, it did seem that "the resolution of past conflicts found a more fortunate pathway." Even though there was a restriction in the degree to which Mary accepted her feminine role, because of her view of femininity as a castrated inferior state, she was more comfortable with herself after analysis. Clearly, the view of women as inferior had a defensive meaning, to some extent, manifested in Mary's contrast of herself to the "ditsy women" or the girls who teased their hair. Yet there were many indications that Mary did not enact the role of a defective individual. She had friends and went to social events such as dances and parties even though the references to these events were minimized in our discussions. She did well in school and was less defensive with her parents. She seemed to be functioning at an appropriate developmental level, and it appeared that her avoidance of more detailed exploration of the positive oedipal conflicts reflected age-appropriate defenses of early adolescence. In other words, to use the terminology of Abrams's key questions for assessing a young patient's readiness for terminating treatment, a variety of specific drive-derivatives had become manifest and the direction of the restructuring was manifested by more appropriate defenses.

Mary's references to missing me were veiled and at times spoken in mocking jest. Her humor served as a defense to disguise as well as to acknowledge her insight (similar to situations previously described by Hoffman, 1989, and Richards, 1990). She communicated that she had insight into her competitive feelings, her feelings of attachment, and her need to defensively avoid acknowledging them. Van Dam, Heinicke, and Shane (1975) state that "age appropriate defenses may come into play in the termination phase itself" (p. 444). In fact, Mary's defensive mocking, while communicating her understanding of a variety of feelings, including her attachment to me, became evident and was understood concurrently with our discussions of the meaning of termination. Furthermore, analysis of the transference in Mary's beginning "adolescent revolt against the analysis" (A. Freud, 1971) allowed for greater analysis of the oedipal conflict.

Van Dam et al. (1975) as well as Sandler, Kennedy, and Tyson (1980) discuss the idea that the patient's relationship to the analyst is more of a "real" relationship for the child than it is for the adult and that the transference quality is less intense. Thus, when termination of the analysis of a young person is discussed, "the theme of severing the relationship to the real person of the analyst arises in full force" (Van Dam et al., 1975, p. 469). This motif did not occur in Mary's case; her separation from me did not seem to have the qualities of separating from a "real relationship." In contrast, this case material demonstrates that the focus in Mary's analysis was a result of conceptualizing transference, as in the adult model as suggested by Chused (1988). Mary's reactions to the termination were analyzed as displacements from the original objects. For example, she compared "not thinking" about leaving me to "not thinking" about leaving her parents for camp. Chused criticizes those child analysts who have stressed the concept of the "real relationship" in child analysis and maintains that this emphasis leads to an avoidance of the full development of a transference neurosis in the treatment of children and adolescents. Chused proposes that a neutral stance by the analyst who treats children and adolescents, but including those modifications that take into account the developmental differences between children and adults, will lead to a fuller experience of the transference and a greater working through of the neurotic problems.

It may be difficult in any particular situation to assess the thoroughness with which an analysis has been conducted and the appropriateness of the timing of termination. Francis (Panel, 1969) states:

> Adolescence is noteworthy [because w]here the pathological state is primarily neurotic in nature the analysis may be ended much like a successful adult analysis [but w]here character disturbances are being treated, the analysis may not be 'ended' but interrupted at strategic points, to be resumed or continued later at times of need [p. 195].

Francis and Waelder-Hall also maintain that "when the origins of the neurotic conflict are uncovered and worked through and developmental forces have taken over, termination is in order" (p. 196).

It seems to me that in actual practice such clear-cut distinctions are difficult, if at all possible, to demonstrate. A more realistic approach to the problem of termination in early adolescence is similar to the approach to termination of *any* analysis. According to Brenner (1976):

> Psychic conflict that results from infantile wishes never disappears . . . [but] can only be altered, either by analysis or by any other means. They can never be eradicated. . . . the goal of analysis is a limited one . . . to achieve the greatest degree of beneficial alteration of psychic conflict that one can achieve in that particular case by analytic means [p. 174].

The course of Mary's analysis is consonant with the literature. In early adolescence the achievements of the analytic method may be limited because of concealment and other developmentally appropriate defenses to ward off incestuous fantasies. Mary entered analysis with a self-image in which she described herself as "weird." Gradually, we were able to understand the important childhood determinants of this self-image. As a result of the analysis and an alteration of Mary's rigid defensive withdrawal, positive oedipal conflicts became more prominent and could be analyzed, even though a residual problem in fully accepting her femininity remained.

References

Abrams, S. (1978), Termination in child analysis. In: *Child Analysis and Therapy*, ed. J. Glenn. New York: Aronson.

Brenner, C. (1976), *Psychoanalytic Technique and Psychic Conflict*. New York: International Universities Press.

Chused, J. F. (1988), The transference neurosis in child analysis. The Psychoanalytic Study of the Child, 43:51–81.

Freud, A. (1971), Problems of termination in child analysis. The Writings of Anna Freud, Vol. 7. New York: International Universities Press, pp. 3 to 21.

Harley, M. (1970), On some problems of technique in the analysis of early adolescents. The Psychoanalytic Study of the Child, 25:99–121. New Haven, CT: Yale University Press.

Hoffman, L. (1989). The psychoanalytic process and the development of insight in child analysis: A case study. Psychoanal. Quart., 57:63–80.

Katan, A. (1937), The role of "displacement" in agoraphobia. Internat. J. Psycho-Anal., 32:41–50, 1951.

Lomonaco, S. & Karush, R. K. (1990), A pilot retrospective study of twenty-four supervised child analytic cases at The New York Psychoanalytic Institute. Presented at the Child and Adolescent Committee of the American Psychoanalytic Association.

Panel (1969), Problems of termination in child analysis. R. Kohrman, reporter. J. Amer. Psychoanal. Ass., 17:191–205.

Reich, A. (1950), On the termination of analysis. International J. Psychoanal., 231:179–183.

Richards, A. K. (1990), A terrible joke: Humor in the analysis of a young woman. Presented at annual meeting of The American Psychoanalytic Association. New York City.

Ritvo, S. (1976), Adolescent to woman. J. Amer. Psychoanal. Ass., 24:127–137.

Sandler, J., Kennedy, H. & Tyson, R. L. (1980), The Technique of Child Analysis. Cambridge, MA: Harvard University Press.

Spruiell, V. (1979), Alterations in the ego-ideal in girls in mid-adolescence. In: Female Adolescent Development, ed. M. Sugar. New York: Brunner/Mazel, pp. 310–329.

Van Dam, H., Heinicke, C. M. & Shane, M. (1975), On termination of child analysis. The Psychoanalytic Study of the Child, 30:443–474. New Haven, CT: Yale University Press.

6

An Early Adolescent Girl Ends Her Analysis

Lilo Plaschkes

"Will you still need me, will you still feed me, when I'm 64?"

I first saw Anna, at her request, when she was nine. She was worried and had a secret: she preferred her aunt's friend to her own mother— the aunt who lived in Colorado and whom Anna had visited. She also was concerned that "things happen to me without my knowing." For example, she got off the bus at the wrong stop, and she didn't know how that happened. This poised, articulate, mature-looking nine-year-old youngster told me that she felt relieved after the first sessions. On meeting her parents I learned of difficulties Anna had not been able to reveal: nocturnal enuresis was frequent and Anna had severe stomachaches and body aches with no medical etiology.She had few friends. Psychological testing at school indicated that she was intelligent but functioning below her capacity.

From the evaluation I concluded that Anna had not resolved her reaction to the loss of her baby brother, who had died when only a few weeks old when Anna was three. Moreover, Anna experienced guilt and anger at her parents' adopting a boy when Anna was five. She saw the adoption as evidence that her parents preferred boys. Both the death and the adoption had profound impact on her development.

At the age of three, Anna's magical thinking had, it seemed, influenced her to believe that her aggression had played a role in her brother's death. Guilt and anger turned against herself had produced somatic symptoms. Moreover, her ambivalence toward her mother increasingly interfered with Anna's gender identification.

117

Anna's preoedipal conflict about her aggression and fear of object loss had interfered with her oedipal conflict and resolution. I recommended analysis because I saw that Anna had a well-structured personality but had developed internalized conflicts and neurotic symptoms and was developing characterological problems.

Historical Background

Anna's middle-class parents were concerned and empathic people. They had moved from the west coast because the father had a six-year appointment to teach biology at a university. At the time of the referral they were still very grieved at the loss of their infant son six years earlier. They were content with their adopted son, then four years old.

Anna's birth and early development appeared to be normal. She was considered a bright, alert, active, and friendly child; she had grandparents, uncles, and aunts who valued and liked her. Anna said, and this was confirmed by her parents, that she had looked forward to having a sibling when her brother was born. After his death at a few weeks of age, Anna was distractible in nursery school. In first grade she had difficulty learning; she cried a lot and had trouble making friends. All this became progressively worse when she was about eight years old. Although toilet trained by the age of two and a half, Anna began sporadic bed-wetting after the loss of the infant brother. The enuresis had been increasing during the past year, along with hypochondriacal fears. At the time of the evaluation Anna was bossy and complained of being teased by her peers; clearly, she provoked some of the mistreatment.

Characteristic Features of This Analysis

Although initially eager, when I recommended analysis, Anna was reluctant, but worried about the enuresis and anxious about her body and had somatic complaints. She attended sessions regularly and spoke freely. She wrote poems, told me her dreams, and sometimes used doll play and read stories. She did not want me to meet with her parents and at the beginning of her treatment practically forbade it. I did, however, have sporadic contact with them, both in office consultations and by telephone. Later, Anna was less adamant about my meetings or contact with her parents but felt very strongly that this was her treatment and her life and she wanted it kept private.

Anna's frequently angry, defiant, and oppositional affect and behavior reflected a defense against positive feelings and wishes for closeness. Some of her anger toward me and disappointment with me reflected transference feelings that stemmed from disappointment with her mother for not having supplied her with security, relief from anxiety, and "a perfect body and brain." Her insecurity was related to her feeling that her parents had abandoned her at the age of three, with their trips to the hospital and their depression after the baby's death. Anna felt responsible for her grieving parents. Her narcissistic hurt that they adopted a baby boy when she was five years old was profound. Anna's feelings and conviction were that being a girl was inferior because she lacked a penis. The depressive affect resulting from the alleged loss was extreme, in spite of her feminine gender identification. Her defenses included externalization of her conflicts, displacement, and, at times, projection of her negative self-perception onto me. A positive transference gradually emerged, but her disillusionments often came quickly. Moodiness and moods were very much the material of her analytic treatment and were a distressing problem at home at the beginning.

During the second year of analysis, Anna sometimes saw herself as a fortune teller who foretold her future: "It's going to be bad. There will be much disaster. When I'm 21 I will die. On the other hand, if I don't die at 22 I will marry at 62 and die at the age of 99. I will have 17 children. Some of them will die and some of them will be kidnapped. Some will burn down in the house." These contrasted with some optimistic predictions that she wrote in a diary at the end of her analysis.

The First Year of the Analysis

Anna gave very clear indications of some of her concerns during the first months of treatment. She asked, "Did my parents tell you about my urinary infection? I had a bath with my brother and he kicked me just there. Then I screamed and my brother threw up and my parents came and now I have a bad cold. I need some water." She had read a story, she told me, about an orphan girl. It was the girl's mother's birthday and Anna said, "I get mixed up between birthdays and death days. I guess because of my baby brother. I think this is the day of his death." In another session Anna said, "Everyone wonders why they adopted a boy, that is, my parents, when he died. If I had died they wouldn't have had another baby I bet."

Anna also liked to play with the dollhouse and toys and make up stories, which mainly involved children who were orphaned, adopted, treated badly, or very angry. Her longings to be a small child and to be taken care of conflicted with her wishes to be grown-up and identify with her caretaking mother. Anna also felt guilty: whenever she had a good time, she would have to add trouble and pain. For example, following a day in which she had had a good time at a birthday party, she told me that she was going to be sick again.

Rivalry with her brother emerged in many forms, very clearly in envy of his penis. One day she came into a session in a very good and cheerful mood and wrapped herself in a curtain. She said, "Guess what I'm doing?" Following my neutral response she said, "I'm playing secrets, surprises, hiding. The game was king and queen beds but they slept separately. But sometimes they do sleep together," she said, "to make babies." Anna spoke about how little boys can move their penises when they are little but when they get to be about 10 years of age they can't do that anymore because the penis gets too big and heavy.

Early in Anna's treatment, it was clear that oedipal themes and concerns had been shaped by preoedipal influences, and the analytic material reflected the interests of a much younger child. For example, Anna was preoccupied for a time with wishes and requests that focused on who had the bigger or the better. Both in her behavior at home and within the transference, Anna displayed longings for safety, closeness, and nurturance.

As the analysis progressed, Anna reported a "bad dream about something old-fashioned," she said, "in the past, like in the book *Little House on the Prairie*," which she was reading to me. It had something to do with her grandmother. She said to me, "You were in the dream but I don't remember." Then she looked completely uninterested. I said, "What was in your past history that you dreamt?" She replied, "I don't remember" and went on reading aloud from her book. I said, "I will soon know the story as well as you do," because she kept repeating the same part of the story. "Except," I said, "I am missing the beginning and the ending and the place in the middle. One just has to imagine them, or you'll have to tell me one of these days. Like the pieces in your dream." Anna said, "Oh wait. I do remember. In fact I'm remembering it right now. It wasn't the little house on the prairie; it was my parents' house, and they were all dead." Then she said she had to leave and she would tell me tomorrow, that is, if she remembered.

During the following day's session material emerged with aggressive feelings and some warm feelings toward her father. Anna said she didn't like being angry at her parents. She was in an angry mood and screamed at me. I described to her the way in which her anger was displaced from her parents to me, and this was the way we began to understand her moods. As Anna began to understand her anger towards me as a displacement, she moved into a more positive transference.

In the swings of progressions and regressions in the analysis the oedipal material was becoming more dominant and heightening Anna's anxiety. She was more competitive with me and made derogatory comments about me, declaring that her father understood her much better than I did. She made similar comments about her mother. She reported that she generally was kinder to her father than to her mother and that she got along better with her father. They had a special relationship. She also told me that her mother was more critical of the clothes she wore and that her father admired her much more.

Anna began a session saying that something awful had happened: she had wet her bed again the previous night. She hadn't slept at all. She was bothered that just several days before she had told me how well she was doing and how happy she was with my helping her. She said maybe her sleeplessness was a punishment for showing off (she had told her father that she was doing well too). I commented that she was disappointed with herself and she agreed. She said, "I'm angry at myself." Then she said, "I slept before I wet the bed and then I had a dream." Her dream was that she was on a skateboard skating better than all her friends and showing everybody how well she was doing. She almost bumped into someone but moved away. Then she crashed into some glass. "I don't know how it went further. What does it all mean?" She began to cry and said, "Don't you know what it means?" with a sense of frustration. "Don't you know anything about me?" I suggested that she was angry with herself and disappointed because I couldn't make her perfect and that she was also angry with me because I'm not perfect. Punishing herself for her success was one way of denigrating our work together.

In a session soon after Anna said, "Listen, I'm going to read you a story that I read all night. It helped me the night after that dream. It's about a princess who had all kinds of doctors and physicians and psychiatrists and geologists. They tried to find a cure. Imagine, no one knew." I said, "What was wrong with her?" She said in a friendly, laughing way, "I'll tell you. She was a princess and when she was born an aunt was jealous of her and hexed her, and she had to float all night. Not only at night but all the time. And they were trying to kill her."

The next day Anna said, "I have some more ideas about the story. It's a Nancy Drew mystery. The girl's name is George; but funny, George is a girl this time." In the following period we were able to work on themes of her knowing and not knowing, leaving things out, surprises, and how she externalized conflict onto me, feeling that I don't know anything. She said, "Can't you see? I have shoes on, not sneakers. Actually I'm angry at you. You told me I could get angry at you. What should I do? Should I get angry at my mother, my father, my brother? They did nothing. I'm furious at you. You make up all these things all the time and you invent ideas. What am I supposed to do? Maybe I know what you said and maybe I don't know what you said."

I think it is clear from this material that Anna's phallic, narcissistic, and oedipal wishes had caused her much anxiety; she felt that she was defective as a girl, that it was her mother's fault—her mother had hexed her. She had choices of regressing to illness and to bed-wetting as solutions. Wishing to be a boy was a bisexual solution, but her better way was to avoid seeing and thinking and knowing. We were able to work further on the defense of knowing/not knowing and also on her fear of what she was going to find out—maybe, thought Anna, she actually had been given a penis so that she was once lovable like her brothers. On the other hand, she said, she really liked being a girl, and her father and she had a very good relationship and her father liked her as a girl.

The wish to be a girl, conflicting with the fear that without a penis she was unlovable, was Anna's dilemma. We were also able in the transference to explore her anger at her mother and her projection of her self-perception onto me. The following material is illustrative: During one session Anna took a glass of water in her hand and said she could see witches in it. She looked at me and said she had mesmerized herself and then told me of course it was an act. I waited and said something about her feeling that she was hexed in this room and that she could hex me. She said, "It's because I don't like you." I commented on her mood change and said that when she came into her session in a bad mood, she wished I could change this and make it into a good mood and a good feeling and she wouldn't have to worry so much. She started smiling and said, "I'll tell you something about the school play I'm in."

At the end of the first year and in part of the second, although there were still many preoedipal issues in the transference, themes of rivalry with her mother and secrets (sexual and bedroom) were prevalent.

The Second Year of the Analysis

Anna, now between the ages of 11 and 12, began dealing with many more concerns about her femininity. This development was impeded by guilt about what she thought her aggression had done and particularly by guilt about her jealousy of her infant brother and, more disguised, of her adopted brother. She had once commented, "If I get angry about my brother, it will mean that I didn't want this brother" (that is, the adopted brother). She was concerned about her anger at her mother—and me, in the transference. Also, since she feared that her ambivalent feelings toward her infant brother had magically resulted in his death, she was afraid to experience anger toward her adopted brother. Anna was becoming aware that she had secret feelings and fears. Anger at her mother and her perception that her mother would have preferred her as a boy had interfered with identification with her mother. In stark contrast, she liked to be a girl and liked having boyfriends. She enjoyed positive feelings for boys and also happily engaged in competition with them. She introduced one session by saying, "I've seen Sophia Loren on TV. Sophia Loren is prettier than my mother, and also Sophia Loren has a baby out of wedlock. Sophia Loren has hair like mine, exactly the same color."

Many analysts feel that children are not able to experience a full flowering transference neurosis. Chused (this volume) suggests that this may result from gratification in the analytic situation, a departure from neutrality that early child analysts felt was required in order to keep a child engaged in analytic work. Anna clearly demonstrated evidence of a transference neurosis that seemed crystallized in this phase of the analysis. She continued to be puzzled about why she got angry only at me and not at her friends or at her parents; changes of feeling about me were another puzzle for her. She became angry when I didn't figure things out quickly. However, she also told me that she was glad she was in treatment, that she and I could figure things out together, and that she was lucky she could tell me things.

Anna thought that God punished her by not letting her have a good time and that God would not allow her wishes to come true. One of her wishes was to be a good, kind, loving person. She didn't like her feelings of anger and jealousy. Anna then talked about the

movie *Ordinary People* and about the boy who felt so guilty because
he had allowed his brother to drown. At that time she also brought
in a new symptom that she called "anemia," by which she meant
insomnia. There was also material suggesting masturbation and
masturbation fantasies and daydreams. One morning Anna wrote a
poem:

Bedtime

Night is the time when you're all alone,
and you hear the ringing of the telephone,
you don't answer,
let it ring on and on and on
and let your thoughts slide away
until it becomes another day.

A preadolescent feeling appeared in Anna's talk of herself as an
Amazon woman. This led to her talking about a boy named Michael,
whom she liked very much and for whom she had a number of
rivals. She spoke of how she'd like to be a lady and said that while
she sometimes felt like a lady, at other times she felt like an Amazon
woman. Then she said, "But wait a minute. I have a poem that I have
to tell you. I'm going to read it to you." This was from Robert Louis
Stevenson's *The Land of the Counterpane*. Suddenly she said, "You
know something? Nobody will marry me. I'm not pretty and I'm
bad. I think I'll have to adopt a child." For a moment Anna felt that
she could not compete successfully. Then she said that next year she
didn't need to come anymore because things were pretty good.
These themes had clearly created anxiety for her and she defensively
talked of terminating treatment.

What was the secret that Anna had in her mind that she wanted to
run away from? Anna brought in a poetry book and read a Words-
worth poem that, she said, told a sad story about seven children who
had died and were in a graveyard. "This is sad," she said, "but I like
it. It's about a sister longing for her dead brother. Isn't that sad?" I
said, "Yes, it sounds like a sister who knew her brother well and
she's longing for him." "Yes," she agreed. I commented, "I guess
one could also write a poem about a brother one didn't know so
well." Anna replied, "I guess so." Suddenly she said, "I have an
aunt who died of a brain tumor." I said, "By the time you were eight
two people died in your life." Anna replied, "Actually three." The
third was Zobo, a guinea pig. She told me about this guinea pig in

elaborate detail. "I'm not blaming Dad, but when I came home from school, Dad had left a note that Zobo was in a plastic bag and may not be quite dead. . . . I'm not saying that M [her adopted brother] killed him, but I saw the turtle liquid on his skin, and my brother may have given the turtle liquid to the guinea pig by accident. Zobo was little and the turtle loved him. But Zobo may have licked the turtle liquid and died." She said if she had been home he would not have died (because she was like his mommy and took good care of him). But she had had to go to school. I said, "What a worry." She said, "I cried so much. I had a big burial but I wasn't allowed to put him in the park." Anna didn't want any more pets. "No more pets," she said, "because they die" and mumbled, "people too." I said, "Yes, pets die and people die. I guess sometimes one could say no more people." She smiled and said, "My brother likes animals and he likes to stroke them. He likes to stroke himself. I don't know why I said that," she said. "He doesn't show his feelings so much. I wrote a poem, a lullaby, for Zobo. I'll bring it for you, the lullaby I mean. And I'll read it to you. Would you like that?" "Yes," I said. "Like you read me the poem about the sister missing her brother."

It is particularly interesting how Anna's conflicts were inextricably interwoven with typical issues of adolescent development. She wore her hair short and said that she hated it short and curly, that her mother's hair also was too short. "It looks like a boy. I like it long because girls' hair is long and prettier." She also added that she had other things to show off now: she was, she said, very good at drawing—not that she wanted to boast. She made a drawing to show me how well she had been doing.

Her body, however, was a source of dismay to Anna. "It's getting skinny and ugly." Then she said, "I'm less moody now. I can make my moods go, and I can sometimes make them come." Anna said she was embarrassed to go and see her doctor. She was uncomfortable seeing a male doctor, and she hated the cold stethoscope on her body. She said, "I think I'm getting what girls get. You know what I mean [meaning her menstruation]."

Anna told me how her conscience bothered her. I said, "I know. I hear how angry your conscience is." "Exactly," she replied. "When I was little I was so angry at my mother. I thought she didn't take care of my baby brother. It was my father who fed him all the time and looked after him. But it's always the woman one feels sorry for. It's hard to understand, but I just feel so angry. It's like it's happening here right now, this minute. I'm *never* angry at my parents like that. Only at *you*."

The Termination Phase in the Third Year of the Analysis

During the last six months of the analysis Anna had begun to talk about how well things had been going at school. She now had friends. She thought that maybe after the summer she would not want to return to analysis. She discussed this with her parents, and they agreed. I spoke with her parents on the telephone and confirmed that they felt Anna was making good progress at home and at school. Hence, we decided that it would be a good plan for her to finish her treatment in the summer. The reports from Anna as well as from her parents were that she was not moody; she was doing her work; there were far fewer complaints about her friends, both boys and girls: she was getting along well. What follows is some material from the last six months of the analysis.

Anna came in one day saying, "Again, I have the same feeling. I don't know if I did something without knowing it. I *could* have. For example, I may have forgotten my glasses at school or at home." I said, "But to have things happen without knowing sounds like some secret wish or misdeed that was long buried away." We had discussed her concerns about secrets and secret wishes previously. At this point she was feeling mostly positive about her work with me and was more involved in trying to figure out things for herself and taking responsibility for her thinking and her impulses.

In response to my comments about her secret wishes she became anxious, and we saw again one of her angry outbursts. She said, "I want to fight with you. I never stopped fighting. I told my father that most of what you say doesn't make sense." She was frantically biting her nails. "Do your parents know what you're angry about?" I wondered. She said, "No. Because I'm only angry with you. Because I hate you more than anyone else in the world. I'm never mean to anyone but you. I only hate you. I'd like to kill you. You think you're God." I said, "If I were God I'd make your brain grow fast so that you would not have to wait until you were 14, like you said your Mom did before she was able to use her brain. And that would save you a lot of worries at school." She said, "How do you know what God does?" I said, "You said you thought I was God. I was only imagining what God might do. God also punishes, and maybe you think I should punish you for wanting to kill me—you know, like the wrath of God." There was a long silence. She then told me how mad she was at her teacher for making her worry about an assignment. However, she said, she wasn't mean on purpose. "It's only you who are. I don't answer her or talk to her like I do with you." Then suddenly she mellowed and made a painting of a woman's face, an angry face. At first she thought it looked like me. Then she said, "No, it looks like my mother." Anna was relieved when she became aware, on many different occasions, of her displacement of anger from her mother to me. As she became more tolerant of her ambivalent feelings for her mother, she experienced less guilt and became generally freer in affective expression.

Anna worried that sometimes she was too greedy, particularly about presents. She started to describe her relationship with me as generally very positive and tried to give me gifts. On one level, this was a defense against her wish to take from me, as a way of holding on. Although the negative transference was still quite operative, externalization of her superego prohibitions and conflicts onto me occurred frequently. In this way too she was able to keep me with her. At times her angry feelings toward me also had the quality of a wish to individuate from her mother, accompanied by the anxiety that Blos (1979) describes as the adolescent's anxiety about regression toward the preoedipal mother and preoedipal needs. This, I surmised, was somewhat more intense in Anna's situation because of her very strong ambivalence and negative feelings toward her mother in her preoedipal years.

Identification with me and with the analytic work was also prominent in this phase. Anna asked, "How does one work with children who won't talk but will only play?" I wondered what *she* would do. She didn't know but she thought I would know because I had helped her; then she added, "You know, I'm a very difficult person. I'm like my mother in the sense that I have a temper like her. I get angry like her and I easily lose my temper."

Anna also began to show more insight into her moods and behavior. She could say, "I guess I'm in a bad mood because I'm tired" or "I haven't slept well." When she was nervous she wished I would make it all better and soothe it away like I used to when I read her stories or listened to her read me a story. But then she added, "When we did that I used to worry that we were wasting time." One thing that still worried her a lot was that she had a secret she hadn't told me. We had talked about secrets, but this one she felt the most concerned about. "Or," she said, "maybe I never quite thought of it before." We discussed her secret and her right to privacy and agreed that everybody has things to keep private but that sometimes she might *want* to tell the private things, as she had actually already done. She said, "But what am I doing here if I have to keep things private from you?" Then she said, "Well, next year I won't come anymore." Anna talked about her guilt feelings; she said she wanted to keep some things private but maybe there was something she still wanted to talk about. Some of this ambivalence had to do with concerns that were revealed later in the treatment; the rest reflected her growing independence and maturation. We worked repeatedly and from a variety of perspectives on Anna's resistance within the transference—in particular, her wish, at times, to have me treat her either as a baby or as a grown-up person. I also addressed the conflict that interfered with her developmental progress into preadolescence.

One day Anna said she felt very grumpy and that she "must be worrying about something." We tried to think of what that could be. The only thing she could think of was that she had read a story about a girl who hit her baby doll and she herself had done that after learning that a boy whom she had liked went out with another girl. She said, "If I had a baby, I might hit the baby too" and then quickly changed the topic to something about school, the theme of which was that a lady whose little baby had had a heart operation brought cake and coffee. The baby was two days old and lived. Anna said, "If my baby brother had been operated on, he might be alive now because the people that operated on him were dumb, because they had operated on his bowels and they burst out blood." Her immediate association was to the people who were coming to her birthday party and how her parents had been very generous about the party. She feared that at her party her friends might divide into pairs and be obnoxious. She said, "I'll burn their butts if they do that." And then she said she was reminded of a story about child abuse in which a baby was burned with an iron. This theme of aggression continued with her questions about why children didn't fight back or hurt their mothers back when they were abandoned or abused. But maybe, she thought, even though they've been hurt, they do love their mothers and also they might be scared to get hurt again in return. I thought we were beginning to deal with the question of intentionality and with her perception as a three-year-old of her own aggression and that of her mother.

Later that week a boy hit Anna's finger and broke it, and she had to wear a cast; she was very upset and in pain. She came in one morning saying that she was able to have a bath, and she was excited that people could write things on her cast. She then talked about the boy who had injured her: he didn't seem sorry; he wouldn't even write on her cast. That offended her. She kept worrying and questioning whether he had done it intentionally to hurt her or whether it was an accident; she thought maybe he had done it on purpose. While discussing this Anna said, "I want to tell you a poem." The poem was by Langston Hughes. "It's very nice. He was a black poet." It was a poem about a mother's words to her son. "Maybe," Anna said, "he wrote it as if it were himself." She characterized the metaphor in the poem, "Life is no crystal stair," as very gloomy. She then asked, "What's an autobiography?" She had to write one; it could be fictional. "Do you think I can begin when I was three years old? I don't want to write about my baby brother. It should only be about two pages long." Then she went back to the poem and said that in class they had discussed the character of the mother. Anna said, "I think the mother's character is a gloomy one. That mother had lots of gloomy feelings. I have lots of gloomy feelings. There are gloomy feelings between Mom and me about my brother [the one who died]. But I don't know how to begin with it. I know. I'll begin when I was three, or should I say something about what I was like before I was three? But I don't really know what happened then. I don't want to make fiction out of it. It's all so important. I think I'll tell my teacher that I'll write about my brother who died, not about my adopted brother, however."

While telling me about the gloomy feelings, Anna looked at a plant bulb on my desk and said, "Oh, look, it's growing. When will it blossom? Oh, I can't wait for my birthday, my bat mitzvah. Maybe the plant will flower on my birthday. Maybe I'll bring you luck. You never know." At this point much of the analysis focused on her concern about the cast coming off and what they would find underneath; at first she was afraid that they would cut too much, that they would cut her arm in the process of taking the cast off and she'd be injured. She was also concerned about how it would look. Continuing to look at the flower, which was in two parts, Anna said, "We'll have a flower newborn and a little finger newborn. Isn't that a funny thought?" She said that she considered her left hand a girl and her right hand a boy. It was her right hand that was in a cast. She said, "I'm so worried about the doctor cutting it off." A boy at school had told her it could happen.

There was an interesting combination here of Anna's aggression against the newborn baby and her identification with the baby. In addition, her castration fears were reactivated. I reminded her of a dream she once had in which she smashed a glass. I said it would have to be an angry doctor who would smash her arm. She looked at the flower again and said, "I guess a flower can be both a boy and a girl. It can be masculine and feminine. That flower seems to be." Here we talked about how when she was a little girl and her baby brother was born, she saw that he had a penis and wished she had one too. She felt that was what her parents wanted, particularly when they adopted a boy later on. "And you felt that if you'd had that maybe they wouldn't have adopted a boy," I said. She smiled and said, "You know Eva's brother had two fingers. He had to have one cut off. And now he has an injured leg. And I also wish something would happen to A [the boy who had hurt her arm]. I wish a part of him would drop off. Of course I mean his arm, not his penis," she said laughingly.

We again talked about her feelings when she was a little girl and how she had wished she had a penis like her baby brother. I mentioned that she might have been so angry that she even wished she could have gotten rid of his penis, adding, "You probably don't remember that. You certainly could have wished for a penis like your little brother had when you were three." Anna said, "Why do you think I don't remember? Maybe I do." She added laughingly, "No, really I don't." I said, "Maybe you do and your memory remembers. And now it feels like wanting to hurt A's body for hurting your little finger." She looked at me angrily and said, "Don't stare at me like that." I said, "Well, let's wait for tomorrow and see what's under the cast." She smiled and said she would be on time and show me. However the cast had to stay on for another week.

This exchange underlines Anna's own equation between finger and penis, and her guilt about her frightening aggressive and destructive impulses and her need at that time to externalize it. At the same time a bisexual theme, although dealing with her envy and identification with her brother, seemed also to have a component of preadolescent bisexuality.

Anna came in the next day, looked at the flower, and said, "The flower is waiting until next week for the leaves to come out." I agreed, and she said, "The flower is like me, like a ballet dancer. That's what my teacher said about me when I was in second or third grade. I did so much better then." She said she had been more graceful then than she is now. I said I had a fantasy about a plant, about her left and her right hand, but it's a boy and a girl plant and it has both boy and girl things. She giggled and said, "You're disgusting." After a silence she asked, "Did you ever see the film called *Darling*?" I said no and Anna continued: "There were two girls in it. They were 12 years old and they were discussing who did it first. One of them said she had already done it. Isn't that disgusting? I don't think I could do that."

The following week the cast actually did came off and Anna was concerned that the skin of her finger was too soft. She said, "Look at that, and don't say that stupid thing about boys and girls and their wanting penises. It's silly. It's silly but it's funny." I said, "It's possible that you could have wanted such a thing." She said, "Why

do you think I *might* have? What makes you think I don't now?''
And she laughed.

Anna's anger at her mother was still intense and she was working
this through in the transference. At those times in sessions when she
was most vulnerable and anxious, when she was concerned about
her aggression, there was what seemed to be a regression that
blurred her perception of our separateness. However, at this point in
the treatment she was able to regain and maintain a sense of our
separate selves and to contain her anxiety and aggression, recognizing them as her own impulses. For example, Anna came in one
morning and said a teacher at school was in a coma; she was living
alone, and Anna worried about how awful that must be. Nobody
would find her. I asked her if she worried about me sometimes. She
said, ''Oh yes. It's very creepy sometimes. I ring the bell and I
wonder what's happened to you. I never know. Will you be there?
You could have been killed. You could have been hurt. There could
be blood all over the floor.''

Anna attempted to change the subject and said, ''You always
want everything perfect. It irritates me. You worry about the rug—it
shouldn't be spoiled. The chair—it can't be sat on. And the flower
isn't straight.'' Then she interjected, ''I can't stand it when I see a
speck on someone's coat on the bus. I can't bear it when they look at
me. I think they're staring at me. It's funny. When I look at you it
looks like you have two bunches of hair [her current hairstyle].'' She
then looked irritated and said, ''Look at your face. You're staring at
me.'' I said that she was interchanging me with herself: she didn't
like the specks on the rug and she thought I didn't; she worried
about her finger not being perfect and thought I wasn't perfect; then
I suddenly had her hairstyle. However, neither of us got to be boys.
She laughed and said, ''Don't tell me about the flowers and the left
hand and the right hand. I already know that.'' Then she smiled.
Thus, her defensive need to deny our separateness was manifested.

Anna also seemed to fear that I would discover her secret wishes
and thoughts, and this fear was displayed in the transference
material. She had secret angry wishes, or had had some in the past,
wishes alluded to but not yet addressed directly in the analysis. A
few sessions later she was again afraid I might not be there. She had
a fantasy that something would happen to me and that she would
come for her session and there would be blood all over and she'd
have to call the police. She then read material from school that had
to do with sharks. She discussed some of her fears about sharks
biting and hurting people. She didn't know who would have hurt
me. Anna was feeling guilty and worried that she had looked at

something secret at home (some letters her parents had) and had read some private information. She talked about how angry she felt at herself and how she was afraid her anger would harm me. She told me that she had spent a lot of time thinking about her mother and father and how sad it was for them when her brother died and they were all alone and how hard it must have been for them. She also acknowledged that it had been difficult for her as well.

Anna was beginning to be interested in child development and was learning in school about what children do at different ages, particularly in the area of language development and the milestones reached before the age of three. She interviewed me for a project. She told me that children between the ages of four and five like their voices on tape because they're not so clear whereas older people's voices are clear but they're more shy. Between the ages of 7 and 13, she said, children are very self-conscious, girls in particular, because they fear that their voices will not sound good. Anna then told me that she was growing up, she was doing well at school, she was having lots more fun, and she didn't spoil things for herself because she didn't feel so bad about herself anymore. She had many more friends, she continued, and was getting along pretty well with her parents. She had told her parents that she would like to stop coming after July. She also said she now liked being a girl. (Anna liked boys and told many stories about boy and girl interactions at school.) She said, "You know I'm really serious now about stopping. I like you. It's no offense to you, but I don't think I'll need to come anymore next year."

Soon after, Anna spent a series of sessions with the book Mommie Dearest. It made her cry when she thought about how sad it was for the daughter to feel so lonely because she had such a difficult mother. The mother needed the daughter to love her. Anna felt sad. "You know I like sad things. But I also think how sad my mother was." She was clearly identifying with both mother and daughter. I said, "It must have been hard for the daughter to feel she had to help her mother feel better; in other words, to be mommy to Mommy. I wonder how the daughter felt about that in the story?" She said, "What do you mean?" I said, "Well, what if the daughter felt very angry? It's hard to be angry at a mother who's also upset." Anna replied, "Well, that's just tough luck. That's her problem."

Anna spoke a great deal about her mother. She said it would have been hard for her if her mother had been a writer because it would have been difficult for Anna to be creative in writing, which she felt she now was; she liked writing and got very good grades. It would be fine if her mother were a doctor because she would still want to help children, and both she and her mother would be famous.

Anna was now trying hard to take responsibility for her own wishes and impulses. She announced one morning, "I am late. I didn't know the time. I won't bring a watch and you can't make me." I said it seemed that she felt that I was making her responsible for something that she felt that I, as a grown-up, was responsible for. She said, "Well, you're supposed to make me bring a watch." Then she corrected herself and said, "Well, let me think about it. Not really. It's my responsibility. You're not downstairs to know the time and you're not my mother." We discussed how at times she wanted to be taken care of and other times she wanted to be very grown-up. Thus, Anna was expressing a developmental conflict of early adolescence although it had resonance with her conflicts during the first year of analysis.

Robert Kabcenell (1990, personal communication) has referred to the way in which transference in a child analysis occurs not only with reference to the early parental relationship but also to aspects of the relationship with the analyst that are present at the very beginning of treatment. This was the case with Anna. When I asked how she would feel about not coming anymore, she said that in some ways she was pleased and in other ways she thought she might miss telling me things. Then she joked and said she would miss reading stories to someone. It was exciting coming here, she said, because we went from day to day not knowing what would happen next—not only in the stories but also in her life. As she was leaving, she said, "I have to sing a song" and sang the Beatle songs "Don't Walk Out of the Door," "I'll Be All Alone," "Listen to My Song." I said, "It sounds like a goodby song." She went on singing, "Will you still need me, will you still feed men when I'm 64?"

Anna decided that before she ended her treatment she would like to write a "diary" predicting her future. She also thought she would leave it with me so that I could see it. If she became famous, then I could say that she and I had been friends. She said that she had never told me that she had been a very pretty baby and that everybody had liked her so much. "Sometimes people thought I was a boy because I wore blue clothes." When she has children, she predicted, she will dress them in blue because that is really her favorite color. Anna said that when she was a baby, a woman in the park had given her some jewelry; she had taken it and played with it. She had very little hair then. "But look at me now. I have lots of hair," she said, displaying her hair. Anna often brought clothes that she had bought to show me and discussed her friends—both boys and girls.

This analytic material demonstrates how, as she reflected about ending her analysis, Anna viewed her own life from babyhood on and how in her associations she described herself as an admired child, in her favorite color (blue—a boy's color but now hers), with jewelry that had been given to her, not taken away. Instead of being deprived of something—hair—she now had lots of it. This reflected not only her integration of her now positive perception of herself as a girl but also her sense of herself in past, present, and future.

Anna was very quiet during our last session. She talked about how in a way she was practicing what it would be like when she would no longer see me. But she would still think about me. She said that when she was grown-up she would let me know what she was doing, and she reminded me that she might become famous and that I would recognize her and remember that she and I had seen each other for a long time. Together we reviewed her "diary" of the future and talked about how she now felt there was an optimistic future for her.

Anna thought of earlier times. It had been difficult when she was younger because at that time she felt so bad and so guilty. She had thought she didn't deserve to do well because she felt she had been angry about her little brother. She had feared that she would grow up to be a bad and angry mother—that she would feel just as she felt toward her own mother. She talked about how hard it had been to feel that she had to take care of her parents. She could not feel it was all right to be a little girl and have them take care of her because nothing seemed safe. She remembered how she had thought that her future was so gloomy and how she had liked gloomy and sad things. But now she was excited about her future and how well she was doing.

About ten minutes before the end of the session Anna started looking at a book. She said she was reading a sad story; then she said, "Actually I'm a bit sad. I'm in a sad mood altogether. But I really don't want to be sad around you." I wondered about that, and she said, "I guess it's time for me to go to school." We spoke about how it was a little easier to feel a bit sad than to turn the sadness into angry feelings and how, as she grew older, she would become even more able to do that. She shook hands with me, she wished me well, and I wished her well.

Discussion

Anna, at three, had been faced with confirmation of her magical thinking regarding her angry feelings and ambivalent feelings toward the new baby and her mother and father. The termination phase of her analysis highlighted Anna's feelings that her parents had been neglectful and cruel to the baby by allowing him to die, and to her by not protecting her. She had internalized these perceptions and felt that she was doomed to be a bad, cruel, and neglectful mother. This fear, a secret that she had harbored unconsciously, finally emerged at the end of her analysis, freeing her to see her future optimistically and constructively.

It noteworthy that in the early part of the treatment Anna talked of houses burning down, children being killed, death, and destruction; her predictions of her future included death, destruction, and human frailties. While these subjects were included in her worldview at the conclusion of treatment, Anna was still able to imagine a productive, creative life for herself. She was able to free herself from her concern that her destructive wishes were harmful, and she was relieved of the burden of feeling that being a parent would be a risky business. When these fears were resolved, her feminine development was able to proceed. Her ambivalence toward her mother had the normative features of a preadolescent girl's, but her anger, rage, and fears that her mother did not love her *because* she was a girl no longer interfered with her own vision of herself. She now had a positive relationship with her mother, along with a more accurate perception of me. The idealization that remained at the end of Anna's treatment was part of what is typically present in normal early adolescent development. Anna also demonstrated a more balanced view of her father. She was now charming and flirtatious with him and felt a special closeness with him. With her brother she was at times more playful than before and at other times still rather maternal, in a big-sisterly fashion. As the ending of treatment approached, Anna's insistence on immediate interventions and responses from me was minimized; she had become less anxious.

Because both child analysis and child development are dynamic processes, several questions arise: To what extent do we find resolution of transference neurosis in child analysis? I think the relationship between child and analyst is preserved by the child, by identification and internalization. What is the fate of the punitive superego? Loewald (1962) reminds us that "conscience speaks to us from the viewpoint of an inner future, whether it tells us what we should do or how we should behave in the future or whether it judges past and present deeds, thoughts and feelings," (p. 265). Because of the resolution of the transference neurosis, Anna judged her past, present, and future with a much modified and kinder superego.

I raise the possibility that a youngster who has been in analysis may have a keener sense of past, present, and future than a child who has not. For most children, early childhood is experienced as far away, almost as another world. How does analysis of transference influence the child's subjective sense of time? Does analysis make possible a greater sense of childhood, as a distant, yet important experience in these children?

Anna appears to have experienced a transference neurosis, most passionately expressed in the negative transference, a feature that Chused (this volume) describes vividly. Anna also, in the early part of her analysis, experienced in the relationship with the analyst the longings for infantile object relationships, that is, dependency needs and wishes. Willie Hoffer (1950) describes the transference neurosis in adults and its resolution: "Painful actuality in the transference situation becomes transformed into memories of the past, and with it the patient's actual infantile relations towards his analyst will gradually become past and will relieve him from much actual suffering" (p. 195). Anna had memories from her early childhood; she also expressed memories from the early part of her analysis. She was able to resolve her negative transference, as evidenced by her improved relationship with her mother and with me in the termination phase of the treatment. New faith and hope made possible a future in which the impact of her childhood trauma could be resolved; her growth now included the new relationship with me as the analyst. Anna used me less as a real object than many children whom I have treated. This may have been related to her active involvement with her family, her peers, and her teachers. She identified with me as we worked analytically, motivated also by her wish to rid herself of the discomfort of her problems. She also used her relationship with me as many preadolescent girls do—to discuss clothes, appearance, boyfriends, as if we were simply friends. This too was a characteristic of the last phase of her analysis.

At the end of treatment Anna showed creative interests and talents and a wish to be unique, most apparent in her narrative of her future. Her past from the age of three years on she felt she had "told" in her analysis. Anna's fantasy predictions reflect active mastery and an identification with creativity and the helping professions. What follows is Anna's fantasy prediction of her life:

At 15 years of age, chairman of the Student Council for stopping drug abuse in school.

At 17, go to Harvard.

At 23, Yale, major pediatrics.

At 27, receive M.D.

At 29, marry a lawyer.

At 30, fly to Africa, save 59 children's lives.

At 32, have twin boys, named Paul and Simon.

At 35, open school for nursing to train for working with retarded children. Also at 35, have baby girl, Cassandra.

At 36, husband wins famous law case and gets an award of $50,000.

At 38, adopt two retarded children, called Bettina and Arthur.

At 40, figure out cure for mental illness.

At 45, get book published on children's health.

At 47, interview on abused children on TV.

At 48, both twins get accepted to Yale.

At 51, buy big new house in country.

At 53, Cassandra marries a ballet dancer.

At 65, Cassandra has art exhibition of her paintings of modern art. Also at 65, both retarded children learn to weave Persian rugs.

At 67, Cassandra has a baby boy, Daniel.

At 68, Simon marries a Chinese girl and moves to China.

At 69, Paul composes some pieces, becomes famous, like a new Beethoven.

At 73, I retire but continue writing books on mentally retarded and how to help them.

At 74, my husband retires.

At 76, retarded daughter marries painter and has a baby girl, Laura.

At 77, Simon has twins, called Lydia and Peter. (I had to have one sad thing happen. On the other hand, I had enough sad things until I was 12 years old, but I guess the retarded children are kind of sad things.)

At 84, myself and granddaughter invent a cure for cancer.

At 91, myself and granddaughter invent a cure for MS. And then something dramatic—my grandson invents a time machine but it blows up.

References

Blos, P. (1979), *The Adolescent Passage.* New York: International Universities Press.

Hoffer, W. (1950), Psychological criteria for the termination of treatment. *Internat. J. Psycho-Anal.,* 31:194–195.

Loewald, H. (1962), Superego and time. *Internat. J. Psycho-Anal.,* 43:264–268.

Midadolescence

Jaap Ubbels discusses the termination phase of John, whose five-year analysis began when he was 16. During this period, John grappled with his long-cherished notion that a great artistic talent had been inhibited by his psychological distress. Thus the typical disillusionment of adolescence, in which infantile wishes are both transformed and relinquished, was intensified by John's conflicts, by developmental issues, by wishes for narcissistic perfection, and by the belief shared by John and his parents that a hidden talent would emerge at the conclusion of treatment.

John exhibited a persistent silence during his analytic sessions as the conclusion of treatment approached. His parents were anxious about his apparent apathy and his avoidance of his schoolwork. By his behavior, John communicated his fear and desperation to both his parents and his analyst.

John met with his analyst three months after the treatment ended and was able to speak of external gains that could not be expressed during the final phase of treatment. The analyst felt that John used the termination and posttermination periods for progressive growth.

John's case demonstrates both neurotic conflict and substantial developmental delay and the analyst's work with the "holding environment" until the patient was able to analyze material within the transference.

7

Developmental Issues in the Termination of Analysis in Adolescence

Jaap Ubbels

"I am no longer afraid of you."

This is a study of John, a young man whose five-year analysis terminated when he was 17. The essential issues with which he grappled were characterized by van der Leeuw (1958) in the following way:

> In the analysis the patient had to learn how to be active, productive and creative, in spite of feeling helpless and having aggressive impulses. This is a problem dominating our whole life from the cradle to the grave, but it is of course particularly pressing in this earliest phase of a young ego organization. This feeling of helplessness is a very deep injury of a person's narcissism [pp. 368–369].

John Munder Ross (1979), a researcher of the early father–son relationship, elaborating on van der Leeuw's statement, believed that the powerlessness of the small boy toward the active, productive mother is mitigated by his identification with a father perceived as nurturing and creative. Blos (1984) emphasized the great significance of this early dyadic or preoedipal relationship between father and son, identifying it as the basis of the negative oedipus complex, from which the ego ideal emerges following its resolution at the end of adolescence. He stated that the dyadic father complex of the boy

This case report was written as part of the systematic investigation of the termination of child and adolescent analysis by the Child Department of the Psycho-Analytic Institute of the Dutch Psycho-Analytical Society. Amsterdam, The Netherlands.

plays a central role in the formation of the neurosis of the man, and disturbances in the resolution of this early tie in adolescence are frequent and not often recognized. John's analysis brings into focus—in poignant magnification—these developmental difficulties of the son.

In this report on the termination of John's analysis I would like to emphasize three issues that arise in the termination of child and adolescent analysis. The first is developmental delay, prominent in this case. The second is a shift in technique that occurs after substantial work has been accomplished in the "holding environment" and after developmental issues have been addressed extensively. Part of this shift occurs once an analytic process has been established, that is, when there is evidence of transference neurosis. Finally, we have the question of infantile trauma in the sense of a phase-specific developmental disorder that is reflected in unconscious fantasy. This relates, in some sense, to Kris's (1956) notion of "the personal myth."

John's History

John was 12 when his treatment began. He was the eldest of three children in a family living in a provincial town in The Netherlands. His father enjoyed a good deal of respect in this small town: he was a successful shopkeeper, active in community life, and, in his leisure time, quite a creditable hand at drawing. John's mother was also very interested in the visual arts, and both parents had high hopes for John in the field of art. Because of difficulties of their own they tried to form a bond with John through prematurely encouraging and making demands of him. His mother started toilet training John before his first birthday, and as soon as John was able to hold a pencil, his father attempted to give him drawing lessons. When he was a kindergartner, John was worshipped by his parents as a child prodigy. According to his parents John still met their expectations to a degree at age five: he could paint nicely and had taught himself to read. After that he appeared increasingly less capable, which was no mean disappointment to his father in particular. After the birth of his sister, when John was three, and his brother, when John was five, John appeared downcast. A series of persistent childhood neurotic symptoms developed: difficulty in falling asleep, nighttime anxieties, and nocturnal enuresis. Serious learning disorders became evident when John was in elementary school; he appeared fatigued and sullen. When John was brought for treatment at 12, the family situation was one of intense turmoil. The previous year John's father had suffered a serious illness, from which recovery was slow: he was haggard and worn-out. John's mother could no longer tolerate her husband's presence, and as soon as John was settled into analysis, she proceeded vigorously with a divorce.

At the beginning of the analysis I encountered a tired-looking boy, cowering and dejected, who felt betrayed by his parents. At times feeling desperate, John would become completely absorbed in fantasies in which he took revenge on his parents. He viewed his world as alternately horrifying, grim, and threatening. At school John was a poor pupil. Among peers he was the lowest in the pecking order; he did not dare to ride his bike for fear of having an accident or being molested.

John welcomed the daily attention and the feeling of protection that analysis offered him: the analysis was a last resort. At times he arrived for his appointment long before the scheduled hour. At 12, John still felt like a small, helpless child between his quarreling parents. He told me explicitly that he wanted to stay small because he was too afraid of growing up.

John's Analysis

Early in treatment I represented the strong ideal father for John. But sometimes, without being really aware of it, he hurled at me the reproaches he did not dare to feel, let alone express, toward his father. At the end of the first year of analysis, when John began to ask for my admiration of his drawings, we were able to understand his profound anger over my neutrality as the result of his viewing me as his father, from whom no amount of admiration would feel sufficient. John's feeling humiliated and ridiculed when explicit admiration was not forthcoming also reflected early feelings in relation to his father. Only with painstaking work was John able to understand that these symptoms were, in part, an effort to restore his damaged self-esteem.

John's early-rooted ambivalent conflicts, the struggle for power, and the regulation of his self-esteem were primarily expressed in relation to his father, to whom John felt strong attachment. John had been furious with his father, who meekly (in John's view) allowed himself to be sent away by John's mother. John wanted to remain loyal to his father and feared losing his father's love. For a significant part of the analysis John's anger at his mother was much more accessible than his anger toward his father. In his mother's eyes John was the grown son who could be a better man for her than her husband had been. An abrupt end came to this situation when John's mother's boyfriend began to visit regularly. John then felt small and humiliated and anxious about his sexual fantasies of his mother and her boyfriend.

As we worked on John's feelings of humiliation, it became clear that John was aware that he was not the artist for whom his parents had hoped. He experienced it as a horrible injustice that he would not get the fame and recognition that he had anticipated in his early years. In the transference a pattern of coercion and ridicule emerged: "Us artists, you don't know the first thing about us . . . I know your type, Ubbels, deep down inside you secretly believe you're an artist. We artists see right through that." At the end of such sessions full of scorn and contempt, John sometimes managed to express some amount of the terrible pain and humiliation caused by his father's constant disappointment and criticism of his drawing. The analysis gradually offered John an opportunity to tolerate his rage and his destructive wishes.

At the end of the third year of analysis, John's father once again fell seriously ill; he recovered slowly following major surgery. During his illness John was intensely frightened; he felt guilty about his anger toward his father, whose illness threatened to spoil John's vacation.

It was difficult for John to tolerate it when I tried to help him identify some of his conflictual feelings toward his father: fright, concern, and—particularly—fury. "No one looks as healthy as my father," John commented. Unconsciously, he mimicked his father: emulating a sick man, John sprawled in his chair, complaining of fatigue. He announced that he was depressed and drew his jacket up over his ears to sleep during his session. At that point I suggested to John that his behavior was telling me that this was what he observed in his father, now and even much earlier.

This intervention was followed by John's expression of regret that his father had not been available to him as a model or partner in youthful activities: his father did not swim, bike, or skate, and he generally conveyed to John the idea that he was too tired to participate in physical activities that interested his son. Contact between father and son took place primarily in the shadowy area of the father's artistic aspirations, to which he devoted himself entirely since being disabled by his illness.

John wanted to share in what he perceived as his father's greatness; for John there remained no other possibility than imitation. His father could hardly serve as a model for silent, adaptive, ego-syntonic identifications. I was impressed by how fascinated John was by his father's artistic skill. John told me in great detail about the series of self-portraits his father was making. "If anyone so much as puts a scratch on them, I'll kill him," John said. He cherished a memory from the time before his sister was born: one summery day John was outside in the yard at his father's feet while his pregnant mother walked around the yard. Full of admiration, John watched his father draw the trees and flowers. As John recalled this, he demonstrated exactly how his father's eyes had moved rapidly up and down, how his father's hand had flown across the drawing paper. John feared that in recounting the image it might be damaged or lost, as if it were a painting that could be scratched.

I interpreted to John the conflict between the feelings of the small boy who had admired his father intensely and adored his powerful mother who produced children but who had felt exasperated with having to do what was expected of him as a son, never quite reaching the goals he had established for himself or those his parents had set forth for him.

John began to recognize how empty he would feel if he were to give up his artistic fantasies. He needed his father's love to protect himself from what Winnicott termed "unthinkable anxieties." "I'm such a nitwit, just a zilch, empty," he complained sadly.

John's gradually increasing tolerance for feelings of rage and helplessness preceded his growing aware of a sense of shame, which emerged particularly in relation to his own narcissistic demands. I considered his increasing capacity to experience shame to be an important indicator of John's emotional growth.

It was during the third and fourth years of the analysis, when John was a midadolescent, that he no longer felt depressed much of the time. Gradually, things were going better for John at school and in other areas of his life. He had grown to a height of six feet, with a strong, graceful body, of which he was proud. His constricted world began to enlarge; although still fearful of getting lost, he took a train trip to a nearby city and went hiking with a friend for several days. The modest dimensions of these steps show how much John's development had been delayed. John, who had not previously exhibited sustained interests of his own, now responded to his father's encouragement to cultivate the hobby of collecting Chinese curiosa. He joined a judo club and continued with it for some time. In this way, John had more opportunities to maintain his identity and demonstrated a higher level of general functioning.

This turn for the better, however, brought back the high hopes of John's parents, and sometimes John talked about how the disparity between these hopes and his present attainments deepened his feeling of desperation. "How can I ever become a full-grown man? I still have so much to do, and when I think about where I am now and what I still have to do, I get so scared that I might be on the wrong track," he lamented.

Both in the outer world and in the inner psychic world, John's life had become somewhat calmer. He had found a grip and acquired more hope and trust; the balance between regressive and progressive wishes more nearly approached equilibrium. The analysis occupied an important place in John's experience, and his neurotic conflicts were now primarily expressed in the analysis. A transference neurosis, defined as "the concentration of the child's conflicts, repressed infantile wishes, fantasies, . . . on the person of the therapist, with the relative diminution of their manifestation elsewhere" (Sandler, Kennedy, and Tyson, 1975, p. 427) had come to full-blown development.

On the other hand, it could be observed in the analytic situation that John had not yet confronted, with full intensity, the essential challenges of adolescence. Like a late latency child, John continued to idealize his father and derive part of his self-image from his father's fantasied greatness. A thrust into adolescence, a second separation–individuation from infantile objects, and a de-idealization of his omnipotent father with the formation of an adolescent ego ideal (Blos, 1979, pp. 319–369) had not yet emerged fully. This was John's position at age 15½.

The Termination Phase

In my view, the final phase of John's analysis focused on John's seeing the possibility to terminate as a challenge that helped his progressive development. With termination in view, a further working through of the transference neurosis opened possibilities for John to initiate separation processes necessary for his continuing development.

The theme of termination first appeared in the analysis when John's mother told him that, in her opinion, he might as well stop treatment because things were going much better for him. John's mother's attitude to the analysis had changed once she began to live with her boyfriend. For her, John's analysis represented the failure of her marriage, the trauma of the divorce; the end of the analysis meant a farewell to and separation from a painful past. For John, the reverse was true. In the transference he could attempt to enact the illusion that the "happy family" of his childhood had remained intact so that he could repress aggressive, destructive fantasies.

I told John clearly and directly that of course an end would come to the analysis, but only when he was ready for it and at his own pace. I also said that there was still a considerable amount of work to be done in the analysis. John was ambivalent: he felt that I was supporting him, and at the same time he was full of reproach because he felt I wanted to hold onto him. "And with a man like you I don't get one step further," he complained.

John spoke, with much affect and detail, about his feeling that everything was always against him in life: the perpetual feeling of not being good enough, all those feelings of imperfection related to his early speech therapy and to the other treatable medical conditions, his failure to exhibit the artistic talent for which his parents had hoped, the difficulties of his parents' marriage, his father's illness, and his parents' divorce. The analysis could not change reality, he said, and precisely because of the analysis he had begun to realize how truly difficult everything had been. At the same time, John felt supported by his mother's attitude: she felt that things were going well for him, showed her confidence in his abilities, and took him seriously.

In the following months John began to grapple with issues of adolescent development that he had previously avoided. At times he preferred to sit in the high window seat of my office so that he could look down on me and the rest of the world. He lectured me on the birds that he saw skimming past the window. At the end of the session we were both surprised to see how much he knew about them. "Learned it from the nice, young father of a friend of mine, completely different from those dusty old stuffed birds in my father's studio," John commented.

But in a later session John again praised his father's great knowledge; for John, his father was a walking encyclopedia. I suggested to him that he felt compelled to keep it that way by remaining small and lacking knowledge himself but that we also saw in the analysis how he was starting to outgrow this trusted protective jacket. John experienced this as a challenge he wanted to accept immediately. He wanted to play checkers with me, rummy cup, to show that he was a match for me. "I'll beat you because I'm young and strong and you're old . . . I've had enough of that old bullshit of yours."

Just like a typical adolescent, John would expound on philosophical subjects and thoroughly enjoyed disparaging adults. This philosophizing was an indication of his progressive development, and it helped him to organize a set of defenses. Our work at enabling John to tolerate a wide range of painful affects and experience them within the transference was partly responsible for this change. For John, who in the early phase of treatment had exhibited an almost concrete-operational manner of thinking, philosophizing was also a practical opportunity to understand and think about more difficult interpretations that appealed to a more abstract level of thinking.

I always tried to formulate my interpretations in terms of the accessible affect of the highest level of conflict so that they served John's self-image and defenses (integration), which supported his further development. I tried to avoid interpretations that John, whose ego strengths were still somewhat tenuous, might perceive as seductive, hurting, or shameful (Edgcumbe, 1988).

A series of brief segments from the final months of John's treatment give an indication of issues with which John struggled at that time; our dealing with these matters permitted further development once the issue of termination had emerged (Novick, 1988).

Session 750

John cradled his head in his arms, fed up. For four years he had been "shooting the crap" with his analyst because his parents were getting divorced. Angry, he grabbed a pencil to draw a cartoon. He imagined that he was a world-famous cartoonist who drew a comic strip about flying eyes with eagle claws attacking each other with hatchets. I acknowledged John's pride in being able to express his fantasies so freely. Feeling encouraged, he told me his version of "Pittsville", giving graphic descriptions of the tenements. He promptly made an improvement to his cartoon—one eye became the good eye that would defeat the evil eye, forever. I interpreted the cartoon as an indication that John felt that his uninhibited fantasies were an evil he needed to conquer.

Session 756

John met a few pupils from a local high school just outside of the building where the analysis took place; he felt terribly embarrassed. Going to a psychiatrist meant that you must have killed your father, mother, or thrown your sister from the window, he said. He felt like a convicted criminal who had fouled the city with his graffiti. He compared himself with Hitler: power fascinated him. He imagined that he would have to report to his concentration camp guard/ analyst for years. I interpreted John's fear of never being able to become a grown man if he could not equal his father. All he had left, I said, was to have fantasies about being a terrible criminal, which made him so unhappy. John denied feelings of devastation, which he had clearly experienced on some level.

Session 765

"What would you do if a pit bull terrier attacked you?" John asked as he observed me closely to see my reaction to this effort to frighten me. "You just watch out for my mother," he continued. "She shoved a newspaper into a dog owner's hands to clean up the shit his dog had left in the doorway." I interpreted John's admiration for his mother's competence and his fear, as a boy, of being no match for this woman who had sent his father away. John reacted with angry, growling noises. "Oh, of course, you want to be a pitbull terrier yourself," I added. John flared up, agitated, and stood as if he were about to pounce on me. He expressed fantasies of how he would overwhelm, humiliate, hurt me. In earlier sessions we had worked at John's conflict over his loving feelings toward me, and it became clear that part of his aggressive stance was his way of demonstrating his manliness to me, for which he had hoped for fatherly recognition. In his behavior John portrayed a masturbation fantasy in which he identified with his phallic mother and got even with his beloved father. As John's ambivalence toward his father became more intense within the transference, John expressed a fear that my concerned, sometimes protective attitude toward him might make him feel 'too dependent' on me. John's mother had deprived him of his father, and now, by suggesting that he consider ending his treatment, she was depriving him of me. John expressed a wish to be in analysis as long as Woody Allen. Nevertheless, he skipped the following session. Later I interpreted his difficulty tolerating support from a man while at the same time longing for such feeling.

The Last Stage of the Termination Phase

In the final phase of the analysis John could experience pregenital drive derivatives more genuinely and in their full intensity. With this his sense of self grew, evidenced also in the greater intensity and differentiation of a variety of feelings, of which a sense of shame was prominent. John could now accept the developmental challenge to form his own identity.

Issues of activity–passivity reappeared in the terminal phase. Underlying the passive stance were fantasies about the idealized child who remained united with his parents; John's repeated queries of whether I liked his sweater, or his hair, were examples of this. These fantasies protected John from the fear of becoming a man and acknowledging his sexual and aggressive wishes. Interpretation of John's defensive use of passivity led to John's associations, indirect at first, to masturbatory fantasies. He spoke of a tingling in his nose when he saw pretty girls and wondered if I had had similar experiences. John's associations led to girls who "look nice but make a fool out of you." With further work at this material, there was a diminution of John's anxieties over masturbatory fantasies, which, while still charged with a regressive cast, were able to serve his development as an object-oriented experiment in his imagination. John no longer avoided contact with girls.

Before the summer vacation of the fifth year of analysis, John stated emphatically that he wanted to end treatment. He summarized a series of motives: he could manage by himself now, he got along well with his stepfather, and he felt supported by him. And he wanted more time to study for final exams in the upcoming year. John expressed his feelings in this way: "I used to be terrified; I had the feeling that I had to go to the analysis or else terrible things would happen—as if the world would come to an end. The analysis has made me much less anxious . . . I'm sick and tired of always being that pathetic little kid who is under treatment and can't do anything himself." (Since age six John had experienced a variety of examinations for physical symptoms that had yielded little more than a reinforcement of his feeling of being somehow defective.) "I am through talking with you . . . and I am no longer afraid of you," he added.

After the vacation John said that at first things had gone just fine but halfway through he had gotten a nervous feeling that he could have talked to me endlessly—so he was glad to be back after all. In the following weeks John was often silent and periodically expressed a wish to end treatment before his final exams. The only reason to stay in treatment, he sometimes felt, was his great fear that he would not pass the exams. "Shall I stop right now, before my exams, or right afterward?" he worried. John had conflicted feelings about maintaining contact with me, in order to benefit from some fantasied magical influence of mine, and feeling free to move away and function independently.

During this time, John's social activities increased. He had a steady girlfriend and proudly showed me a photograph of her. When he heard about the divorce of her parents and about an accident that her brother had, John was upset. His feelings about his own parents' divorce reemerged as he spoke of his mother's "terrible unfaithfulness." At times he continued to resist being aware of his anxious and angry feelings toward his mother, and these feelings were experienced in relation to me in the transference.

One day John grumbled about his mother, who set "too many rules," and about his girlfriend, who had been ill-tempered for several days. With a mixture of trepidation and pride John told me that he had spent the night with his girlfriend in her bed; he had not come home that night and he had not called. Then, vehemently, John shouted, "Don't expect me to tell you anything more about it. None of my friends would ever dream of talking about something like that with their father. I'd be afraid that you would laugh at me; you're an old-fashioned prick who *thinks* that you should screw your girlfriend if you are in love, and boy, are we in love! When I *think* that you are married and have children and I haven't even started yet, it gives me such a horrible feeling of devastation. If you say one more single word about it, Ubbels, I'll sock you, because I'm not afraid of you anymore."

I told John that it seemed as if he first had to feel that he destroyed me before he could get any further himself: "As if the two of us couldn't rest assured that you, in your way, will develop into a grown man." John looked at me, grateful and a bit embarrassed. A little later John said, "It would be pretty extreme to castrate you, but everything lies in extremes with me; it would make that awful difference between us a lot smaller; I'm always such a clumsy, bungling oaf."

In his fear that his anger would harm me, John had not dared to end the analysis. Now he feared that if he stayed in analysis any longer, his yearning for tenderness would divest him of his so recently acquired and vulnerable manliness. John had attained a level at which he could at least endure this conflict for some time without regressing to the desire for unconditional paternal love and subjugation to his father's greatness.

John began to show an energetic wish to compete successfully with me in the transference, but also with his father. At school he made efforts to pass his final examinations and made realistic plans for his future. He no longer allowed himself to be led only by a tyrannical self-image. An ego ideal that set attainable goals was becoming prominent. The previously described difficulties would remain a weak point in John's character, but their overpowering inhibiting influence on his development had diminished significantly. During this phase, in which he expressed repeatedly that he felt ready to end treatment, John had intense and ambivalent feelings; he was anxious and hovered between progression and regression.

After 4½ years of treatment, when John again mentioned his wish to bring our work to a close, I said that since he was so in favor of it, it seemed a good idea to me too for him to try being on his own. We agreed to a termination date three months later.

In these final months John was able to work with reconstructive material with respect to the significance of the birth of his siblings. Previously, his typical reaction had been one of denial, telling me how nice things had been with his father during his early childhood. Now his sense of being left abruptly by his father after the birth of his siblings, who did not have learning disorders and who grew up to be father's "favorites," emerged sharply in his perceptions.

To John and to his parents the end of the analysis also meant the end of the illusion that behind the neurotic inhibitions lay a great talent. Reality now became inescapable, and the disillusionment seemed to come from the outside world: his girlfriend left him, he was not accepted at a secondary school for which he desired admission, and his father was hospitalized again.

During the final months of the analysis, John regressed into a stubborn, silent state. At school, he avoided doing his work. His parents were very worried—understandably so, in view of John's resignation and apathy. But they were also dismayed now that the reality of John's difficulties and his limited possibilities could no longer be brushed aside. His parents viewed John as depressed, but in the analysis a more defiant, silent resignation predominated.

At first I tried to let John see that this was his way of taking revenge, because he was so disappointed and angry that the analysis was coming to an end without reality having been magically changed. I suggested to him that in this way he wanted to force me to keep him in treatment. When John showed scarcely any reaction to my interventions except for an increased sullenness, I realized that he was also letting me share in his fear and desperation. Sometimes he expressed these feelings in their full magnitude: John would grip his head and say that he thought he was going crazy because everything was draining out of his head.

At great length, I put into words for John his feeling that everything had always been against him in life, starting with the birth of his siblings and ending with the divorce of his parents. I discussed with John how his obstinately woeful attitude of doing nothing used to be the only way he had of coping and of communicating his utter desperation to his parents. I added that he now had other ways to master his feelings. "Do you think it's so strange that I have a hard time stopping after I could come to see you for so long?" he asked bitterly, not unaware that he wanted me to share the desperation he felt. I continued to state clearly that we could understand his intense reaction to our joint decision to end the analysis and that I was still of the opinion that he was now at a point at which he could go on without me. I did offer John the opportunity to postpone the termination date, if he wanted to, so that we would have more time to work through the emotions aroused by the termination.

But for John there was absolutely no question of postponing the termination. He brought forward arguments that I felt were a confirmation of our earlier decision. "I trust you and that's why everything that I think and feel always comes out here. But I'm getting sick and tired of you knowing everything about me. I want to keep those things to myself and solve them myself." The last weeks of the analysis brought little change in John's silent attitude. His parents strongly urged me to offer John occasional appoinments following termination, but John refused. "When I see you, I get the feeling I'm meeting someone I just had a long talk with this morning in the museum. We've said all there is to say."

In a session three months following termination, John exuberantly told me that he had passed his final exams with good marks in languages and mediocre marks in sciences. He had enrolled in a graphic arts program at a vocational-technical school in the fall. Things had gone well for him since the termination of the analysis; he had felt much more energetic and was relieved and happy. I noticed that he spoke with shame about having been in analysis for so long.

Discussion

An important consideration for me in assessing John's readiness to terminate treatment was that in the transference his fear of his sadistic fantasies, his anger and jealousy, and the menacing emptiness left by the destruction of the idealized father–son unity had been worked through to a considerable degree. During the final year of analysis, with termination in sight, John had acquired sufficient ego strength to dare to separate himself from me. One aspect of

John's wish to leave treatment was his feeling that being independent of me would permit him to feel more like an adult. I wanted to take care not to enact the role of the exacting, disparaging father by insisting that John continue in treatment at a time when he wanted very much to separate.

With respect to the emergence of countertransference feelings, I suspected that I was unconsciously defending myself against sadistic fantasies and related guilt. From early in his treatment John had demanded an endless amount of admiration for what were often mediocre accomplishments, which he exhibited to me in a masochistic manner, in this way unconsciously inviting me to humiliate and denigrate him.

Separation, surely with an adolescent as seriously neurotically handicapped as John, is a struggle filled with jubilation, doubts, and fears—for both patient and analyst. I do not know how John as a young adult now looks back on his analysis and his experience with termination. In fact, I am not aware of any literature in which the protagonist in the drama of the termination of a child analysis looks back and speaks out.

During the termination phase of the analysis John threatened to reenact the infantile trauma, to be the son who could not satisfy the expectations and the demands of the father. But ultimately John showed himself to be capable of better conflict solution, of a more adaptive mastery of his feeling of desperation.

Was the infantile trauma worked through in this analysis at the level of the unconscious fantasy as organizer of character development? Several factors show that this occurred during the termination phase of John's analysis: John was able to put his fantasies of fame into a more realistic perspective and could better tolerate his limitations and his feelings of helplessness; his defenses against aggression were much less rigid; he no longer denied aspects of the painful past and he was able to use reconstructive material; he took the initiative himself to end his analysis and he was the one who set the pace; and, finally, John became able to use his capacities in a productive and creative manner.

References

Blos, P. (1979), *The Genealogy of the Ego-Ideal, The Adolescent Passage.* New York: International Universities Press.

——— (1984), Son and father. *J. Amer. Psychoanal. Asnn.*, 32:301–324.

Edgcumbe, R. (1988), Interpretation in clinical work with adolescents. Presented at the weekend conference of the British Psycho-Analytical Society, London.

Kris, E. (1956), The personal myth. *J. Amer. Psychoanal. Asnn.*, 4:653–681.

Munder Ross, J. (1979), Fathering: A review of some psychoanalytic contributions on paternity. *Internat. J. Psycho-Anal.*, 60:317–327.

Novick, J. (1988), The timing of termination. *Internat. Rev. Psycho-Anal.*, 307–319.

Sandler, J., Kennedy, H. & Tyson, R. (1975), Discussion on transference. The *Psychoanalytic Study of the Child*, 30:409–441. New Haven, CT: Yale University Press.

van der Leeuw, P. J. (1958), The pre-oedipal phase of the male. *The Psychoanalytic Study of the Child*, 13:352–375. New York: International Universities Press.

Late Adolescence

In chapter 8, Judith Yanof describes the termination of the analysis of an adolescent girl, Cindy, who began four-and-a-half year psychoanalysis when she was 14 years old. The termination phase lasted a year and divided itself naturally into two parts. In the first seven months, Cindy struggled with the question of whether to go to an out-of-town college and leave her analysis. During this phase she had a long period of renewed symptoms. The second phase, of five months' duration, began when a termination date was established. The focus of this phase was her mourning for the end of her analysis and her separation from the analyst.

Although the analyst considered the psychoanalysis successful, Cindy did not develop a full-fledged oedipal transference neurosis during the termination phase, nor did she fully analyze an idealizing transference. These two factors raise the question of the adolescent's capacity to disengage fully from the analyst before the adolescent has taken the developmental step of fully disengaging

from the parents. Other papers in the adolescent psychoanalytic literature report a high frequency of unilateral
and interrupted terminations in adolescent analyses.
Flight, regression, and terminating without giving up the
idealized version of the analyst are all ways of avoiding
disengagement.

Paul Kay discusses Gary, who at 18 terminated his
analysis, with his analyst's consent, before he left for
college. Two years of treatment had involved work with
neurotic conflict and developmental delay. An intense
maternal transference provided the early arena for work
with Gary's substantial resistance. Following the initial
phase, Gary reported two manifest incest dreams, both of
which provided significant opportunity for continuing
exploration of intrapsychic conflict.

When the initial treatment ended, Gary and his analyst
agreed that substantial work had been accomplished.
Gary returned to analysis on several occasions following
termination. These renewed efforts were not planned and
allowed Gary to explore, in greater depth, his conflicts
over disengagement from his analyst. While the literature
of child analysis refers to efforts of adolescents to return
for further work during college vacations, Gary's case is
unique in presenting details of clinical process when such
work is resumed in a totally unplanned fashion. The
ambiguity that exists in termination of analysis is emphasized, and Gary's case illuminates specific difficulties in
work with late adolescents.

Ann, Ruth Frenkel's patient, ended her analysis during
her first semester at junior college, a school close to home
that was selected so that her analysis could continue, if
indicated, following her graduation from high school.
The initial diagnostic impression was of hysterical neurosis. Ann exhibited school phobia at the onset of treatment and pseudo-cyesis during the first extended interruption the following summer. Following detailed
exploration of preoedipal and oedipal issues, the termination phase of Ann's analysis occupied about five
months, with the most intense work occurring during the
final month. Ann's decision to end analysis earlier than
anticipated is explored from varying perspectives, including structural changes, the state of transference,

wishes for autonomy, and the developmental stage that was attained. Countertransference issues are also addressed.

8

Singing Harmony: Termination in an Adolescent Analysis

Judith A. Yanof

> *"Singing harmony is doing my own thing,*
> *like being my own person."*

One of the major tasks adolescents face is disengaging from their parents. On a psychic level this means withdrawing from the parents the infantile feelings, conflicts, and emotional investment associated with early childhood. At the same time, adolescents must prepare to live independently, finding new relationships outside the family that will not only substitute for but be of a different kind from the old ones. This process of disengagement is painful and has been likened to mourning (A. Freud, 1958; Wolfenstein, 1966). It is also tumultuous.

Within a short period of time the adolescent is beset by major changes in her body and, with them, the awakening of strong instinctual urges, both sexual and aggressive. Besieged by these feelings, the adolescent distances herself both emotionally and physically from the parents, who cannot safely remain the objects of these feelings. However, the incestuous objects are also the omnipotent and aggrandized parents of early childhood upon whom the child has come to depend for her security and self-esteem. Relinquishing these objects to rely largely on inner resources is experienced as a major loss. It is not surprising, then, that the process of disengagement creates much conflict.

When adolescents come to analysis this central task of separation is almost always disrupted. Often, conflict over separation or the symptoms arising from it are the main reason that the adolescent has been brought to treatment. This conflict will affect no aspect of the treatment more profoundly than termination.

161

Termination itself is a disengagement, a disengagement from the analyst who has become invested with the multileveled attachments of the early infantile objects. Termination in adult analysis has been likened to the normal developmental process of adolescent separation (Rangell, 1966; Miller, 1965; Novick, 1982). However, when adolescents terminate they must separate from both their parents and their analyst at the same time. It may not be possible to disengage totally from the analyst before the disengagement from their parents is consolidated, that is, before the adolescent is truly independent.

The literature on adolescent analysis has called attention to the frequency of "premature termination" and "unilateral termination" among adolescents in analysis. According to Jack Novick: "The usual experience of termination for adolescents is that of a premature termination. Unless met with great skill, tact, and strength, adolescents, in relation to their families and to the therapist, tend either to run away or to subtly provoke the adult to throw them out" (Novick, 1982, p. 334). A unilateral termination is a consequence of the conflict of disengagement; it is the adolescent's premature flight from an object who stirs up too many conflicted longings. In a similar way some adolescents try to disengage from their parents by physically leaving home or by cutting themselves off emotionally from their parents' influence. On the other hand, some adolescents deal with the conflict of disengagement by a pathological regression. Instead of giving up their childhood objects, they remain infantile themselves, hold on to their infantile attachments, turn away from the outside world, and renounce their autonomy.

In this chapter I discuss the case of an adolescent named Cindy, whom I saw for 4½ years in psychoanalysis, four times a week, from age 14 to age 19. She was very gifted in her capacity to think analytically and had what I believe to be a successful analysis. During the analysis, Cindy had sustained periods of intense transference in which her conflicts were organized primarily around the analyst. Yet, unlike many successful adult analysands, Cindy terminated without having developed a full-fledged oedipal transference neurosis and without fully analyzing an idealizing transference. For this reason, Cindy's analysis drew my attention to the adolescent's capacity to disengage fully from the analyst. This capacity relates to the question: What is a successful adolescent termination?

Background

Cindy was brought to see me by her parents in the middle of her eighth-grade year, when she had just turned fourteen. Although her parents had been concerned about Cindy's unhappiness for many years, her refusal to do her homework precipitated their decision to seek treatment. Her parents astutely observed that their daughter "did not seem to want to grow up." They reported that in the face of difficult assignments Cindy threw up her hands, inviting her parents to take over, but then rejected all help. Her parents also complained of Cindy's chronic belief that she was being cheated in the family, her jealousy of her sister, her unwillingness to cooperate, her refusal to take responsibility for her disappointments, and her tantrums when she felt frustrated. Cindy was the older of two girls; her sister, Julia, was 16 months younger. At the time of the initial consultation, Cindy was the sister who had not yet reached menarche.

At 14 Cindy was a beautiful, quiet, and compliant girl who looked more like a latency-age child than an adolescent. I learned over time that this presentation was a source of great distress to Cindy; yet her internal conflicts did not permit her to relinquish the plain hairdo, barrettes, and childish styles that made her look younger.

It became clear to me that Cindy felt isolated and inadequate within her peer group and that she was having great difficulty loosening the ties with her parents. Although she engaged in enormous struggles with both her parents, especially mother, she did not feel at all able to make her own decisions or manage her independence. I recommended psychoanalysis because her chronic conflicts about growing up were interfering with her ability to disengage from her parents and move into adolescence.

Although Cindy's parents described her early years as uneventful, it was clear that Cindy felt abandoned and displaced when Julia was born. She tried to hide her intense jealousy of Julia and her bitter resentment of her mother. She covered her feelings of loss and hurt by subtly devaluing her mother, and then turned to her father for affection, despite intense competition from her sister. Father played many fantasy games with his daughters that Cindy found exciting and special. As she grew older she complained that father was intrusive and intolerant of her independence. Still, she tried to avoid any criticism from him.

Cindy's main companion throughout her childhood was her younger sister. In many ways Cindy relied on Julia as if Julia were the older sister. This reliance on the family to the exclusion of outside relationships was practiced by the entire family.

Cindy experienced her parents as wanting her to be good, proper, and nice at all times. She could not reconcile this with her own inner feelings; she felt that she had to wear a "mask" with others and that others wore a mask as well. Her own feelings were experienced as bad, dangerous, and potentially explosive. She dealt with them by jumbling them into confusion, discarding them as soon as possible, and projecting them outside herself. She often didn't know what she felt and tried to read the thoughts and feelings of others in order to discover what she "should" feel. In adapting herself to others' expectations, she relinquished her own autonomy. Thinking for herself or thinking differently from her family seemed to her the equivalent of an aggressive act. However, the ease with which she gave up her own agenda—and her difficulty even *knowing* her own agenda—made her fearful of control by others and frightened of intimacy. As she approached adolescence, with its developmental demand for increased autonomous functioning, Cindy began to flounder.

The Analysis

Cindy began her analysis with the magical expectation that I would "fix" her. She presented herself as a victim and hoped that I would become her strong and protecting ally. At the same time, potential closeness in the relationship frightened her. Because she felt that she needed me, she feared that I would control her. She was unable to assert her needs in the relationship and was convinced that if I knew her real feelings I would want nothing to do with her. Cindy interpreted my neutrality as a sign that I didn't care for her. As we explored these concerns, she became more able to tolerate her own feelings and more trusting that I was willing to hear them.

As the analysis deepened Cindy began to talk to me about early and important "secrets." She told me that she had played with Barbie dolls ever since she was a little girl, and this had continued until the analysis began. Throughout her childhood she would secretly seclude herself in her room for hours. There she would enact elaborate fantasies that embarrassed and sexually aroused her. Her parents viewed this doll play as "babyish," but Cindy's fear was that the fantasy play would become so seductive that it would keep her from joining her friends and from experiencing real life. She enacted masturbatory fantasies of oedipal rivalries and sadomaso-chistic conflict with her Barbie dolls. Cindy gave up her Barbie dolls when she began her analysis, feeling that she had overcome an addiction.

Cindy also revealed with great difficulty that her father made her uncomfortable by not changing his behavior with her as she pro-gressed from childhood to adolescence. He would continue to kiss

her on the lips and lie down in bed with her. She would get upset
and wonder if he were experiencing sexual feelings toward her. If he
were, she reasoned, that made him a pervert, and if not, it was she
who was perverted for thinking such bad things about him.

Discussions around this issue were very charged. Cindy could
barely bring herself to tell me what was on her mind, insisting that
I guess, a practice that "cleared" her of some degree of responsibility. Since she needed to believe that feelings were coming from him
alone, she was very accusatory toward her father, whom she
sometimes imagined was a bad, frightening man. Then she became
terrified that I might actually intervene and punish him. Simultaneously, she was furious that I did nothing to protect her and that I,
in essence, abandoned her the way she felt her mother had. In the
countertransference I felt a pressure to act on her behalf because she
was so intensely distressed and seemed so helpless. She was
struggling to avoid her emerging sexual feelings and the revival of
incestuous oedipal fantasies. At the same time, she was recapitu-
lating an old childhood dilemma in which she had turned to her
father for love but then felt overstimulated, unprotected, and unable
to extricate herself from the situation. Instead of intervening with
her family, I worked with her to help her understand her feelings so
that she could feel empowered to improve the situation for herself.
As we talked it became clear that she clung to old ways of relating to
her father because she felt she still needed this closeness with him.
This was a prime example of her conviction that she must please the
other person at all costs lest she lose the relationship forever.
Analyzing this aspect of her relationship with her father brought
great relief, eventually enabling her to handle the situation by
dealing with father directly.

Cindy became very committed to the analytic process. She shifted
to me the idealized view she had had of her parents, enabling her to
loosen her ties with them. Seeing them in a more realistic light, she
felt less threatened by them and less threatened by being different
from them. In the analytic work itself she used less externalization
and developed a good capacity for self-reflection and insight.

Much of the central portion of the analysis focused on Cindy's
disappointment and anger at her mother, which largely stemmed
from her early years. Cindy associated her acute sense of abandonment with the birth of Julia; she also felt excluded from the special
relationship that her mother had with her father. She remembered
how envious she was that her mother got to have babies while she
had nothing. In her Barbie fantasies, getting more and more babies
was a prominent theme, as was killing the pregnant Barbies. In this

way Cindy became aware of how angry she had been as a child. She often pictured herself as a little girl with a cookie, clutching it tightly because she felt she had so little of anything good but knowing she would lose her friends if she didn't share it.

Cindy remembered feeling as a little girl that her mother was "off in another world." She was haunted by a recurrent nightmare of her mother with an immobile, impenetrable face. Cindy vividly reenacted aspects of this powerful negative maternal transference in our relationship. She often seemed to be saying to me that she felt uncared for and that she hoped and expected that I could make up for it. She became hurt and angry when this didn't happen in her analysis, crying angrily and stamping her feet. Yet she was able to work with these feelings in the transference.

This material was repeatedly reworked in the transference and led the way to a more consistent emergence of oedipal material. Cindy talked increasingly about her sexual fantasies and increasingly saw herself as a sexual person. The transference shifted. She now saw me as a figure who was pushing her to grow up before she was ready and who was also letting things get out of control. She associated growing up with leaving home, going down a steep hill, careening out of control, and getting stuck at the bottom, unable to get back up. As incestuous feelings and sexual fantasies came into the analysis, Cindy became quite anxious. It was as if I were seductively encouraging such feelings but then leaving her alone with them while she felt totally out of control. This transference combined aspects of her "too-exciting" oedipal father and of her "unprotective" oedipal mother who didn't seem to see what was too exciting. Moreover, in this externalizing transference Cindy could repudiate her intense incestuous sexual feelings by attributing them to me.

As oedipal material repeatedly came into the analysis, Cindy backed away from it through the typical use of her customary defenses. Often, she presented herself in the transference as a little girl and wanted me to intervene to make her life better. It was most difficult for her to examine her competitive feelings about me. She would "forget" to tell me about the growing, independent, sexual part of herself. Increasingly, she began to feel that I would be angry with her if I knew about these things.

In spite of this, Cindy made many gains inside and outside her analysis. To a great extent she had disengaged from her parents, handled her own life more responsibly, and had become more autonomous. She was well connected to her inner life and had intimate friendships. It was at this point in the analysis that Cindy first mentioned termination.

The process of termination, which took about a year, fell naturally into two phases. The first phase covered a period of seven months, from September to March of Cindy's senior year of high school. During this time Cindy struggled with the issue of whether to go to an out-of-town college and leave analysis; during this phase she had a long period of renewed symptoms. The second phase was ushered in by Cindy's acceptance at the college of her choice in March and included the last five months of the analysis. In this phase the ending of the analysis and separation from the analyst became the focus of her analytic work. In both phases of the termination, Cindy accomplished significant working through and conflict resolution, described in detail in the following pages.

Termination: Phase I

Cindy first alluded to termination in the summer after her junior year. She reported a dream in which she was in a building, half-built. On the floors were puddles with "every imaginable gross fungus and bug in them." She had to walk through this mess barefoot. In her associations to the dream she said that the building represented herself, not completed, not fully grown. "Sexually, I am afraid to jump in and get my feet wet!" she quipped. Cindy went on to say that she had another year to resolve the main problem that still troubled her: her avoidance of a sexual relationship. In this way she defined for herself what remained incomplete in her analysis, and she stated that she had given herself a year to finish the work, coinciding with the amount of time remaining before she left for college. Nevertheless, she worried that she wouldn't be ready to leave by then.

I thought Cindy's assessment of her level of development was an accurate one. She saw having a boyfriend as a developmental task she needed to complete to be like her friends. She was anxious around boys and afraid of going on dates and "lost interest" whenever a young man became interested in her. I thought that these were manifestations of unresolved sexual, primarily oedipal, conflict. I too hoped this could be resolved before her treatment ended.

Cindy saw the ending of her analysis as inseparably bound to her going off to college. It is very common for late adolescents to bring up termination in conjunction with this milestone. It requires analytic work to help them separate and assess the two issues. As in her dream, Cindy would have liked to complete her analysis without having to go through the "yukky" stuff that remained, which included the "yukky" stuff between us. Therefore, Cindy's interest in termination at this point was, in part, a resistance. At the same time, Cindy experienced significant conflict about leaving analysis and quickly expressed doubt that she would ever finish.

For Cindy, leaving analysis, like other steps of independence, took on the meaning of an aggressive act that had to be hidden within a socially appropriate goal. On another level going away to college was part of Cindy's ego ideal, something she had dreamed about for years. During the next months Cindy struggled with all these issues in her analysis.

In autumn of her senior year Cindy began to have difficulty doing her schoolwork. This was the symptom that had originally precipitated her wish to begin treatment. However, after the first year it had remained in the background, only occasionally causing her difficulty. Now the symptom returned with great intensity. Cindy was blocked about writing and would put off studying until she had no time to do it properly. She hated herself for her behavior because she knew her first semester grades would be important to the college admissions committees. She wondered whether she would be smart enough to get into a good school.

On one level this refusal to do her schoolwork was the unconscious and unstated side of her conflict about leaving home and leaving analysis. If she couldn't do her work she couldn't go to college. Cindy was quite aware that she was frightened at the thought of going away to school and that home seemed to her a safe haven.

Cindy's father was very invested in her doing well at school. He was the one she went to for help whereas her mother was completely uninvolved. When Cindy didn't do her work, she and her father became embroiled in screaming battles. She could make her father lose control, scream, or even cry. Cindy became aware that as horrible as these battles were, she was drawn to them when she felt empty and unable to work. They were similar to the Barbie doll play: although "babyish," they kept Cindy engaged in a sadomasochistic, exciting interaction that was hard to give up.

In the fall Cindy's mother became depressed. Cindy had originally denied the significance of the situation, but reality became inescapable. One day she burst into tears, saying, "I think it's her menopause. She's lost her period, and she feels like she's losing her femininity. That seems very important to her. It makes me feel bad and guilty . . . How can I talk to her about my period if she's lost hers?" Cindy then associated to finding out her class rank that day. She had gone from 35th to 28th while her good friend Helen had gone from 28th to 33rd. "It's like we traded places." I said to Cindy, "I wonder if you feel that it's your growing up and coming into your own womanhood that is taking something away from your mother, like trading places with Helen in class rank." Later in the session I pointed out to Cindy that she always said her good marks were just "luck," as if she had nothing to do with them. That would only make sense if she were worried that being responsible for her good marks was akin to taking them away from someone else. Cindy felt ashamed of her competitive wishes. She confused them with her angry rages when she wanted her mother's attention. Now she felt as if her mother were disappearing all over again, as if, perhaps, she were making her mother disappear.

In early winter Cindy's procrastination about completing her college applications precipitated a crisis. Cindy's father called to let me know that Cindy wasn't at all prepared for college. He said that it was obvious from her behavior that she needed to continue in analysis. He thought she should apply to a prep school for an extra year of high school. Cindy was terribly distressed by her father's assessment of the situation, yet she was not certain herself that he was incorrect. She felt her father saw her as the Titanic, a sinking ship. She also feared that her father would take control over her life and "suck [her] up like a vacuum cleaner." It was humiliating to be "held back" with her younger sister.

This crisis gave Cindy and me another opportunity to consider her going to college as a separate issue from her leaving the analysis. She had several options, including one she had never really considered: going to college nearby and continuing her analysis. I pointed out to her that she had been acting as if the decision were not hers to make. By letting things get out of control she wouldn't have to decide: she had invited her father to take over. Part of her might have wished for this because she was afraid of making the decision: afraid of staying, afraid of going.

I interpreted to Cindy that by trying to involve me in her decision, she felt reassured that she still had my full attention. Cindy had always associated growing up with "turning her back" on her mother and losing her. Cindy responded by setting to work on her college applications. She felt very strongly that she wanted to go to an out-of-town school; if it didn't work out, then she could come back to analysis.

This crisis was followed by a session in which Cindy reported two dreams that graphically presented her dilemma. In the first dream Marc asked her to the prom. She had to buy a dress, so she went shopping with her father. She tried on a beautiful, long black dress.

It was tight-fitting and had an exceptionally beautiful lining that felt good, although it couldn't be seen from the outside. It looked very attractive on her, but it was "too mature." It was a dress for a woman, not a girl. Her father liked it, but he knew nothing about clothes. She needed her mother to say it was okay, but her mother wasn't around. The dress was strapless, and Cindy worried that she couldn't hold it up on her own.

In her associations to the dream Cindy said that she was afraid that she could not hold things up on her own in college. She felt that the dream meant that she was looking for her mother's permission and support to grow up and feel sexual. Mother's depression made her feel that mother wasn't there. Cindy felt that the lining was related to her analysis: it represented what was inside of her, which was both black and white, both good and bad, and which she was still not completely comfortable about showing.

In the second dream Cindy's mother had all sorts of delicacies but was saving them for herself and her husband. Cindy felt excluded and realized that she was no longer little and special. It was no longer the way it would have been if she were still her mother's little girl. She associated to reading about animals who would kill their young if the young didn't leave the nest once they were fully grown.

I interpreted to Cindy that she had a terrible dilemma. She didn't feel she had mother's permission to go off to college, that is, to be a separate, sexual woman. This was because she felt she was stealing her mother's womanhood and leaving her mother in ruin. At the same time she didn't feel she could remain a special little girl, her old solution, because she was too big for the nest and unwanted there. I went on to interpret that I thought she might be having similar feelings about me: she seemed to be waiting for my explicit permission to leave analysis, but at the same time she was feeling a need to stay very close to me. This longing seemed to exaggerate all the old feelings she had of being an outsider with me, not special enough or important enough to me. As in the dreams, both staying and going felt dangerous.

One day in the midst of this work Cindy entered my office with great excitement. She had brought me her favorite book from childhood, which she had hunted for in the library. (This was no small task since she had not remembered the title or the author.) She explained to me that she had been thinking about this book more and more in the last weeks and wanted me to see it.

The story was about a duchess who was baking bread one day. For some reason she had put too much yeast in the dough, and the bread began to rise out of control. The loaf became so large that she was caught on top, too high to reach her husband and children. The only way the family could get back together was to begin eating the enormous loaf. The last page shows the family reunited and happy but transformed into fat, roly-poly figures. As I read the book I thought that this regressive solution to separation, eating one's way back to mother, had obviously been a compelling fantasy of her childhood. The fantasy was now revived with the stress of having to look forward.

What felt out of control was further elaborated in that session. Cindy told me that she hadn't gotten her period since the summer, and it made her worry that she couldn't have children when she grew up. She went on to tell me, albeit with great embarrassment, that she had masturbated over the weekend with the fantasy that a man was out of control sexually. He had a fat wife but he didn't like her. He needed so much sex that he impregnated many women and had many families, but the children knew nothing because on the surface the parents acted normally.

Cindy recognized the man in her fantasy as her childhood version of her father, someone exciting and scary but who looked normal on the surface. At first she placed herself as the innocent child who knew nothing. Yet she easily recognized that a part of herself was also the fat woman who indulged in food, as well as the out-of-control man who indulged in sex. Cindy's fear of an out-of-control incestuous relationship made her avoid men, stop her period, and regress by eating her way back to mother.

Cindy continued to do a lot of analytic work, linking up her childhood Barbie doll fantasies, her present masturbatory fantasies, and her concerns about sexuality. One night she had the image of a little girl riding a huge horse and immediately became frightened that she would go into a coma and get stuck there. She linked this to her childhood Barbie story that Ken, Barbie's boyfriend, would become interested in Skipper, Barbie's sexually immature sister. Ken would have a huge penis and when he had intercourse with Skipper, it would hurt her permanently but would also feel good. Cindy said the coma reminded her of Sleeping Beauty, who did not grow up as a punishment for doing something forbidden. Sometimes she had the fantasy that she would be kept locked in a dark castle by a mean witch so she could never grow up. Sometimes she thought I was the witch and would keep her in analysis forever. I told her that she thought I would be very angry with her for her forbidden wishes and would try to keep her from growing up and taking my place.

Cindy associated to a recent fear that she would look into a boy's eyes and their gazes would lock. She would then be under the boy's control and have to do everything he wished. This fantasy "kept her under control" sexually but revived her old fear that she would lose her autonomy and couldn't hold on to herself in a close relationship.

The first phase of the termination was now at an end. It had been characterized by a sustained analytic alliance and a progressive working through of oedipal conflicts. Although Cindy had strong oedipal transference reactions to me at this time, a sustained and full-fledged competitive transference neurosis did not develop.

At this time Cindy wrote a poem that pleased her. It was about the passing of winter and the coming of spring. Although the air was still cold and nothing had yet come into bloom, she knew spring would arrive because she could feel the earth give way beneath her feet. In this very sensuous poem she symbolically anticipated her own blossoming. She knew it not from outside signs, but from a reliance on her inner feelings; these had come to be the more dependable indicators. I interpreted the poem to mean that Cindy was feeling increasingly better about relying on her own resources.

Termination: Phase II

When Cindy was accepted to the college of her choice, she was very happy. To her, the college acceptance made it concrete and unequivocal that she was ending her analysis. At this time (in March) she began to talk about a termination date. Because there was now "no turning back," the final five months of analysis were markedly different in quality. Separation and mourning became the focus of her work. She translated her continued psychological growth into her outside behavior by becoming increasingly more adult and responsible.

Cindy also began to date a boy. She was enormously relieved that she met a boy whom she really liked and to whom she felt sexually attracted. Rob was, like many adolescent choices, an "impossible" choice. He was very different from Cindy; part of a "fast," popular crowd, he was uninterested in going to college and was not at all self-reflective. However, in certain ways he fulfilled Cindy's ego ideal. Well liked, he had a spontaneity and freedom with others that Cindy greatly envied. Rather than being cautious and afraid of life, he was daring to the point of being reckless. In this way he captured the essence of the scary father of Cindy's childhood.

In her relationship with Rob, Cindy reworked some of her superego development. Rob and his ways challenged her overly strict superego. Cindy had to redefine right and wrong. When the relationship was over, she did not suffer enormously and felt that the sexual aspect of the relationship had been positive.

Cindy chose a termination date that was four months hence: she wanted to continue to see me until my summer vacation, which would begin a month before she was to leave for college. Cindy enthusiastically presented her plan for the summer. She wanted to apply to a college summer program near home, where she would live in the dormitory and take academic courses. This would help prepare her for college: she could live on her own, study, and talk to me about any problems that might arise. This plan placed her termination at the usual time we took our summer break, and very close to her actual departure for college. On both counts there was the risk that her feelings about termination could be lost, in either the ordinary feelings around a summer break or in the extraordinary feelings about leaving for college. Nevertheless, as we discussed the date at some length, I became convinced that it was important to let Cindy make this decision. Her plan was an attempt to have a trial run at being away from her family while still having her analysis—an attempt to differentiate her separation from her parents from the separation from me.

Several days before Cindy left home for her summer program, she had the following dream. "I am in a hotel. My parents leave the room to eat dinner. A man comes into the room and rapes me. My parents thought it would be safe because it was someone I knew."

Interestingly, Cindy had "no thoughts" about this dream. For someone who had come to take a very active role in analyzing her own feelings, this was highly unusual. To me it meant that the anticipated step toward independence threatened her and threw her back into a passive position in the analysis. In the dream she was again a child, a child whose parents had left her unprotected. Perhaps this dream was a warning to her about the dangers of being independent. As I felt tempted to jump in and help her work on the dream, I recognized my old countertransference response to her helpless presentation.

At summer school Cindy initially became attached to her roommate in a way that was reminiscent of the relationship she once had with her younger sister. She was surprised at her feelings of great love as well as intense envy. She was angry that she followed her roommate so unquestioningly and allowed her to break the ice for her in new situations. She was able to see that she tried to hide the intensity of her anger and competitive feelings even from herself by becoming dependent and little with respect to her roommate. Unlike in the past, however, Cindy was able to tolerate her intense envy and rage. Because of her analytic work, she could shift to a more equal relationship with her roommate. It was clear to me that these feelings belonged in the transference but were displaced onto the roommate. My attempts to bring them into the transference were not successful.

In the final months of the analysis, Cindy became palpably sad that it was coming to an end. This feeling arose in almost every session. Cindy was aware that she could get in touch with me if she needed to, and at times she felt sure that she would see me again. However, she said quite perceptively that she would miss the analytic work we were doing and just seeing me would not be the same. She felt distressed that new issues continued to arise and that the work never seemed finished. She came to the sad conclusion that she would have to continue the work but she would have to do it on her own. I helped her to understand that this was the way all analyses ended and that she would take the self-understanding part with her.

At the same time, Cindy began to miss sessions with me and come late. She would then berate herself for not using the remaining time she had with me more wisely. She became aware that she did this to avoid feeling discomfort about leaving. It reminded her of an earlier phase of the analysis when she would withdraw during the last minutes of the session, knowing she would not have time to finish everything she had to say and not wanting to be interrupted. Cindy also got into several scrapes from which she seemed to want me to bail her out. This again was reminiscent of our earlier work together. During this termination phase, however, she could easily see that she was presenting herself to me as not ready to leave, even though that was not the case.

Cindy dreamed she was on a bus trip with a very smart girl. She had fallen asleep on the girl's shoulder, like she used to fall asleep on her sister's shoulder in the car. Then the girl got a call from Yale and left abruptly. She interpreted the dream as follows: "Dr. Yanof, you are the smart girl and I was feeling very close to you. Suddenly you left, however, for something academically special. It was your career you had really been interested in and not me all along." I pointed out the obvious reversal in the dream. Cindy could see that she still had to hide her own aspirations and wishes to separate.

Our final sessions together were very moving. Cindy said that her analysis reminded her of the Velveteen Rabbit or an old beloved teddy bear, something that she once desperately needed but could now be discarded. She said, "Or maybe you pack it away and take it out for a hug occasionally when you need to, but it is not the same as when it was part of your life." She then broke into tears: "I am growing up and it feels so sad—wonderful and terrible at the same time." On one occasion when Cindy talked in a particularly sad way about analysis being like an old doll that needed to be discarded, I asked if she too felt like an old discarded teddy bear. She burst into tears and said that if she were not doing analysis with me she couldn't possibly be that important to me anymore. She knew this really wasn't true, yet she felt it all the same. She imagined someone would take her place and get my love. Then she laughed and said, "Someone named Julia."

In the final weeks of analysis there was much discussion of the central role I had come to play in Cindy's life and of the issue of her own autonomy. In one session she reported the following dream: "I was watching an opera with my family and you were on stage singing an aria. It was your swan song. The opera was about a separation. A father was telling his son that he was too young to leave home. The son was saying that he had to grow up. But when you were singing, I couldn't understand the words. They were in another language—Yiddish or something."

The dream saddened Cindy because it was about our upcoming separation. "You were still trying to tell me things, but I couldn't get all there was to get." The impending separation elicited thoughts about my death (the swan song) as well as a heightened perception of our differences (we couldn't even speak the same language). The dream also meant to Cindy that I would no longer be there to tell her things. In the dream the image of me as an idealized protector who would tell her everything to keep her safe was beginning to fade.

Cindy continued to focus on how she would fare on her own. She dreamed she was in a beautiful strapless gown; it made her breasts look large, and she felt aroused and very positive about her femininity. This is how she wanted to feel, but sometimes she was not sure she could rely on her own resources. It was as if I had opened the book to the right page and she still couldn't find what she needed to know. "You and I have woven a cloth together, but I worry that it will unravel if I am not seeing you."

In the last dream that Cindy reported in her analysis, she was in church with her family, standing between her sister and her father. She began to sing harmony. Her father and sister attacked her for singing harmony in church. At first she was upset but then she decided that there was really nothing wrong with what she was doing. So she went ahead and sang harmony. Eventually, she had to move to another pew because of her family's objections, but nobody else seemed to mind.

Cindy interpreted the dream as follows: "Singing harmony is doing my own thing, like being my own person. I feel sad because it feels to me that in order to do my own thing I have to lose my family. But in the dream I do find a place for myself and I do find my own voice. You have helped me find it."

Follow-up

Cindy has seen me several times in the three years since her analysis ended. She is now in her senior year of college and is doing very well. She was involved for several years with a young man in a relationship that was mutually caring and satisfying. She also studied abroad. Whatever distress she felt prior to our meetings was minor and quickly passed after she saw me. It was obvious that she continued to do much self-analytic work on her own. The only symptom that still bothers Cindy is that in unfamiliar situations she often feels that she cannot be spontaneous lest she offend someone. This inhibition makes her feel inauthentic and is reminiscent of the way she used to feel most of the time.

Cindy has continued to grow in the postanalytic period. She has not needed to be in analysis to continue her psychological growth. It is clear that I continue to play a role at this point in her life and that she has not entirely disengaged from me.

Discussion

In considering termination in adolescent analysis, as in child analysis, the analyst must assess whether enough analytic work has been accomplished to allow the adolescent to return to the path of normal development. Anna Freud (1970) wrote, "Children are in urgent need of analytic therapy when normal progressive development is arrested or has been slowed up significantly. . . . From this follows that they should be considered cured as soon as the developmental forces have been set free again and are ready to take over" (p. 14).

When Cindy terminated her analysis, I felt that she had achieved a return to the path of normal development. Through her work in analysis she had largely disengaged from her parents. She could now live away from home, manage her life responsibly, and make relationships outside her family that would sustain her.

The sexual conflicts that had preoccupied Cindy for so long and had made adolescence seem so terrifying had been well analyzed. As a result, she had given up her defensive regression and had become more comfortable as a sexual person. The analysis of her aggressive conflicts gave Cindy an increased ability to tolerate her anger and an increased understanding of the sources of her rage. This freed her to separate from her parents without feeling that she would destroy them. The analysis also addressed an early core issue: the suppression of her autonomy.

Cindy experienced the birth of her sister, when she was just 16 months old, as a profound loss. This early rupture from her mother occurred just as she was in the late practicing/early rapprochement phase of separation–individuation. Instead of consolidating a pleasure in her progressive exploration away from mother, Cindy felt her mother had pulled the rug out from under her. She turned to a very overstimulating relationship with her father in an attempt to deal with her sense of loss, but it left her feeling out of control and frightened. Thus, the earlier issues left her vulnerable to unusually intense oedipal conflicts.

Termination is not merely the ending of analysis but an essential phase in which substantial work continues to be accomplished. (Buxbaum, 1950; Ekstein, 1965; Miller, 1965; Ticho, 1972; Novick, 1982). At the time Cindy began termination, she was, as she put it, "a building, half-built."

Novick (1982) has referred to the interval between the broaching of the topic of termination and the setting of the date as "the incubation period." This is equivalent to what I have called the first phase of Cindy's termination. During this phase there were substantial progressive and regressive forces at work simultaneously. This is characteristic of analytic work in adolescence. Peter Blos (1980) writes that because adolescence is a time of actual psychic restructuring, regressive phenomena and powerful developmental thrusts are always intertwined within the same processes.

During the first phase of termination Cindy became symptomatic, as she had been in the beginning of her analysis. She regressively dug in her heels, as if to say to me and to her parents that she wasn't ready to leave home or analysis. At the same time, a developmental thrust carried her forward in her analysis. The degree of synthesis during this time contributed to the fast pace of the analytic work and led to the resolution of conflict. The analytic alliance was never stronger, and Cindy was fully identified with the analytic task. These features carried over into the final phase of termination as well. Cindy's wish to go to an out-of-town college was an external factor that seemed to motivate her to move forward with her analytic work.

During Cindy's analysis there were long periods of sustained transference, both negative and positive, that could be interpreted and worked through. This was not dissimilar to an adult analysis. Nevertheless, the working through and resolution of a full-fledged competitive transference was not part of the termination. During the terminal phase, Cindy's intense feelings of competition and envy were displaced onto her roommate; her oedipal feelings toward her mother were worked on in the analysis but not in the analytic transference. At the same time, Cindy maintained her view of me as an idealized maternal substitute. She could grow psychologically and separate physically, but this did not involve a de-idealization of me or a disillusionment with the analysis or its accomplishments. Believing in me, she could believe in herself. In this sense the termination was different from terminations in many successful adult analyses.

That Cindy did not disengage fully was confirmed in her continued, though occasional, contact with me after analysis. She used these meetings to maintain contact and to keep me informed of the self-analytic work that she continued to do on her own. Once, after challenging something I had said, Cindy expressed amazement that she had trusted me so completely: "Suppose I wake up one day and find out that Freud was all wrong? Then where will I be?"

This question suggests what Cindy needs to do in order to disengage from me. She must learn to feel comfortable even when psychologically untethered from me. This work is intimately connected to the residual autonomy issues that still disturb Cindy. Whether she can complete her work on her own, as she has started, or whether it will require future treatment remained unclear at our last meeting.

My impression is that it is often the case that adolescents may not be able to disengage totally from the analyst before normal development has allowed them to become truly independent of their parents.

Peter Blos (1980) states that the "nature of the adolescent transference is essentially different from that of adulthood because the transference neurosis remains in statu nascendi until the end of adolescence" (p. 148). In the idealizing transference of adolescence there are always elements of identification with the real person of the analyst because development is in progress. These elements become part of a transference cure and are not fully analyzed (Blos, 1980). Rudolf Ekstein (1983) comments on how often the treatment of an adolescent does not reach "the end point of the process" and that adolescents are often treated with both intermissions and interruptions.

The literature on adolescent analysis suggests that adolescents frequently interrupt their treatment prematurely. I believe this is common for adolescents who have dealt with the conflict of disengagement from their parents by flight. Yet it is not common for those who, like Cindy, have dealt with this conflict by regression. During an analysis, patients reenact with the analyst the central conflicts that have made disengagement problematic; they repeat with the analyst the maladaptive solutions of the past. Thus, adolescents who flee and those who regress behave differently in their analyses, using different defensive measures to deal with their emerging conflicts. However, flight, regression, and termination with the idealized version of the analyst intact are all ways of avoiding disengagement.

In Cindy's case, early issues around autonomy predisposed her to the difficulty of fully disengaging from the analyst at termination. Of course, Cindy is not unique in this respect. Many adolescents who come into analysis have difficult early issues that disrupt their ability to disengage from their parents.

I would like to conclude this chapter by reflecting on my own experience during the terminal phase of Cindy's analysis. I tried throughout this period to assume a neutral stance poised between Cindy's wish to go and wish to stay. Whenever possible I analyzed the issues on both sides of her conflict. My neutrality enabled Cindy to struggle with her conflict internally. This stance reminded me of the parents' task during the toddler's late practicing/early rapprochement phase of separation–individuation: at any given moment the parent is called upon to be a willing participant in providing either the attenuated attention necessary for the child who needs to go off and explore on his own or the more focused attention necessary for the child who needs increased closeness and intimacy.

Chused (1982) has stated that when working with patients who, like Cindy, have had difficulties in this phase of separation–individuation, it is the analyst's neutrality that allows an "autonomous practicing" within the analytic relationship. Chused says that without departing from standard analytic technique, the analyst's neutrality provides a "new type of object relationship" that permits the patient gradually to expand "autonomy in a variety of ego functions." I believe that my lack of personal investment in Cindy's final decision about termination and my willingness to accept her choice allowed her to have the freedom to determine what she wanted to do and ultimately supported her autonomy.

My neutrality did not prevent me from having deep emotional responses to Cindy's departure, and these required my own self-analysis. This was particularly true in the second phase of termination, when we both experienced her departure as imminent. The depth of Cindy's sadness was in direct proportion to the amount of work she did to relinquish her attachments to me and to the early infantile objects through the transference. My countertransference response was the feeling of a parent whose child was going off to college: I felt celebratory and, at the same time, sad because I was well aware that I would never again have the same place in her life.

References

Blos, P. (1980), The life cycle as indicated by the nature of the transference in the psychoanalysis of adolescents. *Internat. J. Psycho-Anal.*, 61:145–151.

Buxbaum, E. (1950), Technique of terminating an analysis. *Internat. J. Psycho-Anal.*, 31:184–190.

Chused, J. (1982), The role of analytic neutrality in the use of the child analyst as a new object. *J. Amer. Psychoanal. Assn.*, 30:3–28.

Ekstein, R. (1965), Working through and termination of analysis. *J. Amer. Psychoanal. Assn.*, 13:57–78.

————— (1983), The adolescent self during the process of termination of treatment: Termination, interruption, or intermission? *Adolesc Psychiatry*, 11:125–146.

Freud, A. (1958), Adolescence. *The Psychoanalytic Study of the Child*, 13:255–278. New York: International Universities Press.

————— (1970), Problems of termination in child analysis. *The Writings of Anna Freud*,Vol. 7. New York: International Universities Press.

Miller, I. (1965), On the return of symptoms in the terminal phase of psychoanalysis. *Internat. J. Psycho-Anal.*, 45:487–501.

Novick, J. (1982), Termination: Themes and issues. *Psychoanal. Inq.*, 2:329–365.

Rangell, L. (1966), An overview of the ending of an analysis. In: *Psychoanalysis in the Americas*, ed. R. E. Litman. New York: International Universities Press, pp. 141–173.

Ticho, E. E. (1972), Termination of psychoanalysis: Treatment goals, life goals. *Psychoanal. Quart.*, 41:315–333.

Wolfenstein, M. (1966), How is mourning possible? *The Psychoanalytic Study of the Child*, 21:93–123. New York: International Universities Press.

9

Ambiguity in Termination

Paul Kay

"You've been like a brother to me."

Novick (1976, 1982) has noted the paucity of clinical case material on termination in adolescent analysis and the fact that few adolescents experience mutual termination. He and Burgner (1988) have reported instances of adolescents returning once for further analysis as young adults (who were psychologically adolescent). There are no reports in the literature of an adolescent analysand returning for further analytic work several times after termination during late adolescence.

In this chapter, I present the termination experience of Gary, an adolescent analysand whose work at ending his analysis lasted for several years and consisted of multiple terminations based on both mutual and unilateral decisions. Gary's termination experience was ambiguous in many important respects. That ambiguity provided Gary with the psychological space required to permit substantial working over of both the separation-individuation and termination processes, which occurred simultaneously and were mutually facilitating.

Ambiguity in analysis has long been recognized by analysts as an intrinsic and important part of the analytic situation. Recently, Adler (1989) has written about this subject in connection with transitional phenomena, countertransference, and other aspects of the analytic situation. Here I try to demonstrate the particular value of ambiguity (especially in regard to the posttermination period) with respect to major issues in the termination experience of an adolescent patient. Ambiguity offered the patient an opportunity for the recognition and beginning mastery of important traumatic experiences; for further differentiation of his perceptions of himself from those of important figures in his life; for the ability to appreciate his mother as a separate person who needed him desperately; and, for the continued resolution of those anxieties and conflicts that had prolonged the termination experience. Finally, ambiguity provided the analysand with the opportunity to both defend himself temporarily from those anxieties and conflicts and to adapt to the idea and reality of termination.

The Consultative Phase

Gary, a bright and articulate 16-year-old boy from a middle-class background, sought treatment because of shyness with girls, failure to get along with male contemporaries, concerns about his school work, and his "temper." He stressed his wishes to be independent, successful, more intelligent than other people, and the center of attention. Even as a child, he had been very smart. Gary tended to blame other people, especially his mother, for his troubles. He had enjoyed outwitting two previous therapists by making them end his treatment; he claimed that he had not wanted and did not now want treatment. He thought that the doctor should do all the work although he knew and accepted (intellectually) the basic principle of the patient talking freely. He was usually eager to talk and had been lively and somewhat ingratiating during the consultative phase. At times, he seemed arrogant and boastful. Fluctuating degrees of accurate self-awareness coexisted with the apparent use of denial, projection, isolation, and rationalization. He showed no thought disorder, loss of affect, or reality-testing defect.

Gary's parents were concerned about his rages, which included assaultive and destructive behavior when he did not get his way and jealousy of his 4½-year-old brother. (He also had a year-and-a-half old sister.) His social isolation and erratic functioning in school had also disturbed them for a long time. In addition, his teachers portrayed him as disruptive.

Mother recalled Gary as a sickly child who had not eaten or slept well for the first few years of life; he had vomited after eating, but this stopped when she stopped forcing him to eat. Subsequently, she and Gary had "battled over everything." As a child, Gary had had multiple fears, sucked his thumb, masturbated often, and was accident prone. He wet his bed till age 13. Mother and Gary had

showered together until he was eight, and Gary had often spent time
in the parental bed kissing and hugging both parents. Mother had
encouraged Gary to walk around nude. During his early childhood,
she had often examined his genitals to see if they were all right. She
felt that she had been his adviser, confidante, and dream interpreter.
She had induced Gary and his father to share in the care of the
younger children and other family responsibilities; the care included diapering, feeding, and cooking (chores generally performed
by mothers at the time of Gary's analysis in the late 60s).

Gary's parents had often been on the verge of divorce. Mother, an
obese woman, had often screamed at and physically attacked Gary's
father (a short, slight man) in the presence of the children. Both
parents had had many years of psychotherapy and thought that it
had helped them. Both, especially mother, were eager for Gary to
enter analysis. Their present complaints aside, they anticipated a
glorious future for their adored, indulged son.

I viewed Gary as a youngster with a personality disorder in whom
narcissistic, exhibitionistic, manipulative, sadomasochistic, antiso-
cial, and paranoid elements were prominent. I thought, however,
that he might benefit from psychoanalysis because of his partial
insight, his wish to be independent, and his ability to form what
appeared to be a potentially useful, albeit highly ambivalent, relationship with me. His intelligence, capacity for reflection, articu-
lateness, and memory strengthened my decision. The enthusiastic
conscious support of his parents also contributed significantly to my
decision. I was, on the other hand, concerned about his ability to
tolerate and use productively the inevitable frustrations and regressions in analytic work.

The Analysis

Soon after the analysis began, a formidable resistance emerged in the
form of an intense maternal transference. The resistance arose in the
context of Gary's nearly continuous flow of complaints and frustrations arising out of daily incidents involving his mother, me, peers,
and teachers. When I tried to explore or interpret his increasingly
frequent demands for advice, particularly in relation to dating, he
attacked me verbally, became silent or sleepy, or threw small objects
(made of paper or other harmless material) in my direction. Because
Gary's resistance led to fragmentary verbal and nonverbal communications, the analytic process assumed a disjointed character for a
long time. Complicating the analytic situation very early in the

analysis were the intrusions of Gary's mother, who called to complain about his behavior at home and to ask for my advice on how to deal with him.

Opportunities for interpretive and noninterpretive interventions arose in the context of Gary's frequent frustrations both outside and inside the analytic situation. Sporadic brief periods of analytic work on various interrelated issues began to take place. Externalization was often one of those issues; repeated interpretations of his attacking me in various ways as an attempt to protect himself from painful feelings of frustration, self-criticism, and inferiority gradually led to Gary's acknowledgment that he wished to make me (and other people) "squirm" and "eat [my] heart out," feelings he was experiencing in his relationships with girls in school. I became the rejected, inferior boy and he the superior, rejecting girl. Repeated references, early in the analysis, to his tendency to stress isolated events and experiences, to shift from one subject to another, and to pause for varying periods of time rather than express his thoughts and feelings freely and continuously often led to his expressing anger at his mother's domination and intrusiveness and revealing his spiteful attitude and behavior towards her. His hatred of his mother and siblings and his wish to be rid of all of them emerged in this phase of the analysis.

Gary presented increasingly detailed and emotional reports of how he had felt terrified and confused in the past by his mother's screaming at him and hitting him, threatening to "cut off" his "allowance" when he had displeased her, and treating him as an equal or even someone to lean on. Depending on her mood, she made him feel "superior" or "inferior". He also accused her of making him grow up too fast by treating him as an equal. He felt that he had "missed out" on his childhood. Depending on his mood, Gary feared, hated, loved, idealized, and denigrated his mother.

As the maternal transference unfolded, Gary complained about my "shoving the analysis down [his] throat," as his mother did to him with her ideas. Interventions aimed at stimulating his awareness of his wish to control the analytic situation allowed us to begin to appreciate his attempt to control me (and his mother) in the same way that she, whom he referred to as the "general," had always tried to control both his father and him. For Gary, feeling in control of the analytic situation meant that I was the patient or "servant" and he the "king." But being in control also meant being cruel, like mother, and he disapproved of that trait.

As Gary focused increasingly on his paralyzing and frustrating conflicts about social interaction with girls, the opportunity arose for me to interpret his often desperate, angry demands for me to help him get dates as a reflection of his underlying demand that I treat him as he said his mother did (by advising and directing him or by frustrating and punishing him), despite his strong wish to be independent of me (and of her). The transference resistance at these times began to approach the structure of a transference neurosis.

Gary began to connect his vague and uncertain sense of himself to his mother's paradoxical treatment of him and his blurred perception of their relationship. Essentially, he could not be powerful like his mother since he hated her power over him. Nor did he want to be like his father, whom Gary viewed as "weak." Further illumination of Gary's attempt to define himself resulted from attempts to interpret his motility. My attempts at interpretation led to the emergence of his wish to be athletic and thus different from his parents, whom he regarded contemptuously as unathletic, "fat," and "weak." Later, repeated references to the movements of his hands led to fleeting and vague allusions to masturbation and masturbatory fantasies, as well as his wish to grow up and get married and other apparently healthy strivings.

Feelings of affection for his father and the wish to respect and protect him arose fairly early during this phase of the analysis. Up to this point, Gary had dismissed his father contemptuously as a "jerk" and a "weakling. He had boasted of his ability to "get away with murder" with his father, an attitude that he often displayed toward me in the transference and in school toward his teachers. He wanted his father's possessions and to be the "head of the family," although he referred to himself somewhat disapprovingly as "greedy" in this regard. These old perceptions of his father and the feelings associated with them did not, however, prevent him from beginning to express pride in his father's business achievements. Signs of a beginning friendly relationship with his father appeared.

Gary found it extremely difficult to talk about his sexual life. He felt that he would lose my respect if he did. My repeated interpretation of his fear as a reflection of his own disapproval of his sexual feelings led him gradually to reveal his wish to have "sexual intercourse" with girls. He began to realize that his fear of being rejected by girls had been holding him back from calling them up for dates and that that fear had, itself, arisen partially out of his anxieties about having intercourse with them. His growing interest in and increasing contact with girls led to the emergence of other conflicts, some of which seemed to be connected to his feelings and perceptions about his mother.

In the context of our first vacations, which took place during the last third of his junior year in high school (about eight months after the analysis began), he acknowledged the wish to please me. He wanted to be a "good" patient so that I would "miss" him, although he had been repeatedly and contemptuously dismissing me and the analysis as worthless (and continued to do so subsequently). About this time, he expressed briefly and vaguely the wish to go to an out-of-town college after graduation. He wanted to get away from his mother whom he was increasingly experiencing as "impossible," and start a new life outside his family. It arose in the context of his increasingly painful struggles to develop relationships with his female contemporaries and complaints about his mother and me failing to help him in one way or another. I stressed the importance of the analysis. Gary's wish was soon buried in his daily frustrations.

Prior to the senior year and in the context of wishes to be manly, independent, and free, a new attitude and behavior towards people appeared. He was able to express genuine remorse when he hurt someone (e.g., he apologized to a woman teacher whom he had physically injured (slightly) because she had given him a low grade). Early in his senior year, after 15 months of analysis, Gary began to report progress in his social and academic activities. Increasing socialization with peers of both sexes, the start of his first friendship with a male peer, the beginning of a new and apparently benign relationship with his father, and an improvement in his academic attitudes, behavior, and work constituted the main features of that progress.

The unfolding pervasive maternal transference still constituted a formidable resistance. It did not allow for more than a fragile therapeutic alliance. Gary's persistent and frequent demands, and his denigrating attacks when I did not gratify them, still dominated most sessions. He had become sharply aware, however, of being painfully conflicted about several important and interrelated issues: his persisting and intense fear of being rejected by girls; his inability to establish satisfying relationships with them; his inability to talk about sexual feelings; and, above all, his conflicted dependence on his mother and the possible connections between that dependence, his difficulty with girls (as well as with people generally), and his difficulty in defining himself.

The psychosocial issues were the conscious and behavioral signs of the conflicted underlying and essentially preoedipal tasks of achieving intrapsychic detachment from the maternal representation, self-definition, autonomy, a stable self-esteem, a lessening of his self-centeredness and need for admiration; a realistic and stable sense of himself and other people; and a new and socially acceptable moral code accompanied by behaviors based on it. (Oedipal strivings, mainly of a defensive and compensatory nature, were visible from time to time; they were not, however, in the foreground of his immediate struggles.)

Incest Dreams

The recurrent manifest incest dreams reported in this section were dramatically relevant to Gary's termination experience. They catalyzed the analytic process, and they provided rapid access to Gary's traumatic incestuous experiences, his attempt to define and reduce the self-defeating identification with his mother, and other major related issues. The analysis of these dreams facilitated Gary's separation-individuation journey, making it possible for him to leave the analysis and his family for an out-of-town college.

The first dream appeared in the 15th month of the analysis. Gary had been in a bitter and angry mood because of his failure to call a particular girl for a date (and had been angry at me for failing to help him do so); he was also anxious about a physics test the next day. In the dream, which Gary related at the end of a session with severe embarrassment, his mother was teaching him how to perform sexual intercourse and they had intercourse. He was stunned to have had such a dream because he had been hating her and anxious to escape her domination.

In the next session, Gary was very eager to talk, but not about the relationship of the dream to his frustrations over the physics test and his difficulty in dating the girl who had attracted him. Some of his remarks indicated that in the dream, he had replaced those frustrations with the regressive gratifications available from a mother who seemed to know everything and be able to do everything. But Gary's sustained and highly emotional communications in response to the dream quickly led to the emergence of several major interrelated themes: his (conflicted) wish to be feminine in the sense of having what he perceived as his mother's awesome strength and wisdom; his angry and bitter feelings about her exploitation of him in her attempts to use him as her husband; his cruelty towards women, especially his mother; his attempt to delineate, condemn, and discard various unacceptable tendencies in himself that he attributed to his mother's influence; his tendency to perceive and react to female peers as if they were his mother; his masturbatory experiences and accompanying (sadistic) fantasies; and his need for adoration from girls regardless of how he treated them.

Several months following these painful discoveries, Gary voiced the disturbing realization that, in contrast to his fear of being rejected by girls, he might be causing them to reject him because of his conflicted wish that they kiss his penis. Some time prior to this realization there had been an episode of regression lasting for about two weeks. Much of Gary's old symptomatology recurred in the home, in school, and in the analytic situation. It subsided after interpretations organized mainly around his rage at the girl whom he had not been able to date, his mother, and me—all of whom he had experienced as having bitterly disappointed him.

Six months after the first manifest incest dream Gary reported a second one. Gary had become aware of the connection between his ambivalent attitude towards sexuality and girls and his difficulty in feeling at ease with them. He was pleased with his good grades in school and with the golf clubs which his mother had just given him.

The dream was the same as the first one except for a new detail (which he had forgotten when he first reported the dream): he kisses his mother's "tushie" (buttocks) and genitals. (As with the first manifest incest dream, no specific previous day residue emerged.) Then, Gary revealed for the first time his mother's old and frequent practice of kissing his and his brother's genitals and buttocks in the past and his doing the same to his siblings (in particular, his brother). He interpreted his kissing his mother's buttocks in the dream as his revenge on her because of what she had done to him; also, he felt that he had made himself her equal in this way. He indicated strong feelings of both shame and triumph while reporting his mother's use of him and his use of his brother. In a later session, Gary spoke angrily and bitterly of "getting even" with girls because of how his mother and some girls had treated him (referring to the second incest dream). He thought that treating girls cruelly made him feel strong.

In subsequent sessions, Gary continued the detailed, systematic inventory and condemnation of more unacceptable traits in himself that he attributed to his mother's influence, a practice that he had begun after the first manifest incest dream.

He became increasingly frustrated about inviting a girl to the prom. Whenever he felt that I was failing to help him in this, he would attack me almost as fiercely as he had done in the past. Now, however, his attacks were briefer and far more accessible to analysis. More than once, their analysis led to the explicit and sustained appearance of the father transference (which had emerged intermittently prior to the occurrence of the first manifest incest dream). Gary complained bitterly about his father's neglect of him. For the first time, he expressed intense jealousy of his father's relationship with his brother. He wanted me to be his father. I could then think for him and get him a date for the prom. He could talk to me about sex. He indicated that he had felt hurt and angered at my failure to give him the attention which his father denied him. He thought that, in contrast to his father, he would be a strong one. (The "father transference" consisted of reactions similar to those that Gary had described experiencing with his actual father as well as wishes for an ideal father.)

At one point, I had occasion to suggest that his difficulty in getting a girl to take to the prom might be related to the dream about his mother. He responded by talking about girls "blowing" boys and that he had been having fantasies about girls blowing him when masterbating. In later sessions, he revealed his "disgust" about touching girls. This revelation came after I had had the occasion to interpret his oedipal conflict in connection with the daily frustrations he was experiencing with girls.

In the context of his struggles over his sexual wishes, he referred, from time to time, to his relationship to his teachers. He came to realize that part of his difficulties with them had to do with wanting to be treated as "special." He viewed this as originating in his mother's treatment of him as the man of the house. He connected her treatment of him with his difficulty in working with me. He could not accept my having "good ideas." Only he could have them.

Following the two manifest incest dreams the previous massive resistance in both its verbal and nonverbal forms which was largely based on the maternal transference now rapidly gave way to a relatively strong therapeutic alliance. Gary became a consciously eager, if not proud, participant in the work and showed increasing pleasure in his participation. The dreams and their impact on the analytic process permanently settled my previous doubts about being able to analyze Gary. Gary's resistance did not disappear but it became far more accessible to analysis than before.

The manifest incest dreams arose from the ongoing analytic process and then dramatically catalyzed that process. They provided a natural, relatively comfortable, and rapid means of diminishing Gary's resistance and providing access to issues and experiences that he had had to repudiate. Their analysis allowed Gary to introduce his sexual life into the analysis, a crucial achievement for the success of Gary's struggle to detach himself from his mother intrapsychically, create a new identity for himself, and build new relationships and a new life in general outside the family. There was a marked and sustained lessening of Gary's sexual and social anxieties. He was now able to meet with increasing effectiveness the daily challenges posed by his burgeoning heterosexuality and his expanding social life. These achievements prepared the way for termination.

The Termination Phase

Gary brought up the issue of termination briefly in April shortly before the second manifest incest dream and about the time he began to be concerned about getting a date for the prom in June. He decided to terminate in September when he left for college. At this time and, then, intermittently during April and May, he referred to the issue of termination differently than he had the year before. The reasons which he had given the year before remained essentially the same. Now, however, he was more reflective and candid. He paid homage to the value of the analysis. He showed concern about my possible wish to get rid of him as a "nasty" patient. He alluded to fears of not being ready to be on his own. At this time, he was usually not in the frustrated mood in which he had been when he had initially brought up the idea of termination. (After June, however, Gary's angry denunciation of me and the analysis as worthless and the attempt to disavow his anxiety about termination surfaced repeatedly.)

Also, as previously indicated, marked changes had occurred in the analytic situation when the definitive mutual decision to terminate took place. The therapeutic alliance had become stable. Gary had become involved in the analytic process and had begun to internalize it. He had begun to achieve useful insights (mainly about preoedipal issues). He had developed the ability to form increasingly new and satisfying relationships outside the family with members of both sexes. I accepted his decision about termination and the date he had set for it. I thought (but did not say) that if he developed too much anxiety at college, he could either obtain psychotherapeutic assistance at or near the college or return for more analysis with me. (I did have doubts which I did not express about the strength and stability of Gary's insight, autonomy, capacity for self-analysis, and new tenuous social skills.)

The issue of termination, however, receded quickly from Gary's mind. During the Spring, he seemed oblivious to the forthcoming graduation, my vacation in August, and the termination of the analysis. He was increasingly and painfully preoccupied with inviting a particular girl to the prom and having intercourse with her. His frustration and rage focused more and more on my failure to help him find a way to do this. He harrassed, mocked, and vilified me. During this time, I had several opportunities to suggest that some of his anxieties about H., the young woman whom he wanted to ask to the prom were connected to his guilty wish to take advantage of her sexually.

In the context of acquiring his first steady girlfriend and doing well generally, he said very little about the recent graduation ceremony. He explicitly acknowledged his resistance for the first time saying that he was trying to avoid unpleasant thoughts and concentrating on pleasant ones, something he had been doing for a long time. He hinted at being very disappointed, however, in not winning certain awards at the graduation ceremony.

The issue of detaching himself from his mother was always present and interwoven with his reactions to girls and to me. On one occasion he was furious at his mother for not letting him give a photograph of himself (which he had previously given to her) to a girl whom he liked. In a later session, he noticed that I was chewing gum and asked for some. He seem agitated and refused to talk about his request. Spontaneously, I gave him a stick. Later, he said that one of his "faults" was that he needed too much "loving." I said that since he could not get my love, he wanted a substitute in the form of my gum, that he wanted my love more than ever now because of his failure to get what he wanted from a girlfriend., Gary smiled. After a pause, he said that his parents wanted him to be a psychiatrist, but he preferred to be a "Civics" teacher. He wondered how I remembered so much.

In a subsequent session, he wanted me to write something in his yearbook. He had brought it to the session. I said that his request was natural but if he could talk about it, we might find out something important. He became annoyed at me. When I said that he might be worried about feeling close to me, he became embarrassed. Then he acknowledged wanting a "remembrance" from me because he would be leaving for college pretty soon. This wish represented his first explicit acknowledgment of possible anxieties about termination.

Several sessions later, Gary indicated a concern about missing sessions because of a brief trip he was planning. When I pointed out that he seemed troubled about being away from me, he reported a dream from the previous night: a girl had asked him for some gum in order to get close to him; he gave it to her and invited her into his room; when he touched her, she ran out screaming. He had masturbated after the dream with fantasies in which he told her that he loved her and would marry her in order to seduce her; then he had intercourse with her. Gary thought that the girl's coming to him showed that he was "powerful." After I said that the dream and other communications from him indicated that getting close to a girl could feel dangerous to him, he talked about being a "Pied Piper." He compared the girl in the dream to a rat who had followed him into a room where music was playing; then, he thought that he was a rat in the sense of deceiving her. He paused and referred to his acne. I said that he might be worried about being punished for doing something to the girl in the dream and wanting to do something similar to the girls in his waking life. He said that when he has acne he hurts himself by digging into his skin in order to remove the pus heads. He thought of himself as the "rat who attacks" and remembered that in the dream the girl ran out screaming. This, he thought, was also his punishment.

Gary wondered why he was working so hard and persistently on the dream and related fantasies in the next session. Previously, he realized, he would mention a dream and then quickly avoid associating to it. He noted that his interest in particular girls was brief too: one date and it was "all over." I said that he feared that there might be something sexual in our relationship. He wondered if our relationship was like having intercourse. Smiling, he said that he worked in the analysis in "spurts;" he also did his homework in "spurts."

In later sessions and in the context of feeling angry at one of the girls in whom he was interested and by whom he felt frustrated socially and sexually, Gary praised his work in his father's business. He had been working there a few hours a week. He voiced his admiration of his father's business accomplishments. He began to enjoy spending time with his father and his father's friends. They praised his likeness to his father and his attractiveness as a young man. When his father and the latter's friends talked about sex, however, he was uncomfortable as he was with me. He talked vaguely about "settling down" some day like his father and having a family indicating some pride and pleasure in this anticipation.

In mid-July I told Gary that my vacation was approaching and reminded him that the treatment would end soon afterward. He responded by talking about his mother spending a lot of money on his wardrobe. He did not think that he was ready to be independent and give up the "convenience" of home. He dismissed the analysis angrily and contemptuously, saying he would not miss it. Then he expressed concern about getting along with his roommates in college since he always wanted to have his way. (Here Gary acknowledged explicitly, for the first time, this persistent character trait.) He asserted defiantly that his academic progress was due to his own efforts, not to me. Also, for the first time, he spoke at length of wanting to please his teachers and of how he had antagonized them in the past by being "fresh" and "rowdy."

In another session, Gary was in a sleepy and snarling mood. He took his shoes off. He said he had been quarreling with the lifeguard at the pool. The lifeguard had wanted to throw him out. I said that he was also worried about trying to provoke me. He becaue furious and called me names. I said that we might be able to find out a lot about his suffering if he could put his shoes on and talk about his wish to take them off. After contradicting me vehemently, he put his shoes back on. When he tried to walk, he had difficulty: he had put his shoes on the wrong feet. After he took them off and put them on correctly, he demanded that I tell him the time. If I didn't do that "little thing" for him, he said, he would leave immediately. I said that he might be worried about being weak because he could not get along with girls the way he wanted to and because he was afraid of what was going to happen when he was away at college and on his own. As a result, he was trying to make himself feel strong and independent by being defiant and contemptuous toward me. Sarcastically and belligerently, he shouted that I was wrong.

In the next session Gary was sleepy and refused to talk. I said that his silence could mean that he was trying to be like his powerful mother: when she was frustrated and angry, he had told me, she would withdraw in silence. He admitted feeling devastated recently by the news that a girl whom he knew had just left for college and had not visited him to say good bye. Soon afterward, in the last session before my vacation, he teased me in a friendly way. He complained that I was not helping him with his "shyness" with girls by telling him what to do. Later in the session, I interpreted his teasing as his reaction to my impending vacation and his perception of the approaching end of treatment as a rejection. He said that he didn't want me to help him because that would mean I was dominating him and making him face disturbing ideas. His initial silence, he said, meant that he wanted to be the doctor and that I should do the talking. He tried to link this idea to his mother's alternating between being like a mother and then like a father to him.

Gary seemed to be trying to deny his feelings about our impending separation and to master the anxieties associated with it by reversing our positions. He was trying to do something similar in regard to his fear of separation from his mother. He would do the abandoning and I, as transference mother—as well as his actual mother—would be abandoned.

When I returned from vacation, Gary expressed the wish to solve his own problems so that he wouldn't be "totally unprepared" for college. He seemed pleased to see me. During my vacation he had visited his grandfather, whom he had found restrictive and critical. When Gary had indicated his wish to "pick up" a girl, his grandfather had warned him about "catching a disease." He thought that he needed a "big brother" to lead him like a "baby" so that he would be "normal" and know how to get along with girls. He pressed me to advise him about girls. He thought that part of his difficulty in talking to me about girls was related to his difficulty in talking to me as an older person. When an older person tried to discuss sex with him, he said, he got "jumpy." This fear had "bottled up" our work. Then, he recalled that his aunt once told his mother—in his presence—that "it would be funny seeing Gary make love to a girl." His mother and aunt had laughed. Gary had been deeply hurt and had felt "undying hatred" for both.

Gary talked eagerly about the letter he had sent me while visiting his grandfather; he had wanted to continue our analytic work by recording his experiences. The main part of the letter was about a dream he had had during the visit. In the dream Gary was playing cards with some boys and a woman. He and the boys were losing a lot of money. The woman—Phyllis Diller—was winning everything and laughing. He was very scared; finally, he bet everything on one round and won.

Gary was eager to discuss the dream. Money, he said, was the "dearest thing in [his] life." Taking his money was like "kicking [him] in the groin" and "taking [his] manhood away." He liked Phyllis Diller but feared and hated her in the dream as he did his mother. His associations led to the idea of his mother taking his manhood away by making him bathe, feed, and dress his younger brother and sister. Phyllis Diller also made him think of a boy changing into a girl and of his mother being like a "father" to him, a complaint he had often verbalized before. He objected to his mother's having always excited and frustrated him and his brother. She had also made him feel "lousy" by persuading him to betray his father's confidence.

I acknowledged the analytic work that he had done on his own and now with me. I commented that Phyllis Diller had laughed in the dream and that she was regarded as a comedian. He said that his mother had laughed when he was suffering. Then he laughed. Yesterday, he said, his brother had shouted to his girlfriend (who was visiting him at home) to stay away from the bathroom while Gary was in it so that she wouldn't see his "schmeckel" (Yiddish for penis). I said that he seemed to be worried about his mother doing something to his "schmeckel." After a pause, he said that when he was a little boy his mother had, at times, jokingly threatened to take his "schmeckel" away. She was now doing the same with his brother.

In a subsequent session, Gary was in a reflective, affectionate, and sympathetic mood in regard to his father and me. He brought in two "visions;" he was not sure if they were dreams or fantasies. In one, his mother gave him a fishing rod and reel. It was big and heavy and had a lot of hooks. In the other, he and his father and his father's two brothers carried umbrellas and wore bowlers. The rod made him think of "catching" girls. Mother was like a heavy rod. She held him back from "catching" girls. Mother, he said, had always given him the wrong ideas about girls. She had said that they would take his money away. Now, he realized how wrong she was. "Hooks" reminded him of mother having her "hooks" into everything. The other day she told him what to do about his girlfriend. He had gotten very angry at her. Mother had always "bribed" him with gifts. That's how she got him to be like her. He thought that his "visions" were also connected to his refusal last night to tell his mother the contents of the letter he had typed for his father and to the advice that she had given him about his girlfriend.

Afterward, Gary refused to talk any further about the "visions" unless I mentioned them. I said that he wished me to treat him as his mother did and "sink" my hooks into him. He said that he had to be "prodded" by his mother and teachers or else he would not do any work. He went on to talk about a recent visit to the college he was going to in a few weeks. He had met and liked his roommates. However, he had lied about himself in order to make a good impression and had antagonized one of the students.

Gary felt sad in the next session. His friend J. was leaving today for school. It was like "losing a brother." Gary wished that J. could be his roommate. After noting that there were only three session left, he said bitterly that he had gotten absolutely nothing out of his analysis. I had let him get away with not talking. I wasn't as bad, though, as the therapists whom he had had before me. Gary described in some detail how he, by being silent, had tricked them into appearing to be uninterested. Then he had forced his parents to stop the treatment by complaining of the therapist's lack of interest. Anyway, he had always wanted to solve his own problems. He did not want anyone to know about him or tell him what to do. He had never wanted psychiatric treatment. That was the trouble with this analysis. I said that he had a lot of feelings about the analysis coming to an end and that he was trying to work them out.

In the following session Gary proudly displayed an expensive watch his parents had just given him. Then he referred to his mother's recent dream about him in which a girl loves him very much and gratifies him sexually. He was annoyed at me. He accused me of being uninterested in him and threatened to go to sleep. I said that he seemed to be very impressed by how much other people, like his parents and the girl in his mother's dream, gave him while I gave him nothing. He said that he would like me to give him a lot, the way he and his mother gave to each other. He decided that he had to work (in the analysis) now because it was near the end. He was concerned about his mother "warning" him about sex and resented her need to control his private life: the previous night she had tried to enter his room while he was masturbating. Gary informed me that he had only gotten one thing out of treatment: he could talk about sex without becoming disturbed.

In another session Gary talked about his teachers' hugging him and taking him out for lunch. They had invited him to visit them in the future. Their affectionate attitude and behavior had excited and pleased him. He had asked his mother to invite one of them for dinner. He paused frequently while talking. I said that he might be struggling with some strong feelings about me. Suddenly, he blurted out a request: could he call me up in the future about a "problem" even though he would not be my patient in analysis anymore? I said that he could.

In the next to the last session, Gary was in a sleepy and irritable mood. He expressed the wish to correspond with me about his problems while at school. I said that his wish could be a way of bringing out more important feelings about me. He immediately denied any truth to this and insisted that tomorrow I must answer all his questions. He became arrogant and scornful. He was angry at me for not giving to him (gifts, affection), as his teachers and mother were doing. I didn't seem to care about him. He denounced the analysis as ineffective. I said that he knew we had worked hard on some important problems and with some success but that he was now criticizing me and the analysis because he was very angry at me for not giving him what he wanted. He left snarling.

In the last session of the analysis, just before he left for college,

Gary was initially silent. I said that maybe he wanted me to treat him in a very special way and get the ball rolling as his mother did, and then he would talk. He snarled, "Why don't you?" He disparaged and regretted the analysis. We had, he said, accomplished nothing. I said that he was very angry at me, partially because he was disturbed by feelings other than anger that he had toward me. He responded that on the previous night his mother had asked him whether she had overprotected him. He had said no. He told her that she had given him a lot but that she needed too much praise in return, just as he needed too much praise. That's his remaining problem, he said. How could he get rid of it? He's like Asia needing help from the U.S. The U.S. is his mother. But he wants to have the feeling that he's accomplishing things on his own.

When he left we shook hands. Suddenly, he seemed to choke up; he could barely speak and became tearful. Then, with much feeling, he spluttered, "You've been like a brother to me!" and left quickly. I repeated my willingness to see him again if he wanted me to and again referred to the good work that we had done together. His outburst had surprised and moved me.

In retrospect, the brother transference that had emerged so dramatically when he said good bye was Gary's most nurturing, albeit ambiguous, transference. This was not a real transference, since it was obviously not a repetition of the relationship he had with his younger brother. It was the transference of a wish or fantasy of an ideal nurturing figure, a composite parent-sibling figure. It was, in a sense, both a transference and an externalization. By replacing the mutually exploitative and destructive relationship to his mother (and other family members) with a relationship to an ideal figure who was seen as a contemporary and whom he perceived as getting along well in the real world, he could count on that figure to show him how to grow up in a "normal" way.

The ambiguous brother transference may well have silently facilitated Gary's ability to use the analytic process productively by strengthening the therapeutic alliance. It may also have given him a respite from preoedipal and oedipal struggles, as well as the strength to resolve them. It may have, finally, helped him diminish the resistances generated by the mother and father transferences by providing him with anticipations of a gratifying future instead of confronting him with conflict and frustration. Gary was leaving a quasi-transferential sibling figure in whom he could find a source of strength and hope.

Gary's quasi-transferential figure and his developing wish and ability to analyze himself reflected the beginning internalization of the analyst and the analytic process. These achievements reassured me that our mutual decision to terminate when we did was correct. They represented a useful adaptation to the anxieties of the terminal phase, a sublimation of his feelings for me, and a crucial step towards achieving further intrapsychic detachment from his mother and from me as both a real and a transferential object. The changes in his defensive structure also augured well for the immediate future. His use of denial, externalization, projection, isolation, and rationalization had diminished considerably. Reaction formation, suppression, and repression had largely replaced them. Gary had begun to give up his fantasies of omnipotence and omniscience. Above all, he had become increasingly realistic about himself, his mother, and his life in general, reducing considerably his earlier frantic use of primitive defenses.

Important changes in character structure and other aspects of ego functioning were also taking place, which made termination feasible. Gary's tendencies to torment and be tormented, to dominate and exploit, to be dominated and exploited, and to be self-defeating were beginning to be replaced by the ability to protect himself, to be considerate and express warmth toward others, to receive affection from others, and to succeed. These and other changes of a more profound nature (greater awareness of and control over his feelings, increased ability to integrate feelings, thoughts, and actions and a keener appreciation of inner and outer reality), however tentative, were important indications of Gary's ability to leave the analysis and function satisfactorily on his own.

Finally, Gary's increasingly satisfying and successful involvement with nonincestuous figures, which had begun prior to the terminal phase and was one of the important visible results of his growing intrapsychic detachment from his mother, represented an important behavioral indication that termination was practical, if not necessary. Temporarily contributing to Gary's ability to terminate, in an illusory way, was his persistent need to deny the value of the analysis and attribute the improvement in his functioning only to himself.

All of the foregoing changes reflected, in part, the result of the partial resolution of preoedipal and oedipal conflicts and of the limited transference neurosis.

Posttermination

Gary returned for more analytic work at the end of his freshman year of college. He was pleased with his academic work and social life despite lingering social anxieties and inhibitions. He was eager to see me and tell me about his academic achievements. In the second session he brought up a dream similar in tone, content, and underlying significance to the two manifest incest dreams previously reported—similar, that is, except in several important respects: the absence of his mother, the presence of a new figure, a prostitute, his activity, and his ability to take responsibility for his sexuality. That is, in the dream, Gary "propositions" the prostitute. They have intercourse in her apartment. She "shows [him] things" (positions, techniques). She really loves him.

The dream had occurred about a month before the session. As with the earlier, manifest incest dreams, no specific previous day residue emerged. Gary noted that the prostitute was slender, unlike his fat mother. Still, she taught him just as his mother had in the manifest incest dreams. His mother, he said proudly, had taught him about "life through experience." She knew everything, he said, and she was also very controlling. Then, Gary had difficulty talking and wanted me to "order" him to talk. I said that he was afraid to take responsibility for the dream and for talking about it and that this fear was tied up with guilty feelings about what he wanted his mother and me to do for him. He talked about his excessive dependence on people and, later, about his "forgetfulness." I said that his forgetfulness might be associated with disturbing wishes that he had for his mother. He wondered if all girls made him think of his mother and therefore he could not be at ease with them. The elaboration and working over of these issues dominated the analytic work for about two weeks. (Both of us then went on vacation, and afterward Gary returned to school.)

Gary's way of reporting this quasi-manifest incest dream differed sharply from the two earlier manifest incest dreams. He enjoyed talking about it and gave considerable detail, omitting nothing. He was in a confident, optimistic mood, although not without traces of anxiety.

The manifest content of the dream also differed significantly from the previous manifest incest dreams. The dreamer is clearly active sexually (foreshadowed, perhaps, by the act of revenge in the second manifest incest dream, his gambling victory in the Phyllis Diller dream, and his increasingly active functioning generally in the analysis and in his daily life): he initiates and takes responsibility for the sexual instruction and activity, and his activity is organized, purposeful, and pleasurable. In replacing his mother by a prostitute in the manifest content, Gary has, in effect, made his mother unacceptable to him sexually and replaced her with a nonincestuous partner.

The form of the manifest content of this dream also differs sharply from the two manifest incest dreams in the complexity of the sexual activity. The details of that activity, the mood of pleasurable triumph within the dream and in the dreamer's recounting of it reflected Gary's increasing acceptance of his sexual feelings towards nonincestuous women, his ability to communicate that acceptance to me, and his new crystallizing perception of nonincestuous women as potentially gratifying, if not loving, nurturing, and reliable (in contrast to his perceived unpredictable, exploitative, and frightening mother). As the prostitute in the dream, his mother now represented both the bridge to nonincestuous women and a woman no longer available to him sexually. (Gary had anticipated this pathway to intrapsychic detachment from the maternal representation of psychosexual autonomy early in the analysis by his conscious wish for a girlfriend who was a "tramp.") These changes in the manifest form and content also reflected Gary's increasing consolidation of the incest barrier and the appropriately healthy direction of his psychosexual and social development. His former idealization of his mother as omnipotent and omniscient returned momentarily in the first posttermination phase in response to his anxiety over the wish to replace his mother with a nonincestuous woman.

In this first posttermination period, Gary brought up an important dream, the associations to which facilitated developmentally useful changes involving his drive organization, the resolution of oedipal and preoedipal conflicts, and the resolution of the (mother) transference neurosis.

When Gary resumed treatment at the end of his sophomore year, in the second posttermination phase, he stressed both his need for help and his eagerness to be independent. He had been increasingly successful with girls but still not as successful as he wanted to be. He referred to the lavish gifts his parents had recently given him. Soon afterward he disclosed for the first time that he used to "make" his brother "kiss" his penis. (Previously, he had disclosed only his practice of kissing his brother's penis.) He condemned this practice and, like the other secret incestuous experiences that he had previously reported, quickly relegated it to the past. Then he explored the possibility that his fear of girls had to do not only with the fear of raping them and treating them cruelly in other ways (as in his masturbatory fantasies) but also with his wish to force them to perform fellatio on him.

In a later session, Gary wanted advice about dealing with his mother's objection to his getting more involved sexually with his current girlfriend. Mother also told him that when he leaves for school he'll "break her heart." He became angry at me for not telling him whether or not he was "using" his girlfriend for sex, by now an old concern. I said that not only was he trying to put me in the position of his mother by making me tell him what to do but, at the same time, he wanted me to help him solve an important problem in his life in such a way that he would know how to get along with girls on his own in the future. He responded by trying to figure out if he really liked his girlfriend. Then, he acknowledged that he found her body physically "disgusting," a word that he had used to describe his mother's body.

Gary spoke of a "sexual breakthrough" soon afterward. He had felt his girlfriend's breasts; it was "great." But he was worried about having taken advantage of her. He was also worried about his mother's health: she might need an operation. Gary suddenly asked to use my phone to call his mother. He seemed anxious, and I gave him permission. When no one answered he found it difficult to talk for a while. Then he revealed that at home he had been busy taking care of the family. He seemed to enjoy replacing his mother in that capacity and indicated a sense of pride in being a responsible, sympathetic, and competent son rather than a helplessly victimized one filled with bitterness and hate. This feeling of pride probably represented as much an attempt to diminish his guilt feelings over the possibility that he had taken advantage of his girlfriend as it did a developmental advance. In the context of the impending separation from me, Gary's request to use my phone to call home seemed also to be a way of holding on to me (qua mother and as myself), a denial of the forthcoming separation. Allowing Gary to use my phone instead of interpreting his wish suggests that in this instance I had unconsciously colluded with his transference wishes.

In a later session, in the context of reporting his ability to be freer than ever before in sexual play with his girlfriend, Gary reported a dream about a blonde girl who loved him very much. She kissed and hugged him. Her father, a millionaire, talked to his mother about "buying" him with a lot of money. He did not know what to do; he was both observer and participant in the dream. Gary responded to the dream by referring to his mother's urging him to find a girl from a wealthy and socially prominent family. He enjoyed the idea of his mother making a "deal" for him in the dream. After discussing the advantages and disadvantages of marrying a wealthy girl from the point of view of who would have the "power" in such a marriage, he returned to his concern about using one of his girlfriends for sex. I said that he was struggling with his wish to value the girl for herself and to treat her with respect and his wish to use her sexually. He quickly disapproved of the latter wish.

Gary continued to report amorous adventures with his girlfriend.

At one point I had the opportunity to say that he seemed quite concerned about how much she could give to him rather than vice versa. He acknowledged a concern about his ability to love her. Subsequently, he spoke of wanting me to think better of him and of wanting to feel better about himself. He asserted that he and his girlfriend did love each other. Later he spoke of getting into bed nude with her for the first time. She had kissed his penis. He had wanted her to do it. He had enjoyed the experience for a while and then had tired of it. When he kissed her vagina, he was "disgusted" by the smell. He was disappointed in her body (she had acne and was hairy); the experience was not as good as his fantasies. In a later session, he reported another unusual experience with her: she had kissed him continuously and hadn't wanted to let him go. He had found the experience remarkable.

In the next session Gary was silent and sullen. He complained about my not giving him enough time and advice about getting along with his mother and other people. Then he reported a dream in which he played games with two fellows. One of them died. He had felt sad, cried, and was fearful during the dream. He had wet the bed. The dreams reminded him of the "games" that he though we played with each other: we tried to "trap" each other and as a result we never got anywhere. I said that the dead fellow might refer to me. He was silent. I said that he might be angry at me and feel like killing me not only for going on vacation but also for not giving him what he wanted. He became sarcastic: I shouldn't "flatter" myself; it was his mother whom he could "kill;" they had been fighting a lot.

In the last session before my vacation Gary referred to a recent movie in which a teacher decided to teach his students about life. He had changed them from hippies into serious students and they "adored" him. They gave him a gift when they left him. Gary had been deeply affected by the movie. After the movie he gave his ring to his girlfriend. He felt that he had "clarified" and strengthened their tie. I said that he might be worried about losing me and that this worry might have contributed to his reaction to the movie. Now, for the first time, he wondered out loud if he had been holding back his feelings and thoughts in the analysis in order to hold on to me and if he had forgotten to bring me the check his father had given him because he wanted to see me again.

On my return from vacation Gary stressed how much his girlfriend loved him. She had been away while I was away, and although she had written him frequently, he had seldom responded. He seemed euphoric. I said that he might be anxious about wanting all the love that I could give him without his giving me much in return. Gary responded that the previous night he had thought of me liking him in more than a professional way because of the way in which I had responded to his telephoned inquiry about the time of today's session. Then he stressed his wish to be independent of me and how impressed he was with his girlfriend's loving him as he really was. He had stopped lying to her, he said, in order to make an impression. Then he said that he, like his mother, lived in fantasy: he pretended to be a great athlete or some other famous person. To his mother he was "ideal;" they thought of each other as "perfect." He acknowledged more keenly and ruefully than ever before how much his mother controlled him. Lately, however, she had been talking to him about her painful relationship with his father. Gary could now understand why she feared losing him. He referred to the trouble he had caused his parents in the past by getting them to fight, although he denied feeling responsible for their current fighting.

In the next session Gary reported a dream about a baby who was "crushed" by a train. Earlier in the day he had quarreled with his girlfriend, had felt guilty about hurting her, and had apologized. He felt that she had been "crushed" like a baby. Then he complained about his mother being "mean" to him: she had recently refused to do something for him. He thought that he was growing away from her. He was angry with her. I said that he, as well as his girlfriend, could be represented by the baby in the dream, that he felt crushed, as he had in the past, by his mother's treatment of him. He was silent.

In the next and last session before his return to school for the fall semester, Gary was sad. He was glad to return to school. He thought that his mother would be very lonely, and he stressed his girlfriend's love for him. When I referred to the possibility of his having some difficulty leaving me, he was silent.

The second posttermination period is noteworthy in several respects. Gary could now acknowledge, for the first time, what to him had apparently been the most unacceptable form of his incestuous activity: his aggressive sexual exploitation of his brother. He could also begin to connect it to his masturbatory fantasies and his earlier fear of girls. He translated his fantasy of making or having a girl kiss his penis into a real experience, actively repeating the passive experience of mother (and brother) kissing his penis. In kissing his girlfriend's vagina, he was also identifying with the exploitative mother kissing his penis. He had, in effect, acted out the illusion of mastering his mother's traumatic sexual exploitation of him first with his brother and then with a nonincestuous female. The powerful urge towards mastery involved the compulsion to repeat the pleasurable aspects of the incestuous experiences as well as the wish to achieve mastery through analytic understanding.

For the first time, Gary indicated the beginning of an interest in and empathy toward his mother as a separate person and as one who had been incapacitated by illness, emotional burdens, and loneliness and who desperately needed his assistance and companionship. His pleasure and pride in taking care of her and his siblings seemed, in part, to reflect this new understanding of her and his place in her life and in the rest of his family. His need to exploit girls for social position and power as well as for sexual pleasure could now be understood not only as an identification with his exploitative mother and as an attempt to master the traumatic aspects of that exploitation but also as a conflicted wish to remain under her control and act as her proxy.

Gary's "sexual breakthrough" represented a developmental advance in his ability to detach himself from his mother and brother and form psychosexual attachments to nonincestuous females. The guilt over using women to achieve this and other related aims had expressed itself, to some extent, in his being the good son who was helping his mother at home.

This second posttermination phase illustrates vividly the depth of Gary's feelings about me as a transference and real figure and his need to repudiate or at least reduce them to manageable proportions while, at the same time, trying to find a way of expressing some of them directly. In his relationship to me during this period he was experiencing for the first time someone who, like his girlfriend, was not only accepting him as he was but was also helping him realize his own potentialities in his own way. He and I did not have to idealize each other; therefore, he could begin to acknowledge his dependence on me because he did not have to fear the terrible consequences of the kind of dependence that he had experienced with his mother, that is, mutual entrapment.

The opportunity to feel accepted as he was, to be realistic about himself and others, and to feel safe meant he could acquire realistic rather than magical strength. This new perception of himself was tied up with the fantasy of my having transformed him from being a "hippie" or "clown" into a "serious student" and person. I had inferred this fantasy from his having dwelt with much feeling on the movie in which the teacher transforms a class of "hippies" and "clowns" into serious and successful students. Gary's perception of me had made me too important and, therefore, too dangerous to him. He had to be independent of me as the transference mother (and as myself). He had to turn to someone else, a girlfriend, to give him strength or else he would be the "crushed baby" whose analyst-mother had abandoned him. It was better to be the crusher, the one who did the abandoning.

The third posttermination phase occurred when Gary came home for Thanksgiving in his junior year. He seemed to be in a confident and friendly mood. He said that he had grown quite a bit. He acknowledged for the first time that his mother and grandmother had been sending him many large packages of food, cake, and candy since his freshman year. He reported that his mother had called him "friend" the other day; the word seemed "odd." He was his own boss now and "free of her nagging." He liked his teachers and courses. He was working hard and doing well although residual social difficulties with peers of both sexes, especially with girls, persisted. When I suggested that his dependence on his mother might still be interfering with his ability to date girls, he agreed. For the first time he referred to himself as a "child" in the sense of being dependent on his mother and fearful of her disapproval; he didn't like feeling this way. As before, he wanted advice about his parents, who were fighting and ready to separate. His mother was nervous and cried often, and his brother and sister were hurt by the fighting between their parents.

I tried to link his concerns about getting along with girls with the fear of being dominated and frightened by his mother, as his brother and sister were, and particularly with the struggle over his mother's repeated injunctions to make a good marriage instead of having pleasant dates with girls. He acknowledged that he couldn't think of just dating a girl: he felt he had to marry her (if he liked her). He wondered if he was provoking girls whom he liked so that he could avoid having to marry them? He discussed his belief that his mother was too dependent on him: she had told him that he was her only "friend," her "protector." He was like her "husband," he thought, yet he didn't feel like an "adult." He was aware that his mother had "used" him, and therefore he hadn't been able to grow up. When his parents fought, they treated him like a grown-up and competed for his attention; he remembered that he had gotten them to fight in the past. He left for school soon afterward in a friendly, confident mood.

In this brief third posttermination period, consisting of only a few sessions, Gary acknowledged more directly and fully than ever before the discrete elements of the complex, mutually dependent (preoedipal and oedipal) relationship he had with his mother and the paradoxical ways in which he experienced himself in that relationship. This important acknowledgment was partially based on his newly developed ability to experience her and himself as separate people with separate personalities, histories, and futures. He indicated an increasing degree of empathy and sympathy toward her as well as an understanding of her as a desperately lonely and troubled human being. He could now begin to appreciate and acknowledge her need to control him and to understand that she accomplished this by offering him various gratifications, which he enjoyed receiving albeit with misgivings. He could also now acknowledge that he had been causing his parents to quarrel in an attempt to get them to treat him as an important and separate figure instead of as a pawn or a nuisance. He could take note of what appeared to be his mother's poignant attempt to give him a new and more appropriate place in her life as a "friend." He was not yet ready, however, to integrate this new and "odd" sense of himself into his developing core identity. He still felt, to some extent, like a frightened child in his mother's presence. His increasingly realistic and stable sense of himself, however, allowed him to at least begin to identify the issues underlying these and other experiences and candidly share them with me.

When Gary returned for the fourth and last piece of analytic work during the following Christmas vacation, he was in a good mood. He had been dating a particular girl, and seemed to be casual about his parents' problems. In one session, he was in a subdued mood. He referred to his difficulty in treating girls well and he complained about his parents having used him as a "pawn" in their quarrels.

I said that even though he resented being used by his mother, he had become used to giving to her rather than to other women and that it was hard for him to give up that relationship. He admitted that he now realized that his mother depended upon him completely and referred to her recent repeated statements that she had stayed with his father only for his sake and that without him she would "die." Gary now revealed that she had been calling him several times a week at school since the beginning of his freshman year. He thought that it was all too much. I said that he was worried about betraying his mother and so did not want to get involved with other women. He said that he had never thought of it quite that way, that it might be so. He seemed to be in a pleased and proud mood at the end of the session.

In the next session Gary spoke of having met a girl with whom he had gone further sexually than with any other girl—but not as far as intercourse, despite her encouragement. It had been an unusual and gratifying experience. He shifted to the issue of being independent of me, the treatment, and his mother. He said that he envied his girlfriend's strength and independence; she, not the treatment, had given him strength; he had never had much faith in treatment anyway. Recently, he reported, he had spoken to his mother in an aggressive manner and called her an "octopus." He agreed quickly with my comment that a big part of his difficulty with treatment was that he also saw me as an "octopus."

In the last session of the analysis, Gary seemed to be in a good mood. His mother's recent crying had been the instigating factor in his buying his girlfriend expensive Chanukah and birthday gifts (necklaces and earrings), gifts his mother had originally wanted him to buy for her: she now wanted him to bestow such gifts on his girlfriend, lamenting that she (his mother) had never had a "proper courtship." I said that he must have a lot of feelings about his mother urging him into treating her (indirectly) as a girlfriend. He referred to his mother's repeated description of his girlfriend as someone just like her and mentioned his mother's plan to help his girlfriend learn to cook and assume other responsibilities after they married. Ruefully, yet rather casually, Gary observed that his dependence on his mother was a "bad habit." The session and the analysis came to an end; our good byes were friendly and spontaneous. I told Gary that I thought we had accomplished a lot and I wished him well. He left in a friendly, relaxed, and confident mood.

During this fourth and last posttermination phase, Gary continued to show increasing understanding and appreciation of his mother as a separate and very troubled person who was very dependent on him; he struggled to define and defy the various specific ways in which she had been both seducing and coercing him into satisfying her apparently desperate demands for an inappropriately close relationship with him. His latest solution to the problem of giving up, or at least weakening, his dependence on her (and on me both as a mother transference figure and a "real" object) was to develop an attachment to a girlfriend whom he seemed to experience as an ideal mother-analyst substitute. He experienced his mother's current behavior, her attempt to make his future wife into a replica of herself, as an opportunity she was offering him to give up his attachment to her: he could keep her close to him in the relatively harmless guise of a future wife's domesticity. An important part of this anticipated achievement consisted of Gary's ability to be more comfortable sexually with this girlfriend than with any of his previous girlfriends.

By the end of the posttermination phase, Gary had achieved further resolution of the limited transference neurosis and preoedipal (and oedipal) conflicts which were interwoven with the previously described changes in his use of defenses, his character structure and self—and object relationships. He was preparing himself for the next developmental phase. He had become able to talk candidly about himself with much insight and with a measure of pride and pleasure. Internalization of the analytic process was continuing. I felt certain that he would need further analysis in the future. His developmental achievements, however, permitted a reasonably successful termination of the analysis at this time when he was giving up the most primitive aspects to his tie to his mother and entering young adulthood.

Discussion

Gary's initial vague and conflicted wishes for termination in the first year of the analysis were consistent with both the inherent ambiguities of the analytic situaion and his intense ambivalence toward the analysis which had magnified those ambiguities from the start. That initial unilateral wish to terminate, however, was the self-initiated beginning of a process that culminated spontaneously about a year later in our definitive and mutual decision to terminate. The latter decision, which had also originated with Gary, was now deliberate and thoughtful rather than impulsive and vaguely hopeful. He was now ready and eager to exchange analytic dependence for relative independence and to exchange traumatic, compellingly seductive ties to his mother and other family members for a radically new, exciting, and possibly dangerous life. He had made realistic preparations psychologically for that exchange through the analysis and though ambivalent, he recognized the possibility of returning for further analysis if his anxieties would threaten his delicately balanced autonomy.

From start to finish, the termination process in Gary's experience was marked by ambiguity. The first formal and mutual termination, to begin with, was not a true termination in that it deliberately provided for future analytic work. The subsequent resumptions and terminations, on the other hand, represented the result of Gary's unilateral decisions based on his own assessments of his need for therapy. These flexible arrangements blurred the issues of mutuality and unilaterality. Also, since each posttermination phase involved its own schedule and a separate piece of analytic work, the continuity of both the content and mode of the analytic work throughout the posttermination experience was compromised. Still, because the therapeutic alliance and the crucial issues on which Gary and I continued to work remained the same, the fundamental continuity of the analysis was intact.

The ambiguity of Gary's termination experience was congruent with the ambiguity that, early in the analysis, I had deliberately intensified through many of my broad interventions. These interventions were, in part, a response to Gary's severe, protective ambivalence toward the analysis because of its roots in the mother transference, his powerful urge toward autonomy, and his fragile self-esteem. I was determined to give Gary as much room as possible for autonomous functioning within the analytic situation and to avoid "force-feeding" him which his mother had done literally during his infancy and which she had continued to do figuratively.

The ambiguities of the analytic situation, especially, the total termination experience, gave Gary the crucial psychological space to do the emotional and intellectual experimenting, evaluating, rehearsing, and refueling necessary for entrance into the next developmental phase of young adulthood. Freeing himself from his mother was no small matter for Gary. He needed time and the internal permission (derived from the analysis) to differentiate more fully his mother's body and person from those of his own and, then, from those of women (and men) outside the family. He needed a special world, one that was under his control, as a bridge from an infantile paradise to the unknown, apparently dangerous real world of young adulthood. In that special in-between, transitional world, he could adjust the degree of reality and illusion to the point at which his development based on analytic work could proceed with the necessary degree of comfort.

The in-between world that Gary and I created and used in the analytic situation allowed him to realize, through the transference, that his infantile paradise was a painful, exploitative, sadomasochistic mutual entrapment with his mother and that the real world might, indeed, be quite safe, predictable, and enjoyable if not exciting. Creating a kaleidoscopic world of illusion and reality out of the termination process, especially, in the posttermination period (if not out of the entire analysis) offered Gary a transitional experience in which he had considerable real control (over the scheduling of analytic sessions and, hence, the rate of progress) along with the illusion of control for as long as he needed it. Thus, the termination process was more than a bridge to the new world of young adulthood. It was already part of that world.

Because I had left it up to him to come and go as he pleased after the initial termination, Gary's prolonged, fragmented termination experience superficially resembled demand feeding. It might have kept alive, perhaps, strengthened Gary's demands for gratification in the mother transference. Our relationship, however, had developed into a relatively stable therapeutic alliance, making possible realistic and reasonable decisions and actions, in regard to Gary's repeated return for more analytic work and his ability to work productively. Gary's analytic work and the geographical and psychological space in which that work took place, especially, during the posttermination period allowed him to safely experiment with increasing degrees of autonomy and individuation. He maintained and used the therapeutic alliance until he no longer needed it. He stopped requesting analytic assistance when, with varying degrees of success, he could manage his residual anxieties as well as the developmental and other challenges of his life.

Gary began to use the relationship with a girlfriend and the anticipation of marriage and family life as a solution to and partial sublimation of his ties to his mother and to me (as both a real and transferential figure). He also seemed to be using his academic work as a sublimation of his attachments to his parents and me. His academic and other achievements represented, to some extent, an identification with his father and with me as a real figure.

References

Adler, G. (1989), Transitional phenomena, projection identification and the essential ambiguity of the psychoanalytic situation. *Psychoanal. Quart.*, 58:81–104.

Burgner, M. (1988), Analytic work with adolescents: Terminable and interminable. *Internat. J. Psycho-Anal.*, 69:179–187.

Novick, J. (1976), Termination of treatment in adolescence. *The Psychoanalytic Study of the Child*, 31:389–414. New Haven, CT: Yale University Press.

———— (1982), Termination: Themes and issues. *Psychoanal. Inq.*, 2:329–365.

10

Termination in the Analysis of an Adolescent Girl

Rhoda S. Frenkel

"I grew to the point I should be."

Ann was 18. Ending the session that preceded her last analytic hour, she said, "I grew to the point I should be, and now I can progress normally. I have a lot to learn, but I can now." Thus she rephrased Freud's (1937) well-known adage "Our aim will not be to rub off every peculiarity of human character . . . nor yet to demand that the person . . . shall feel no passions and develop no internal conflicts. The business of analysis is to secure the best possible psychological conditions for the functions of the ego; with that it has discharged its task" (p. 250). By presenting some data relevant to the termination of this case, this paper highlights the similarities of adult and adolescent analysis (Novick, 1976, 1989).

From the beginning, transference issues (transference reactions, transference resistance, and the evolution and relative resolution of the transference neurosis) were the fulcrum for the regressive and progressive flow of the analytic process (Chused, 1988). Thus, the transference provided the vehicle through which preoedipal and oedipal conflicts could be reexperienced and sufficiently worked through to produce insight and structural changes (Hoffman, 1989). These normal tasks of adolescence, the modification of the superego and the vast restructuring of the ego (Adatto, 1958), are necessary in promoting the establishment of a nonincestuous object choice, a critical issue in Ann's case.

The difference between Ann's analysis and adult analysis is more in degree than substance. Ann's analysis was intense but short, and

211

the termination seemed abrupt, although the abruptness may have been more apparent than real. While her total treatment lasted less than two and a half years, Ann was in formal analysis for two years. She was seen four times a week, and aside from the first few weeks and two separate sessions during which her ego seemed overwhelmed by her drives, she used the couch. Her motive for choosing the couch can be found in a more detailed description of the opening and early midphases of our work (Frenkel, in press). While the total termination process covered a five-month period, the final phase occurred in less than a month. Blos (1974) emphasizes the necessity of resolving negative oedipal conflicts in late adolescent males. Significantly, a more definitive resolution of negative oedipal issues was an important aspect of Ann's termination. Although mourning during the final phase, as described by Loewald (1988), was brief, there had been intermittent periods of mourning throughout Ann's analysis. When we decided to terminate at an earlier time than first estimated, I had to agree with Ann's assessment that she was able to proceed with her normal developmental tasks without me.

Clinical Data

The Referral, Evaluation, and Initial Treatment

Ann, the youngest of three children of a homemaker and a wealthy academic, sought treatment just prior to her 16th birthday, complaining of stomach cramps and a fear of "throwing up in class." These symptoms, originally diagnosed as flu and treated supportively, began seven months prior to my initial psychiatric evaluation. Three months later Ann's internist, after ruling out organic etiology, referred her for psychiatric evaluation. An extensive workup had included two hospitalizations and several trials on tranquilizers. Although Ann refused to go to school for the next four months, her parents did not seek consultation with me until the school refused to give Ann credit for the year and suggested that the family get counseling. Her family's complicity in her symptoms was evident in their further two-month delay in having the evaluation completed and their initial refusal to allow Ann to be seen more than once a week despite my strong recommendation for analysis, which was supported by their internist.

Although Ann was a pretty, well-developed teenager, in the initial interviews and treatment sessions she spoke with a soft, wispy voice, dressed in loose-fitting little-girl clothes, and in general had the demeanor of a cheerful, cooperative, latency-age child. She related her complaints with a great deal of laughter and apparent indifference. When this behavior was contrasted with her complaints, she expressed embarrassment. Ann exhibited a capacity for insight in her response to my comment that although she was pleased by the attention at home, she was avoiding attention at school where she was afraid people would stare at her. She told me that she hadn't realized before that the two were indeed connected and it confused her. The diagnostic impression was a classic case of hysterical neurosis.

Despite the limited frequency of sessions, I maintained an analytic stance because Ann's resistances appeared analyzable and because I believed her wish for analysis would, in time, prevail. Subsequently, her symptoms became more global. Rarely leaving her house, Ann withdrew from all her activities and most of her friends, complaining, "I'm afraid of throwing up if I leave home." Long silences filled her sessions as she became reluctant to talk. In order to explore reasons for this change, I encouraged Ann's expressions of her sexual and angry feelings. My behavior, rather than a verbal clarification, had the effect of interpreting her reactions as reflective of a developing negative maternal transference. Thus, more at ease, Ann acknowledged that she had been afraid I would act like her mother by crying or quoting the Bible if she even superficially explored these areas. In the emerging therapeutic alliance, Ann began to acknowledge some anger toward her mother. More important, she stated that her primary concern was to know why, since her preadolescence, she had always been "the third person," always involved in "breaking up" relationships. Quickly losing interest in whomever she "won," she would "drop him" and go on to someone else, never sustaining a relationship for more than a month. Ann wondered if she "just wasn't much for physical expression." In trying to deal with her "third-person problem" she had tried running away, religion, and drugs, all of which seemed to make her worse. She admitted, "The problem is in my head" and explained that she felt like a 15-year-old, as if she had lost a year of her life. With this insight she became eager to pursue her analysis. As Ann focused more on her mother's pathology, and became less hostile to her father, she convinced her father to support her analysis. In this way Ann interfered with the earlier unified parental opposition to the analysis. Although preoedipal and oedipal conflicts were interwoven, oedipal problems seemed predominant, exemplified by her repetitive need to be "the third person," even in the initiation of the analysis. Inability to resolve these issues was preventing her progression through adolescence—hence her feeling that she was still 15.

Overview of Opening and Midphase

Once the analytic situation had been secured, the intensity and pace of our work escalated. The formal recognition of the seriousness of her problem and the assurance of privacy for our communication solidified the therapeutic alliance and provided Ann relief and leeway to be less defensive. In place of the delicate, polite little girl was an earthy, passionate adolescent who expressed her feelings with vigor and explicit language. Now dressed in somewhat revealing jeans and sweater, she exhibited her barely contained sexuality, which was frightening to Ann and her family. As the analytic process gained momentum, perhaps my most important contribution was to avoid interfering with its progress: maintaining an analytic stance with Ann was not easy. She flaunted and rationalized her refusal to go to school, her promiscuity, and her avoidance of birth control. Analytic neutrality was critical in eliminating any manifest reason for her to perceive me as a parent, even a benign one. Her parents, siblings, and friends, who were all older than Ann, eagerly gave her advice. Ann knew very well what she should do and what she wanted to do; her inability to act accordingly led her to seek analysis. Highly motivated, very verbal, and delighted to have someone listen to her, Ann had no difficulty filling the sessions with her associations. My noncritical attitude, interest, and occasional interventions helped foster a positive transference response and an observing ego. From these emerged considerable information about how Ann viewed her family, some developmental history, the identification of the precipitating factors of her current illness, and examples of her poor self-esteem and distorted body image.

Feeling free to complain about her family, Ann described frequent fights with her father in which they deprecated each other, apparently defending against unconscious, mutually incestuous feelings. She berated his "hypocritical" values, stinginess with money, and scant time at home, blaming his neglect and promiscuity for her mother's drinking and the inability of her older brother to function at school or work. In addition, Ann was jealous of her older sister, "Miss Popularity," designated by her father as the perfect daughter. Significantly, he would joke that Ann should share some of her figure with her sister, implying that Ann was overweight, which objectively was not so. Gradually, it became transparent to me that Ann unconsciously was aware that neither her sister nor her mother could compete with her biologic endowments.

As Ann's positive transference feelings increased, her concerns turned to her irregular periods, her need "to be on the pill," and her fears that hormones would turn her into a boy. She thought something was wrong with her body and that she might be a lesbian. I inquired if these fears might relate to feelings she was having about me. Unable to deal directly with the question, she replied that she had been ashamed of coming to see me but now it didn't bother her. Nevertheless, fearful of these libidinal and dependent feelings, she began to search for a new third-person relationship. She began to castigate her mother for driving away her father by her unwillingness to cook, clean house, or sleep with him. Fights at home over her mother's refusal to have sexual relations were followed by Mother's reading aloud from the Bible; Ann couldn't understand why sex after marriage was sinful. With disgust she described her mother's devotion to her sickly brother, who was living at home. Confessing her disappointment that her own symptoms hadn't gotten her mother's attention, she nevertheless expressed anger that her mother rejected health and independence.

When I asked if she had mixed feelings about my attention, she replied that that was different. However, once again acting out to defend against these transference feelings, she immediately became engrossed with a new "third person." During her sessions she monotonously related details of the previous day with her boyfriend. This state of resistance was short-lived: her defenses failed when she became overwhelmed by her instinctual drives, and she fled back to the analytic work. Thus, after seeing the movie *The Exorcist*, she became panic-stricken for several weeks. At first she feared she would be possessed by the devil; then that her boyfriend was the devil. Ultimately, she had to sit up during one of her hours in order to assure herself that I wasn't the devil! Eventually, she began to understand that what she feared was the devilishness in herself—her sexuality. Attempting to avoid her heterosexual feelings, Ann broke up with her boyfriend, complaining that he was too much like her father, too domineering. She also recognized that she had used her boyfriend to avoid feelings for me. For a short time she examined her ambivalence about being analyzed, her wishes and fears not only about being dependent but also about what she would learn about herself. Then she recalled frightening images from the *The Exorcist*. These were followed by memories from age seven of a school phobia and of her sister, who shared her bedroom, slapping her hands for masturbating. While denying any current masturbatory activity, she worried that her early "sinful" behavior had caused her menstrual irregularities and may have changed her body. This activated her anxiety about her homosexual feelings, and she again fled to a new third-person relationship. This pattern of the transference as a fulcrum for the flow of material persisted throughout the analysis.

In the following months we explored questions about Ann's femininity. She was aroused by foreplay but anesthetic during intercourse. This convinced her that something was wrong with her body, a conviction that caused her "to feel low in front of boys." Conflicts about pregnancy appeared in her barely disguised dreams and fantasies of being pregnant and having a child. These wishes contrasted with her conscious disgust with the idea of being pregnant and her plan to adopt a child, rather than bear one. Resisting positive and negative transference feelings, she repeatedly acted out through her involvement with a "third person" and also by being late to her sessions. She canceled one hour to get a pregnancy test. After learning the test was negative, she admitted that she had hoped to get attention from her mother. In addition, she fantasied her father's outrage at her reply to his inquiry about who the father was that he could have his choice of three.

Ann rejected any transference interpretations, but as she became more aware of her unconscious conflicts with respect to her parents and siblings, she became less anxious. She decided to take birth control pills and also resumed her education at a small private school. Increased resistance became evident as Ann displaced her transference feelings onto her teachers at school and her parents delayed payments. As the summer approached she decided to quit analysis for several months "to go camping on my father's property." When a relationship with a much older boy reactivated her fears of "throwing up and being possessed by the devil," she admitted, "The problem is still in my head." She observed that at home and in her sessions she felt like a little girl whereas she acted too grown-up with "guys." Deciding to cancel the camping trip and stay in analysis, she got her parents to bring the payments up to date but maintained her relationship with her boyfriend, vaguely aware that he acted like her father.

Following a summer vacation, we dealt with Ann's pseudocyesis, a potent and final resistance to an emerging transference neurosis and to Ann's total involvement in the analytic process. In contrast to her presenting symptomatology, the pseudocyesis was precipitated by Ann's need to avoid the feelings of intense loss and rejection

occasioned by my absence (Frenkel, in press). Briefly, the pseudocyesis was a condensation of oedipal and preoedipal conflicts, in
which Ann felt that being pregnant proved she was loved. She
admitted that she had stopped taking birth control pills. Thus, just
after our sessions stopped for the summer she believed that she was
pregnant. Despite early signs of pregnancy, Ann refused to have a
pregnancy test; she imagined completing her pregnancy free of all
responsibilities. Since she felt complete, as both the adored and
adoring mother, she no longer needed her boyfriend, her family, or
her analysis. On my return, Ann appeared pregnant. Her preoccupation with being pregnant and her refusal to see an obstetrician
concerned me. In time, my focus on transference interpretations
resulted in her recalling that she had missed her boyfriend and me.
Two hours later her period began. Giving up her symptom allowed
her analysis to continue and her life to progress, which is what she
really wanted.

As the analysis became the central focus in her life, Ann began
dealing more directly with her oedipal conflicts, overtly competing
with her mother by becoming her father's tennis partner. In analyzing why, during a doubles tournament, she froze and forfeited the
match, she remembered that she had been fleetingly appalled when
one of their opponents thought she was her father's mistress. Unable
to deny that both she and her father had erotized their play, she quit
tennis. Instead, she completed her long-delayed driving lessons and
got her license. Now, more frightened by her increasing dependence
on me and angry at a winter break, she renewed a third-person
relationship. But when treatment resumed, she noted, "I won't let
myself enjoy a relationship with a guy, like I'm still saving myself
for Daddy." While ruminating about why she thought her father had
some power over her, Ann recalled an intense attachment to her
brother, 11 years her senior. She also remembered that when she was
7, he left for the army; in a whisper she told me that she had
transferred her affection to his best friend, who, as her baby-sitter,
frequently fondled her. After this recollection, Ann began fighting
with her family. We related her subsequent attempts to fight with me
to her worry that her attachment to me meant that she was homosexual. However, she came to believe that these concerns were just
another way of avoiding feelings for her father. Realizing that her
attachment to her father prevented her from establishing anything
but third-person relationships, she knew that she would have to
renounce it. Depressed at the possibility of losing her father, as she
had been with the loss of the pseudopregnancy, she became furious
with me for "taking him away."

Relinquishing her anger renewed Ann's concerns that her body was deformed, as well as her wish to be a boy, primarily as an attempt to avoid her own sexual feelings, particularly towards her father. After much blocking, she said that what bothered her about being a girl was that her vagina made her feel dirty. I commented that perhaps it was her feelings that made her feel dirty. She replied that the dirtiest word in her vocabulary was *love*. In subsequent months she came to understand that her loving and erotic feelings terrified her, since she had associated them only with incestuous objects (mother, father, and brother) and with the subsequent rejection and/or regression. As she began to give up her infantile fantasies, Ann became aware that she no longer felt "low in front of people," she no longer felt her body was dirty or deformed, her periods became more regular, and her school work improved. After another period of mourning over the renunciation of her childhood aims, she said she could no longer fool herself by playing the third person. Increasingly angry at her parents for using their children to act out their problems, Ann realized she had been encouraged by her parents to remain a child. Following a dream in which she unsuccessfully tried to turn on any light in her house, she complained that her parents had left her in the dark. But she was also angry at me for turning on the lights, for revealing things about her family that she hadn't wanted to see. Worried about her increasing affection for me, she still feared that anyone she truly cared for would reject her.

Termination Phase

As Ann approached termination, she continued working through her anger at her parents not only for their harshness with her when she was younger but for their lack of love for their children and for each other. She mused, "Thinking of the way my parents are—they don't show love and they never did to us—like I'm recreating the same situation with guys I see, where it has to be a fighting relationship, like with my parents." Aware that feeling or revealing any affection in a relationship frightened her, she admitted, "During sex I turn myself off and become cold." Thoughts of caring for her parents, for boyfriends, for me, made her uncomfortable, since she feared being mocked, as she had been in childhood when she showed affection for her parents. Unable to tolerate being hurt, she withdrew from relationships before that could happen. Then she recognized that, aside from relationships within her family, it was *she* who rejected the other person first and that it had been years since she had been hurt.

The following week Ann began her first session by relating a dream of experiencing love with a nonincestuous object. It left her with a sense of wonder and led to our first discussion of termination. She reported, "I can only remember a portion of the dream and then only the feeling, and I can't explain it . . . Some guy was holding me as we were looking through the [well-lit] house [her sister's]. . . . It was a real comfortable feeling, like nothing I've ever shared with a guy before . . . I keep thinking about that feeling . . . so nice I didn't want to get up . . . it was like loving . . . so hard for me to talk of love . . . made me think about how I've related to guys before, not even real, so false . . . the feeling in the dream was really great, the thing was being comfortable with myself, didn't feel low at all. I'm always so worried about how I look to other people, have to look good . . . The feeling was so good, I don't think it would matter what you look like. You feel good and warm from inside . . . don't need the other things, weird . . . all my ideas of a [real] person were in that guy, a personality, and I can't remember what he looked like. [She felt at a loss in trying to describe him and recognized only that he was not like anyone she had ever known.] I looked basically, physically, the same, but I was really different. I've grown. I'm older and younger." By this she meant that her new sense of inner maturity no longer necessitated her acting older and she could be and act her own age.

Ann's first associations to the dream were to having had a good weekend because she had learned a lot. Having her period pleased her. For the first time she noticed that she was growing up and "no longer acted fake around my friends." She was astounded that "it had never occurred to [her] before that parents are supposed to love each other." She felt sorry for her mother, describing her parents' marriage as one "where there was only criticism and no love." She knew that was painful, because her parents had hurt her in the same way. She also realized that when she hated them, it was because she had loved them and they hadn't been able to love her back. Although she was angry with her father, she also felt sorry for him. She noticed over the weekend that her feelings about him had changed: she no longer feared or desired him. She complained that when he was around, all he did was hurt everyone. Ann confirmed this assessment in a telephone conversation with her sister, who had married and moved to another city. Her sister described bitter fights with her father when she became somewhat of a hippie and was no longer "Miss Perfect." In earlier sessions Ann had expressed admiration and envy of the caring relationship she saw in her sister's marriage. In earlier dreams, houses had often represented her own body. This dream in her sister's house seemed to represent her new image of herself: one who was no longer in the dark, no longer involved in conflicts with her parents. In this new place, feeling good about herself, she could express her wish and growing capacity to love and be loved.

For several days she was happy and content. Following another dream in which she was married but there was no sex, I asked if she still had difficulty putting sex and love together without feeling guilty. Avoiding this interpretation, she canceled her next appointment, explaining that her mother had left the car lights on and the battery was dead. Although she realized the canceled hour was resistance to dealing with my intervention, she continued her resistance the next day by broaching the subject of termination for the first time. She said she was tired of feeling like a disturbed person when there wasn't anything wrong with her. She agreed there were still a few problems to be worked out, like not feeling guilty about intimacy and love, but she knew the end of therapy was in sight. She didn't know when the therapy would end, and even thinking about it gave her a sense of panic, which she related to a fear of letting go of her parents and, ultimately, of me: "I just thought about my mother . . . I relate you two pretty close, you taking the place of my mother or a parent." Speaking of her recent sense of estrangement from her parents, she recalled being scared as a child that her need for her mother was so strong. Recalling her old fear of leaving her mother, I asked if she was now afraid of leaving analysis and me, and she agreed.

For several months Ann worked repeatedly with her fear of separation, especially from her mother. Slowly it became clear to her that she associated these fears with her school phobia in the second grade. She recalled concerns about her mother's welfare and specific fears that her mother would die. Following this, with considerable difficulty, she associated to her early childhood masturbatory activity in bed and during her bath and her shame when her sister slapped her. Attempts to explore any thoughts or fantasies she might have had at that time aroused a great deal of blocking. She became transiently depressed, concerned again with "being possessed by the devil" and "throwing up in public." As she went through each of these episodes, she observed that they didn't seem real to her anymore, and she sensed that she was avoiding something she couldn't quite define. This resistance lasted for several weeks. During one session, after she repeated her complaint that she didn't know what she was avoiding, I inquired if her fear of "throwing up" could be a way to avoid her fear of "growing up," of something she couldn't swallow.[1]

The following session Ann became enraged that the previous night her father not only had tried to enter her room without knocking but had also complained that she had locked the door. Although she had been talking with a girlfriend while sitting on her bed, she immediately felt guilty and associated it to masturbating. This led to her vivid recollection of an episode just prior to the beginning of the second grade, when her brother's friend had come to baby-sit for her and her parents had not yet left the house. She began by reporting that the boy sat next to her on the living room floor, slipped his hands into her panties, and played with her vagina. She felt sure that her mother had seen him and was furious that her mother had not stopped him. Then, with a sense of horror, she wondered if maybe it was her father who had been playing with her. As she continued, she thought that she could recall seeing her father, not her mother, but that he was in the next room, and she was not sure whether her father saw her and the baby-sitter or not. Finally, she remembered that while she was being fondled, she had, in fact, enjoyed it and had the fantasy that it was her father who was with her. She then recalled wanting to replace her mother, get rid of her. This reminded her of her surprise that in some recent dreams she had experienced a murderous rage toward a female rival, often thinly disguised as her mother, her sister, or me. When I commented that in the past such feelings were probably concurrent with her concern for her mother's welfare, Ann was able to connect these fantasies with her school phobia.

Able to distinguish more easily between fantasy and reality, between her wishes and her actions, Ann now felt less guilty and more confident. With increased self-esteem, she applied to, and was accepted at, both a local junior college and a more distant state college. Since attending the state college raised conflicts over ending treatment, she decided to matriculate at the junior college in the fall. She marveled at how much she had punished herself unconsciously by doing poorly at school, not studying, getting into trouble, and fighting with her friends—all because of her guilt over sexual feelings and fantasies. However, she was almost despondent

---

[1]Initially, I believed Ann's fear of "throwing up" represented her unconscious compromise formation of a wish for and fear of oral impregnation. While her concerns about birth control pills seem to support this hypothesis, there was no other evidence for it (Frenkel, in press).

at the idea of stopping treatment. She felt dependent on me and was not sufficiently confident of her own analyzing capacity to set a termination date. Jealousy of her mother's exclusive care for her brother, cooking and cleaning just for him, led to her wanting to be my baby. Then, as the summer break approached, she became hurt and angry that I would leave her. Moving away from these preoedipal feelings, she felt nauseated at still wanting her father and hating her mother.

Upset after reading about masturbation in *The Descent of Woman*, Ann became conscious of the fact that, since latency, she had regularly directed a stream of water over her clitoris to achieve orgasm while showering. Having totally repressed the sexual nature of this activity until recently, she believed that an evanescent realization that she had been masturbating helped precipitate her current illness. Initially denying any masturbatory fantasies, she conceded that she occasionally imagined "a guy." Later she was able to recall fantasies of winning her father, which she now viewed as "childish." Noting that her parents slept in separate beds, she connected these fantasies with her guilt over thinking that she had caused her parents' fights. After engaging her father in a couple of fights, she stated, "I'm emotionally retarded for getting all worked up over what he did. I'm just exaggerating to keep myself at home."

Drawing her attention to her feelings about my summer absence, I wondered if the problem wasn't more related to her leaving her mother. She agreed that she had been thinking about her mother, worried over the many times she wished her dead. While exploring this, Ann blurted out, "If she ever comes near me again, I'll kill her." In our early sessions Ann had mentioned with little affect that between the ages of 5 and 10 she often slept with her mother when her father was out of town. Recalling the last time they slept together, she now reexperienced her fury at her mother when she manually probed Ann's anus, explaining that she was trying to remove worms. Afterwards, Ann refused to sleep with her. This was the first time Ann returned to that episode, exclaiming that she knew she did not have worms. Recalling it now, she was disgusted with her mother's actions and duplicity. For some time we talked about her hatred, but Ann ultimately uncovered loving and protective feelings for her mother, including wishes to be a man so she could replace her father. Still incredulous at her mother's actions, she repeatedly asked, "Why did she do that?" My comment that she no longer sounded angry but, rather, bashful led to her recollection of being aroused. Once again she became enraged at "being used." In time, with relief, she understood her concern about being a lesbian and her fear of her affection for me.

Before the summer break Ann said she thought that she still needed her sessions but hoped to be able to end analysis before the end of the year, when she planned to transfer to the state college for the spring semester. During her sessions Ann seemed very comfortable with herself and with me. Her associations flowed freely from past to present with little evidence of resistance. Outside of analysis Ann was involved in making plans to go to college, and although she dated, she was not engrossed in any third-person relationship. Occasionally, she would catch herself becoming provocative with one of her parents but would stop, feeling a little chagrined that she had fallen into her old patterns. Although Ann had not yet established a loving and sexual nonincestuous relationship, she was only 18. Her ability to do some mourning over both the impending holiday and the end of her analysis, without needing an external attachment, seemed to me an indication of her growing inner strength. We tentatively agreed to stop three or four weeks prior to or after the usual winter holiday. No date was set, with the understanding that we would be flexible and would even continue longer if that seemed best. Hours were established for the fall, and Ann was to call if there were conflicts with her new college schedule.

When treatment resumed, Ann missed her first appointment. Later in the day she called wondering when her appointments were, indignant that I had not called her and insistent that no hours had been scheduled. Contradicting herself, she announced in a hostile and haughty manner that she could no longer come at the agreed-upon time because of her college schedule. Furthermore, she saw no need to return at all. I suggested that she sounded troubled, offered an alternative time the next day, and encouraged her to return to explore her feelings. The following day she was very apologetic for her attitude on the phone and puzzled, since she had been feeling quite happy with herself during most of the summer. In analyzing the events during our break and the phone call the previous day, she admitted initially feeling rejected, hurt, and angry at my leaving for vacation. She had wanted to retaliate. "I was really dependent, so emotionally attached to you . . . mainly afraid of doing it on my own, but I got over it. . . . I've found out so much on my own, I felt I didn't need you any more." She felt embarrassed by her childish behavior on the phone, realizing that she had repeated with me her old patterns of trying to anger her father or hurt her mother's feelings. She did not want to stop analysis that way and now looked forward to telling me about her summer.

Ann related how at first she tried to lean on her family but decided she really didn't need them or their approval. Then, on a date with an old boyfriend who was "making passes" at her, she became aware that in the past she would have slept with him just to please him but that she really wasn't attracted to him. "It was neat, because I knew my feelings weren't there, that I can judge what my feelings are . . . I learned a way to solve my own problems." She remarked on how painful it felt when she first realized she didn't need me or her parents. Then, she felt pleased that she no longer craved external advice or support, that she didn't feel stupid or bad. She was surprised and pleased that the students, faculty, and general curriculum at the junior college seemed "normal." Eager to participate in activities with her peers, she marveled at "being who I am, and enjoying it."

Ann no longer felt like a little girl during her sessions, and this reinforced her sense of independence. However, although she had established some pleasurable autonomous functioning, she seemed afraid of losing it if she remained in treatment much longer. I wondered if she was protesting too much about no longer needing me. Thus, when she requested that termination be set for the end of the month, I again asked if she was rushing to avoid facing some of her feelings. She promptly denied this. I questioned if perhaps she wanted to reject me, since my summer absence may have renewed her feelings of being rejected by her parents when she was a child. Disagreeing, she retorted that she hoped I wasn't going to act like a parent, telling her how she felt and what to do and not respecting her feelings about what she knew about herself. Then, more calmly, she agreed that she was a little reluctant to stop but honestly felt that for her to grow, she needed an opportunity to practice independently what she had gained in the analysis. She stated that if she felt a need, she knew she could return and saw no reason to continue beyond the end of the month.

I became aware that Ann was not talking in a provocative manner. No longer a frightened, angry little girl, she was reasoning like an adult. She was listening to me and responding according to what seemed sensible to her, that is, without the need to either please or annoy me. The change was impressive. Ann was ready to stop treatment; I wasn't. She no longer was invested primarily in her analysis. While continuing the analysis might benefit me, by allowing me more time to feel assured of her progress, I sensed it could be detrimental to Ann, threatening her newly won autonomy and raising unnecessary doubts about her judgment. After I agreed, she speculated that perhaps treatment had, in some sense, ended with the summer break. She explained that she knew all of the work had been done but that she had been afraid she wouldn't make it on her own and wanted to be sure that time would be available in the fall if she needed it. She was overjoyed at her successful functioning and was happy to share that with me.

Ann related other changes during the last few weeks of treatment. She no longer felt the need to hate her father and felt free to agree or disagree with him as the occasion warranted. Her analysis was no longer the primary focus of her life. Her thoughts and feelings now centered around her activities at school and her new relationships there. College was a little frightening and confusing, but her peers said that they felt the same way. The work was interesting and not as hard as she had expected. She was a little embarrassed to say she found that she was "boy crazy"; although she was dating a lot, she felt no need to sleep with anyone at the moment. For the first time in her life she regarded herself as special. She felt that sex was special, and she wanted to be really close to a boy before having intimate relations. She no longer dated with the idea of what she could get, but looked forward to sharing. Amazed at who she was and what she was doing, she could barely recall herself at the onset of the analysis. She was grateful to me and sad about leaving. She knew a part of her life had ended, but she was glad it was over. The last hour, after admitting how much she was going to miss analysis, she said, "I know I'll miss you . . . This is like no other relationship I'll ever have; it's a different kind of relationship . . . I'll be sad for a while, but I won't have that much time." She went on to say what a special day it was. "It's like one of the things I needed to accomplish . . . I'm excited about it . . . It shows how far I've come . . . and that I'm moving on to the next step." Hesitatingly, she said that she was really proud of what she had accomplished. I agreed she had reason to be very proud.

Discussion

The termination phase of Ann's analysis was similar to that in adult analysis and a natural progression of the analytic work that preceded it. Like most of the analysis, it was driven by the continuing evolution and relative resolution of the transference neurosis. As outlined earlier, the opening phase of the analysis depicted increasingly intense transference reactions and resistances as the analysis began to occupy more of Ann's mental life and determine her behavior both in and out of the analytic sessions. Ann entered the midphase when the transference neurosis became evident, when the analysis became the center of her life, that is, when most of her previous symptoms and conflicts were reformulated around her feelings about me, specifically when she developed a pseudocyesis in response to a summer break (Frenkel, in press). After this symptom, her last major resistance, was analyzed, Ann's life revolved around her analysis as the transference became the primary determinant of her feelings and actions. During the subsequent analytic work it was through the transference neurosis that oedipal and preoedipal conflicts were reenacted and brought to consciousness, and they were resolved so that restructuring could occur (Hoffman, 1989).

Ann's dream of experiencing love with a nonincestuous object seemed a signal dream for termination (Cavenar and Nash, 1976), indicating structural changes, improved ego functions, and absent or evanescent symptom recurrence. However, the dream raises such questions as whether the object was indeed nonincestuous, why critical genetic material was uncovered only after the dream, and why there was a recurrence of symptoms. The man in the dream seemed nonincestuous, not only from Ann's description that he was like no one she had ever known but also because of the absence of guilt, which allowed her to feel so good. Her subsequent associations support this in her markedly less conflicted, more realistic, and more sympathetic view of her parents. Although the dream was set in her sister's house and Ann had expressed interests in her brother-in-law, in her associations to this dream she and her sister were allies rather than competitors. While the dream signified the presence of structural change, a real developmental progression for Ann, it was one she was unable to maintain consistently. In my opinion her capacity to have the dream enabled the final working through of her core conflicts with the critical recall of the fantasies, affects, and events of her childhood seductions. In my experience, during termination adults frequently uncover more genetic material, and that allows for greater comprehension and resolution of core issues. Because of this, previous symptoms may occur transiently. Strengthening and solidifying structural change is probably an essential element of any termination phase.

In Ann's termination phase no new conflicts emerged, but reworking of these core issues helped in the recovery of previously repressed memories and feelings that added depth and meaning to our understanding of the severity and persistence of Ann's complaint that she was always the "third person." Renouncing her infantile wishes and fears about both her parents allowed her to modify the severity of her superego. No longer overwhelmed by her drives, needing to act them out or defend against them, she could allow her ego to expand and function in an age-appropriate manner. After being housebound for almost a year, in less than two years Ann was able to complete three years of high school, begin college with arrangements to live away from her parents, make new friends, and date in an appropriate manner. The increase, reformation, and reintegration of her ego functioning were remarkable. Adatto (1958) described these changes as a hallmark of adolescent analysis. While maximum ego functioning is certainly a goal in all analyses, because puberty destabilizes the ego, its effective restructuring in an adolescent analysand is even more impressive.

Sufficient resolution of her transference feelings from all levels of development allowed Ann to internalize my analyzing function as part of her ego ideal (Novick, 1976). As she said, she no longer needed my help to find out how she felt or what she should do. Although transference residues remained, the transference neurosis was essentially resolved, since Ann's life no longer centered on her analysis. Thus, in the autumn, although positive and negative transference feelings were evident in Ann's angry and provocative phone call, she was, in contrast to her behavior before analysis and following other holiday absences, asymptomatic, and she rapidly altered her antagonistic stance. Independently, she recognized that she was defending against her wish to see me and that she was acting out her anger at my leaving. She was somewhat chagrined by the recurrence of childish feelings, which she now felt were inappropriate. The distinction between transference feelings and a transference neurosis is important. That some transference feelings for the analyst remain after termination is hardly unusual. Since transference residues can be seen after successful and unsuccessful analyses, their presence, in and of themselves, is not a valid indication of the incompleteness of the analytic work. Throughout the last few weeks, while she freely expressed positive feelings for me and our work, most of Ann's energy and investment had shifted from analysis to challenges at college, new friends, and plans and hopes for the future.

Differences from adult analysis seem most apparent in the sustained intensity and velocity of the analysis. The initial work of overcoming the resistances to secure the analytic situation was slow. By contrast, once established, the analytic process rapidly unfolded, accelerating as if it were propelled by Ann's now-released normal adolescent growth spurt. Her request for an earlier termination date came as a surprise to me. After extensive exploration of her motivations, as well as my own, I decided to agree. As I thought about it, I realized that Ann had been working hard at her analysis all summer while I had been on vacation. She had been preparing to stop; I hadn't. Especially in late adolescence, there was every reason not to continue an essentially regressive process that would threaten and interfere with Ann's newly won autonomy (Adatto, 1966). I believe that the resolution of Ann's negative oedipal conflicts was critical in the resolution of the transference neurosis. This allowed internalization to occur and provided her with the ability to do analytic work in my absence over the summer. According to Blos (1974), the mature ego ideal emerges at the end of adolescence as the heir of the negative Oedipus complex, a development that he feels is a crucial issue in treating adolescent boys. In my opinion it is equally important in adolescent girls, as Ann's analysis seems to demonstrate. Whether this is particular to Ann's analysis or characteristic of adolescent analysis or of every analysis is a question for further study. In my view resolution of positive and negative oedipal conflicts allows for the internalization of both maternal and paternal ideals and is essential in freeing the adolescent from infantile objects (Frenkel, 1988). Loewald (1988) believes the work of mourning is the most important aspect of termination. He describes mourning as the gradual relinquishment of a cherished relationship and its internalization. Periods of mourning occurred throughout Ann's analysis, not only in the termination phase. Mourning is a normal task of adolescence, as well as of analysis. With Ann, as with many adolescents, it was intense but of shorter duration than with many adults, but then, there is less to mourn and a whole adult life to anticipate.

Summary

The termination phase in the analysis of Ann, an adolescent girl, was described within the context of her entire analysis. Similarities with adult analysis seemed greater than the differences, which appeared more quantitative than substantive. A dream of experiencing tender love with a nonincestuous object, indicating that structural changes, as well as an increase in ego function, had occurred and signaled the approach of termination. The dream left Ann with a sense of wonder at her growth and a sense of pleasure with herself. This good, warm feeling markedly contrasted with her earlier feelings of being dirty, sinful, and low. After some regression, fears of separation, and depression over loss of her dependence on the analyst, Ann was able to rework both positive and negative oedipal conflicts, amplifying and solidifying the structural changes. Her transference neurosis facilitated her recalling feelings and fantasies connected to a series of childhood seductions, which resulted in a more complete resolution of her core conflicts, as well as of the transference neurosis itself. Her intensely positive and negative transference feelings were replaced by a more realistic view of me and, more important, of herself. No longer preoccupied with childhood fantasies, she found pleasure in more realistic achievements at school and with friends and resumed her normal developmental progression in my absence. She terminated with some sadness but primarily with a sense of joy and eagerness to explore herself and the world around her. Indeed, I agreed with her expression, "I grew to the point I should be".

References

Adatto, C. (1958), Ego reintegration observed in analysis of late adolescents. *Internat. J. Psycho-Anal.*, 39:172–177.

_____ (1966), On the metamorphosis from adolescence into adulthood. *J. Amer. Psychoanal. Assn.* 14:485–509.

Blos, P. (1974), The genealogy of the ego ideal. *The Psychoanalytic Study of the Child*, 29:43–88. New Haven, CT: Yale University Press.

Cavenar, J. & Nash, J. (1976), The dream as a signal for termination. *J. Amer. Psychoanal. Assn.*, 24:425–436.

Chused, J. (1988), The transference neurosis in child analysis. *The Psychoanalytic Study of the Child*, 43:51–82. New Haven, CT: Yale University Press.

Frenkel, R. (1988), Late adolescence: Spock and the ego-ideal. *Adolescent Psychiatry: Developmental and Clinical Studies*, 15:46–64. Chicago, IL: University of Chicago Press.

_____ (in press), The early abortion of a pseudocyesis: Some observations from the analysis of an adolescent girl. *The Psychoanalytic Study of the Child*, 46. New Haven, CT: Yale University Press.

Freud, S. (1937), Analysis terminable and interminable. *Standard Edition*, 23:216–254. London: Hogarth Press, 1964.

Hoffman, L. (1989), The psychoanalytic process and the development of insight in child analysis: A case study. *Psychoanal. Quart.*, 58:63–80.

Loewald, H. (1988), Termination analyzable and unanalyzable. *The Psychoanalytic Study of the Child*, 43:155–166. New Haven, CT: Yale University Press.

Novick, J. (1976), Termination of treatment in adolescence. *The Psychoanalytic Study of the Child*, 31:389–414. New Haven, CT: Yale University Press.

_____ (1989), The process of termination in child and adolescent analysis: Relevance to adult analysis. Presented at the annual clinical meeting of The Association for Child Psychoanalysis, Philadelphia.

II

Theoretical
Papers

11

The Transference Neurosis in Child Analysis

Judith Fingert Chused

The development of a transference neurosis, manifested by symptoms or the intensification of characteristic, pathological modes of perception and interaction in relation to the analyst, is, I believe, the sine qua non of psychoanalysis. Although every attempt at analysis does not result in a transference neurosis (or an analysis), when a full analytic process occurs, analysis of the transference neurosis is a central element. Many analysts believe it to be the pivotal mutative experience in adult analysis; this, however, is not the general opinion for child analysis. Until recently, most child analysts in the United States (other than the followers of Melanie Klein) saw the child as having a limited capacity to form and sustain a transference neurosis. Although this perception of analysis with children is changing and a growing number of analysts today practice "adult-type" child analysis, there remain many who believe children do not develop transference manifestations and transference neuroses as adults do, in either frequency, endurance, or depth. The determinants of this belief lie both in the preconceptions and political struggles that mark the history of child analysis and in certain characteristics of child analysis itself.

I have not found intense transference manifestations developing

An earlier version of this chapter appeared in The Psychoanalytic Study of the Child, 43:51–81. New Haven, CT: Yale University Press, 1988. Reprinted by permission.

around the person of the analyst unusual in children; quite the contrary, without it I find there is no analysis (though there may be very good psychotherapy). However, if the term *transference neurosis* is limited to the development within the analytic situation of a new neurosis, complete with a new set of symptoms, then I have to agree that this is not a regular occurrence in the analysis of children (or adults). This is the definition recommended by Marjorie Harley (1971). But if *transference neurosis* is broadened to include the intensification of pathological character traits and modes of relating within the analytic setting, with the gradual emergence of regressive, incestuous fantasies, conflicts, and impulses experienced in relation to and centered on the analyst and with the intensity of affect and sense of reality described by Bird (1972), then an analyzable transference neurosis can develop almost as frequently in children as in adults. This definition of transference neurosis is similar to that advanced by Sandler, Kennedy, and Tyson (1975): "By transference neurosis we mean the concentration of the child's conflicts, repressed infantile wishes, fantasies, etc., on the person of the therapist, *with the relative diminution of their manifestations elsewhere*" (p. 427).

If the development and utilization of a transference neurosis can be an integral part of child analysis, then when children *fail* to develop an analyzable transference neurosis, we need to question why this is. After a child has developed sufficient capacity to retain a memory of human interactions and to form an internal mental representation of an object, he has the capacity for transference, to "misperceive" an interaction with one person so that it "feels" the same as with another. And when he has sufficient structural development to sustain intersystemic conflicts (Panel, 1966) and the ego capacity to tolerate (even minimally and only transiently) conflictual feelings, impulses, and fantasies, he can develop a transference neurosis. But whether the child develops a transference neurosis and, if he does, how it is utilized for the work of analysis will depend not only on his level of development and his individual psychopathology but also on the theoretical position of the analyst. The analyst's theory and his expectations, regardless of his neutrality, always influence his perceptions and his technique.

One consequence of the skepticism about transference neurosis in children is that it has led to a discrediting of conflict resolution as the major mutative element in work with children. Although theoretical discussions support conflict resolution as the core therapeutic agent in child analysis, clinical presentations often emphasize other elements, such as the relationship with the analyst as a "real object," as important for the therapeutic efficacy of the work. On occasion this has obfuscated the distinction between child analysis and child psychotherapy, leading analysts of adults to declare that "child analysis isn't really analysis."

Historically, child analysis began with Freud's (1909) analysis of Little Hans, conducted through the child's father. The report of this case opened up a world of possibilities to analysts, who hoped that because children were in close temporal proximity to the origin of their neurotic conflicts, the conflicts would be available for rapid resolution through the analytic method. However, analysts trained in working with adults quickly found the work with children extremely frustrating; Ferenczi (1913) decided that "direct psychoanalytic investigation was therefore impossible" (p. 244) when his attempts with a 5-year-old boy failed because the child was bored and wanted to get back to his toys. Analytic work with children soon became the province of educators and pediatricians. From the start, therapists such as the teacher Hug-Hellmuth (1921, 1924), Anna Freud (1927), and Dorothy Burlingham (1932), whose work Hug-Hellmuth influenced, were sensitive to the unique characteristics of the child and felt that the techniques and tools of adult analysis would have to be modified, specifically, that the relative abstinence and neutrality utilized in adult analyses should be set aside as intolerable to children who would neither participate in nor benefit from analysis under nongratifying conditions. They also believed that since the child was still very attached to and quite dependent on his original objects, his parents, there would be no transference or transference neurosis formed around the person of the analyst. At this time, the difference between the psychic representation of the child's earlier relationship with his parents and the external reality of his present relationship with them was not yet elucidated; the relationship of the past and present were seen as the same and, being currently active, as nontransferable. In addition, the awareness of the developmental need for a positive attachment between mother and child led to a belief among these early child analysts that if analytic work was to enable the child to resume progressive development, a similar type of positive attachment to the analyst was essential.

The work of Melanie Klein and her colleagues, presented in a panel in 1926 and reported in the *International Journal of Psychoanalysis* in 1927, reveals a very different perception of child analysis. But until recently, their work has had little influence on the majority of child analysts in the United States.

It was Anna Freud who had the dominant influence on child

analysis in the United States. Her beliefs, including that it was important for the child *to want* to come to analysis, led child analysts to present themselves as benevolent providers, with gifts, skills, or powers (even omnipotence) the child would value (A. Freud, 1927; Bornstein, 1949). It gradually became apparent that exuberant benevolence was not needed to ensure the child's participation in the analysis. But though the seductions and gratifications that occurred in the early years of child analysis are now no longer sanctioned, many analysts still believe it is important for them to be perceived as a "benevolent object." This has led to a self-perpetuating problem in child analysis: an analyst who believes the child cannot tolerate significant deprivation in analysis can justify the very gratification that interferes with the full development of transference and a transference neurosis. Thus, it is not surprising that in a recent panel (1983) on the reanalysis of child patients those contributors who held this belief found that "a transference neurosis, which requires the ability to contain an internal conflict, does not develop before the end of latency" (p. 684) and that "the transference had not been analyzed" (p. 686).

By the 1950s and 1960s most analysts (Harley, 1986, p. 133) recognized that children had transference reactions to the analyst and that these could be utilized for interpretations and clarifications much as in work with adults. Yet there was still a general feeling that because of the immaturity of the child's psychic structure and the continuing dependence on the parents, transference neurosis as such did not occur with children; that since transference manifestations were so fluid and of such relatively short duration, they did not occupy the same central role in the child's analysis as in the adult's. Only when case reports of fully developed transference neuroses in children began to appear in the analytic literature (Kut, 1953; Fraiberg, 1966; Harley, 1967) did the concept gain more acceptance.

Anna Freud (1965) later modified her position, and her observation that a transference neurosis can develop in children but does not equal the adult variety in every respect (p. 36) is currently quoted or referred to in almost every article on transference neurosis in children. The accuracy of her observations of children's behavior in analysis (their inability to free-associate, the preponderance of aggressive transference reactions, the use of the analyst as a real object, and their tendency to externalization of psychic structures onto the analyst) lends credence to her conclusion that the tranference neurosis is less significant in child analysis than in adult analysis. However, the factors that she described as limiting the development of a transference neurosis in child analysis are also found in adult analyses, and some analysts (Bird, 1972) believe these are the very factors that constitute the transference neurosis. I sense, instead, that the specific limiting factor to the development of a transference neurosis in child analysis arises from the analyst and the child patient automatically responding to each other as *adult* and *child*, falling into customary roles of adult who educates and/or directs, child who learns, complies, or rebels. This is similar to the problem Bird (1972) alludes to in adult analyses when he says, "One of the most serious problems of analysis is the very substantial help which the patient receives directly from the analyst and the analytic situation" (p. 285).

For example, with an intensification of transference, not infrequently a child will create bigger and bigger messes in the office, regressively trying to engage the analyst in a reenactment of anal phase struggles (P. Tyson, 1978, p. 227). It is extraordinarily difficult for the analyst to time his interventions so that the child experiences the impulse but does not become so overwhelmed by the associated affects that he loses the capacity to hear verbal interventions. Children move very fast—objects are broken, guilt escalates, and behavior gets out of control as the attempt to elicit punishment intensifies. A conflict is repeated rather than remembered and verbalized. At this point there is a temptation for the analyst to control the child's behavior and instruct (which often contains superego injunctions). However, if the analyst can provide (and the child receive) the structure necessary to halt regression and support self-observing ego capacities, if he analyzes rather than educates, a new solution based on experience can be forged. Enactment of a conflict, a common occurrence in child analysis, does not always require the interruption of an analytic attitude in the analyst. Abstinence is important not only in its effect on the patient; its effect on the analyst is to permit him to become more an "analyzing" and less a "modifying" force.

Unintentionally, Anna Freud's words (1965) have contributed to a premature closure of the issue of transference neurosis in child analysis. Analysts have yet to explore adequately: (1) What inhibits the full development of transference and a transference neurosis in child patients? (2) In which ways does this inhibition alter the treatment? (3) How, if the development of a transference neurosis with child patients is useful, might it be facilitated? Excellent papers have been written (Sandler et al., 1975; Harley, 1986; R. L. Tyson and P. Tyson, 1986) in which transference and the transference neurosis in children are discussed. Unfortunately, they offer little new understanding as to its infrequent appearance, with Harley's doing just the opposite: looking for something out of the ordinary in the child who does develop a transference neurosis.

In my experience, transference and transference neuroses are not uncommon in the analysis of children, although they do differ in some respects from their adult counterparts. In children, as in adults, oedipal conflicts are a significant feature of the transference neurosis, with these conflicts reflecting not only pathogenic experiences during the oedipal period but also organizing pathology derived from earlier preoedipal phases. When the developmental level of the child's ego functions, including cognitive development, affect tolerance, narcissistic vulnerability, and maturity of defenses, as well as the nature of the child's attachment to his current objects (R. L. Tyson and P. Tyson, 1986), are taken into account, a thoughtful analytic procedure, with strict attention to the analysis of resistance and to countertransference interferences, can lead to a full-blown transference neurosis in the child patient.

I reached this conclusion several years ago when I was analyzing, concurrently, two girls, Sarah (11 years old) and Molly (10 years old), both of whom had an intensely negative transference to me. During the many months when exploration of the determinants of their negative feelings did little to alter their behavior, I had ample time to examine our interactions. Three observations stand out: (1) The negative transference from these children was much more unpleasant than negative transference from adults—they were hypersensitive to and openly critical of my failings, and I, in turn, was sensitive to their comments. (2) Even though there was no evidence of any positive feeling from either child and both spoke of wanting to quit the analysis, material continued to emerge that could be beneficially utilized. (3) My initial response to their negative feelings was less abstinent than with adults. Specifically, my attempts to educate them about transference as a phenomenon were clearly defensive, as were some of my interpretations, which, in retrospect, were intended to dissipate the transference rather than understand it. In both cases, the patients picked up on my defensiveness: one became frightened she had hurt me and went through a brief period of "goodness" with some hypochondriacal obsessing during the sessions; the other became more sullen and withdrawn, as if she experienced my defensiveness as coercive, which, I fear, it was unconsciously intended to be.

With adults one expects negative transference reactions; their absence raises concern about defensive compliance, the possibility of a "good" patient who "loves" analysis but derives no lasting benefit from it. Yet, during training most child analysts are taught to maintain a positive therapeutic alliance with the child patient. They learn that though they should not gratify with the aim of suppressing the child's hostile feelings, they must prevent deprivations that would arouse so much negative affect that active participation in the analytic work ceases (Sandler, Kennedy, and Tyson, 1980).

I was powerless to alter, through any change in my demeanor, Molly's and Sarah's dislike and distrust of me, their perception of me as potentially hurtful instead of helpful. And, with an abstinence dictated as much by the patient as by theory, what began as negative transference went on to become a transference neurosis, similar in that both girls concentrated their rage and feelings of deprivation and injury on me (with an increasingly positive interaction with the outside world) but different in the specific content and course of development. However, in both children the transference neurosis was relatively uncontaminated by any attempt on my part to maintain a therapeutic alliance or be a benevolent "good object."

The analytic process with these two children was interesting. Molly, who had recreated with me the horror of her fourth through sixth years, when she had spent many hours alone in a hospital waiting room while her already depressed and unavailable mother attended to her baby brother, who had leukemia, continued to feel negative about me until termination. However, during the last year she continued in the analysis voluntarily (that is, she no longer begged her parents to let her quit), because she thought it was doing her some good. During the earlier "months of hate," the ideational content of her negative attitude changed several times. Her perception of me as nonempathic and "not too smart" (which developed in the sixth month in response to what had been intended as neutral questions about her drawings and description of a future world) shifted gradually to a quite competitive and aggressively taunting battle over when and what she would talk about, followed by a long period in which I was seen as intrusive and controlling. The associations in this period were to her father and were both provocative of and defensive against the gratification she had experienced when he (in part in response to his wife's preoccupation with their ill son) had begun to spend large amounts of time with Molly, instructing her about intellectual matters in a domineering, impatient manner.

After the termination date was set, Molly's attitude toward me changed dramatically. As we examined the change during our final months together, she was able to talk about her longing to be nurtured and loved by me, her disappointment in me, and her awareness that she could not see me as anything but disappointing—anything more would have been too scary (and too stimulating) and would have made thoughts of the past too painful.

Sarah, on the other hand, had a more abbreviated period of negative feeling about me, though hers was the more intense, with a definite paranoid flavor. In addition to imagining that I was taping the sessions with the aim of blackmailing her, she also feared, for a one-week period, that there was poison gas in the office room and during several other isolated sessions was frightened that I was trying to hypnotize her. What emerged during the course of her analysis was an erotic attachment to her mother, which played itself out in the transference neurosis, complete with perverse sexual fantasies and intense rivalry with the male patient whose hour followed hers.

The analysis of these two girls added to my appreciation of the therapeutic value of analytic abstinence with children. Let me make it clear, however, that by abstinence I do not mean withdrawal or withholding. For along with being abstinent, the child analyst needs to be available, speaking and behaving in a manner that is understandable to the child and that, as nearly as possible, conveys what the analyst intends to convey. Thus, I will tie the shoe (when asked) of a child who has not yet learned to perform this task. On the other hand, I will not offer to tie a child's shoe unsolicited, no matter how often the child trips—and will both interpret the value of "tripping" when that seems appropriate (which may include pointing out the wish to have me offer to help) and try to avoid making interpretations that are really covert suggestions. Similarly, depending on the age of the child, I often answer direct questions—my first name, my age, my dog's name, etc. because with the very young child not to do so seems strange and I can think of no explanation that would make sense at the beginning of an analysis to a child under five or six. As time goes on and the child has a sense of me, I say that I prefer to hear what the child imagines the answer to be, and though this often seems "silly," my refusal to answer becomes another aspect of the analytic situation, like the way I talk, the color of my hair, my clothing, the decor of the office, the toys, and the limits. All these things—physical and behavioral—may become recipients of transference, to be perceived as the child's internal conflicts, wishes, fantasies, and past and present experiences dictate.

With an older child who I feel can better understand, I usually make some statement, in response to questions at the beginning of the analysis, about my not answering, that my interest is, instead, to figure out what led to the question. This not infrequently leads to a "drying up" of the questions, a retaliative refusal to respond to my questions, provocative questions, or battles over why I don't answer—but all this is subject for analysis.

My office provides considerable structure, which helps me and the patient understand the meaning behind the process of our interactions. Each child has a drawer to which no one else is permitted access. Drawings, favorite toys, Lego constructions, whatever, can be kept private in the drawer, but I request that nothing be taken home during the course of treatment. If the child is insistent about taking home his drawings, we analyze it. I do not struggle with him about it or say, "It's okay." Instead, if he takes something home, his "breaking a rule," feeling of guilt, concern about my anger (and, not infrequently, his wish to stimulate it) are analyzed. If the child is worried that another patient or one of my children will go into his drawer and take his stuff, we analyze it. And if the child thinks I am mean, we analyze it. One 4-year-old child, Robert, was so frightened of his rage (which he projected onto me) that he refused to come into my office for three weeks. We had his sessions outside on the street, with Robert inside his car and me talking to him through the window. Later, when he returned to my office (after spending the hours outside repetitively telling me that the car was his and I could not get into it), we spent many months sitting in chairs across from one another, with our legs drawn up, pretending that the floor was an ocean filled with sharks, the chairs our boats, and the backs of the chairs control panels for our defense against the sharks. The sharks had one end in mind—eating us, eating our penises, getting into us—and in this displaced way we explored Robert's fantasies, both feared and wished for. The earlier experience and resolution of Robert's tremendous fear of me had increased his capacity to distinguish reality from fantasy and gave him a sense of control over his fantasies. This, in turn, made possible the full flowering of the shark fantasies and their connection with his own wishes.

Robert's difficulties (insomnia, stool retention, marked separation anxiety, temper tantrums, and rage reactions directed at his younger sister) had begun after the birth of this sister, his only sibling. Robert was the product of his father's second marriage and was much adored by this loud, large, and forceful man, who had lost contact with the children of his first marriage. Robert was terrified that he would lose his father after his sister was born, and he was jealous of his mother having the father's baby. He also wanted to have his adored mommy for himself and to get rid of the baby that his daddy had made. In essence, his fear of the consequences of both his negative and positive oedipal rivalry, of his wish to be pregnant and what that would do to him, had disrupted the course of his development. Some of his wishes and fears about his family members were conscious at the onset of the analysis and others became conscious later—but it was his fear of me, his later identification with me in the shark play, and the connection of the two in the interpretation of the transference that led to Robert's recovery.

During Robert's analysis I often wondered about the therapeutic importance of the reconstructions we made, for example, of his feeling jealous when his mother became pregnant. In general, I am uncertain about the value of reconstruction in child analysis, particularly since a child analyst's investment in the reconstruction of past events can interfere with the development of a transference neurosis in his patients. If an analyst wants verbalized content, ideas, information—and wants it from the child, not the parents— then he needs a patient who is willing not just to talk but also to "tell" things, and not just things he feels an urgency to tell but things he feels the analyst wants to hear. Such a patient needs both to understand what is expected of him and to be willing to provide that. This means that the analyst has conveyed his desire for information *and* created a relationship with the patient (albeit covertly or even unconsciously) in which the latter performs as is expected. In so doing, the analyst deviates from neutrality and abstinence (Hoffer, 1985) with respect to the direction of the analysis and the use of his power to direct it.

I also have some reservation about the value for conflict resolution of "knowing" the reconstructed distant past. The ego that reconstructs has changed markedly since the events reconstructed (Kennedy, 1971); past experience has been overlaid with other experiences which alter the impact and meaning of earlier events—as with the Wolf-Man's primal scene experience (Freud, 1918). In child analysis (but also in work with adults), genetic reconstructions often seem to be for the analyst's benefit, to achieve closure (for example, understanding all the determinants of a particular compromise formation) when closure is impossible, or to reaffirm, for the analyst, the truth of his theories.

The process of reconstruction does increase the child's appreciation of the influence of past events on current thinking, feeling, and functioning, which adds to his understanding of the phenomenon of transference (Furman, 1971). Reconstructions can also lead to reorganization of memories with a beneficial change in both object and self representations. In addition, when a reconstruction leads to the recovery of the associated affect, in particular, affect associated with a recent experience (such as five minutes earlier during the analytic hour), it can significantly enhance a child's ability to self-observe. Useful are the reconstructions/constructions/remembering of immediate past events, as, for example, when a child has a specific thought or feeling (like Robert's fear of me) during the course of analysis and the determinants, in terms of unconscious fantasies or affects (like Robert's wish to cut open my stomach), are constructed from the conscious associations (the shark's wish to eat my insides). In the work with Robert, we eventually articulated his early wish to cut the baby out of his mother and eat it—thus destroying it, turning it into stool, and having this gift from the father for himself. However, I believe it was his experiencing how his wishes in the transference and the associated aggression turned to fear of me, not the knowledge of past fantasies, that was most therapeutic for Robert.

The perception of the analyst as a benevolent object may lead, through identification and/or a wish to please him, to development in many areas, including a cognitive precocity that can enhance intellectual understanding. It may even help the child tolerate his internal conflicts and modify his behavioral and affective response to these conflicts. However, the wish to please neither resolves conflicts nor increases ego autonomy. Nonetheless, the "basic transference" continues to be cited as a useful, if not essential, ingredient of child analysis (Ritvo, 1978, p. 300), with the child turning to the analyst for help as toward a benevolent parental figure. Certainly a perception of the analyst as exclusively aggressive, destructive, or overstimulating will interfere with any analysis, particularly that of a child with immature observing ego functions. But the opposite is also true; a perception of the analyst as exclusively benevolent can contaminate the transference template and dilute the mutative force of anxiety-producing impulses.

Those analysts who believe in the importance of experiencing during the analytic process tend to emphasize the development of as full an analytic transference as possible; shared cognitive understanding seems to be the goal of those who stress the need for a therapeutic alliance strongly rooted in a positive relationship. I sense that without the first (experiential) phase of Strachey's (1934) mutative interpretation, the therapeutic value of the second (interpretive) phase lies largely in strengthening defenses for more adaptive functioning—which, of course, can enhance development. In contrast, the experience of the transference, with an elucidation of defensive behavior and the inadequate and inappropriate compromise formations that wish and fear engender, can lead to therapeutic change even without complete genetic understanding.

When Geleerd (1967, p. 10) speaks of the development, after a period of time in analysis, of verbal ability and self-observation that is far beyond the child's maturation, I feel concern lest the precocious ego development reflects a tendency to intellectualization based on a partial identification with the analyst. Such intellectualization either diminishes the force of the internal conflicts so they can be more successfully repressed or shifts the economic balance by providing more successful defenses (augmented by the auxiliary ego strength of the analyst) without really resolving the conflict. As Abrams (1980) observed, "cognitive growth is stimulated in the analysis of children. . . . Generally, this serves the treatment process, but it may backfire and prove disruptive if a proper balance is not maintained between the freeing of the unconscious, on the one hand, and the stimulation of cognition, on the other . . . there may be a fixing of earlier organizational modes if the therapist fosters submission to an omnipotent id-wisdom; or there may be a further encapsulation of the entrapped unconscious if analysis builds a wall composed of a precocious cognitive system" (p. 306).

A relationship with a benevolent object can have enormous therapeutic power. Analysis is not the only form of child psychotherapy; criteria of analyzability and whether one can or should analyze children with major ego deviations remain important issues for child analysts. I am reminded of Susan, a five-year-old girl I saw in psychotherapy four times a week for two years. Her mother had been severely depressed after Susan's birth, and aside from times of feeding and diaper changes, she had left Susan alone in her crib for the first six months. (The mother was already on lithium when I began treating Susan, and although no longer clinically depressed, she was always anxious and emotionally distant.) Susan's two older siblings occasionally played with her, but basically she had no consistent human contact during early infancy. When I first saw Susan, she had no language. The most striking thing about her, aside from her markedly retarded cognitive development, was the juxtaposition of a warm, seemingly responsive smile and complete unavailability.

Work with Susan was exhausting, frustrating, and ultimately exhilarating. I began treatment by imitating Susan's movements and speech as closely as possible, rolling on the floor, drawing, or bouncing a ball when she did; essentially, I tried to enter her world. With excruciating slowness she began to take notice of me and to express anger when she felt I was "doing it wrong." Perhaps the most dramatic achievement over those two years was her becoming aware of the difference between "you" and "me." Susan went on to many years of treatment with other therapists, including a long stay in a residential treatment center. She is now a young adult and functioning quite well, with a job, an apartment of her own, and a boyfriend—able to communicate not only in English but also in German.

The most successful treatment I have participated in was Susan's, but it was not analysis. I was a very specific person for Susan—an intrusive, benevolent force whose job was to convince her she got more from being with me (even though it made her very mad at times) than from not being with me (even though that meant she was sometimes very sad when I wasn't there). Her therapy clearly contributed to her development—I could see that in the two years we were together—but it was not analysis. Analysis is a quite specific treatment for individuals whose development and function are handicapped primarily by unconscious internal conflicts, not by environmental interferences or by structural deficits, except when the latter are the results of fixations secondary to retreat from conflict. Neurotic individuals also can be helped by learning new ways to deal with conflicts. However, if therapy is aimed at the resolution of conflict (with an underlying assumption that with conflict resolution, development will resume of its own accord), then, to that end, there is nothing so effective as the development of a transference neurosis within the analytic setting. And if an analyst believes that intense transference (or a transference neurosis) is essential for a successful analysis, he needs to learn what interferes with its emergence and what promotes its development.

Many of the techniques of child analysis are based on the same principles as those used in the analysis of adults. Nonetheless, there are some significant differences in how they are employed, differences dictated by (1) the maturity of the child's ego apparatus (including his cognitive skills, his reality testing, his capacity for self-observation, and his system of defenses); (2) the appearance and pressure of drive derivatives; (3) the phase of superego development; and (4) the intensity of current developmental demands. Although the use of the analyst as a new object in a current phase of development can require technical adaptations in child analysis, it should not be cited as a justification for deviations from an abstinent analytic position. The child (and adult) will use the analyst concurrently as a transference object, a "new type" of object to rework preceding phases of development, and an object to fulfill current developmental needs (Chused, 1982). But in all instances the patient's use of the analyst must be dictated by the patient's needs and perceptions—not by the analyst's preconceptions of the patient's needs. The use of the analyst should be determined by the patient's psychic reality, not by the analyst's "real" behavior.

I shall use the analysis of 11-year-old Sarah as illustration. During the course of her treatment she made many references to the deprivation she suffered at her mother's hands. She was highly critical of her mother—not only for being self-indulgent and infantile, but also for being ugly, silly, flirtatious, poorly dressed, and overly made-up. It was clear there was nothing the mother could do that was acceptable to Sarah. Yet it was only after her complaints turned on me, in the transference, that we were able to explore her hunger for her mother's attention, her rage at feeling rejected after her brother was born, as well as the tremendous competitiveness with her mother. During the course of her analysis Sarah entered adolescence. This, as a phenomenon, was fascinating to watch and hear about—in particular, the progression, first, from disgust over boys to a fear, embarrassment, and displacement of her impulses (lots of criticism of "boy-crazy" classmates); then, to a relentless pursuit of boys, a combination of counterphobic behavior and active defense against passive vulnerability; subsequently, to a feeling of terror when one young man began to pursue her; and finally, at the time of termination, to real pleasure in early sexual exploration. Throughout this struggle to establish a feminine identity, her scrutiny of me was intense. She carefully noted my dress, my makeup, my laugh—in a way that is typical of adolescent girls' scrutiny of their mothers. But interposed with this ceaseless, yet relatively objective nonmalevolent scrutiny were repeated hostile attacks, with negative, fantasy-filled observations. All was in the subtleties: her comment "That's an interesting color [pointing to a mauve skirt]; I never thought of wearing it with purple; I wonder, did you try to match your lipstick to your blouse?" had a different feel (and different determinants) than "Yuk, one of my teachers still wears bell-bottoms; that's probably from the '60s; that's when you were young, isn't it? I don't mean to say that you look funny—but quite honestly, it's hard to trust you when you look so, I don't know, weird; I wonder if you're still married or divorced; I heard that women really begin to live in the past when they can't get a man; I don't mean to make you mad, but. . . ." The first seemed an attempt to use me as a new object for identification; the second a transference perception of me as a devalued oedipal rival. At other periods of the analysis, when Sarah became able to mourn the loss of the nurturing mother, she fantasized having me be her mother. This was a hard phase of the analysis; it was difficult to distinguish what was an expression of loss from what was a regressive defense against oedipal feelings. One of the clues I used was how the transference affected her participation in the analytic process: when her words became whining and endlessly repetitive, when she misheard my comments as critical and behaved as if she were too injured to analyze, her complaints of deprivation were understood as a defensive transference resistance against the emergence of oedipal rivalry.

It was clear that many of Sarah's observations about her mother's self-preoccupation and unavailability were correct. However, Sarah needed me as an analyst, not a substitute mother: it was the resolution of conflict which enabled her to use me as a current object for identification (without my ever altering my analytic stance); and it was the resolution of conflict that allowed her to mourn not having a "warm mommy for the little Sarah" and to find two teachers at school for whom she could excel and who treated her as a favorite. That it was two teachers instead of one defended against any impulse to act out her strong erotic attachment to women. This had entered the transference at age 12 when she talked about wanting to touch and kiss me and her fear of being homosexual. Her anxiety was intense during the analysis of these wishes; but before the determinants had been fully explored, her homoerotic concerns disappeared. As she was comfortable with her relationship with these two teachers, I decided not to "push" an exploration of the unconflicted compromise (two objects) she had made in the outside world. Similar decisions are made in the analysis of adults, but usually after a longer period of working through. With children in whom development is still in flux, the analyst may wonder whether to "push" harder to create conflict over what appears to be a potentially pathological solution that might affect future development. Child analysts differ in their belief in the importance of neutrality (and other issues), and their belief affects their analytic stance. I decided it was appropriate to remain abstinent in regard to influencing the direction of the analysis and not to push Sarah to examine issues that troubled primarily me. I hoped this would allow Sarah to feel that the analysis was really hers; that she would return for further work if and when difficulty with intimacy became a problem for her.

My decision was influenced, in part, by an awareness that adolescents are frequently conflicted over assuming responsibility for their actions; they both wish for and fear external influence—and are very sensitive to it. I believe an important developmental goal in adolescence is the achievement of comfort with self-determined action (even if it is only relatively autonomous with respect to unconscious determinants). Others differ; for example, Harley (1970) recommended that masculine, phallic behavior be reinforced during the analysis of passive adolescent males.

Adaptations of technique dictated by the specific needs and developmental stage of the child are to be distinguished from modifications which can distort or even disrupt the analytic process, such as interventions aimed at changing the patient's environment or explanations given to correct the child's sexual misconceptions without first analyzing the underlying fantasies (Harley, 1986, p. 130). However, justifications for "adaptations" must not blind the analyst to any potential interference with the development and understanding of the transference.

The child's relationship with his parents cannot be ignored, and frequently it necessitates behavior in the child analyst that differs from his behavior with families of adult patients. The child's attachment to his analyst may lead to jealousy and guilt in the parents and loyalty conflicts in the child, which can distort the expression of the transference or lead parents to withdraw the child from treatment prematurely. Parental support of the analysis is essential. Thus, after an initial evaluation, even if I feel the child will need analysis, I often meet with the parents alone for several months (not seeing the child at all during this period so as not to contaminate the eventual analytic relationship) and try to alleviate their guilt (to prevent a defensive denial of the need for treatment) and help them understand what it means for a child to have internal conflicts. During this time I support their wishes to do what they can to make the child less troubled, but I try to help them understand why environmental changes are often not effective.

The experience of the analyst as available and nonjudgmental can diminish the tendency to undermine treatment that develops in some parents. In addition, even if a child is consciously antagonistic toward analysis, therapist, or parents, he is much more accepting of treatment if he believes parents and analyst are allied in supporting it. Five-year-old Annie quite proudly told me that thinking some-times gave her a headache, like her father had from work, but that her mother said I was probably trying to get her to think so I could discover things about her. With that she handed me the picture she had colored and said, "You discover this!"

To repeat: the major goal with parents is to get them to support the analysis. Once sufficient data are obtained for a complete diagnostic evaluation, there is usually little need for information from the parents concerning the child's behavior or daily life—the analytic work is enough. Although parents may need to be seen at regular intervals to ensure their continuing support, one should not yield to parental requests for advice or information in a way that could undermine the child's trust or contaminate the transference. But even when the analyst is abstinent with the parents, just the fact of their knowing each other will influence the child's productions; however, I have yet to see this create unanalyzable difficulties, even with adolescents.

The external reality of the child's relationship with his parents and the analyst's psychic response (including, but not limited to, countertransference) to this relationship can interfere with the analysis. For example, many child analysts (Geleerd, 1967, pp. 43–44, 201, 304) move their interpretative focus too rapidly to the parents, deflecting the child's attention from the transference with interventions that sound like defensive displacements or premature genetic interpretations (and which would certainly be so labeled if the patient were an adult). This tendency may be a reaction formation against unconscious competition with the parents. Parents can be rivalrous with the analyst while, at the same time, wanting him to take over. Single parents, or those who are self-preoccupied or insecure in their parenting, may want the analyst to parent. When the analyst feels drawn into that role, he may defend against it by referring back to the parents whenever strong affective responses become manifest in the transference. This deflection of affect can be disruptive to the development of a transference neurosis.

The relationship with the parents of the past—both real and fantasized versions—are "transferred" to the parents of the present; when they contribute to pathological interactions, the presence of a transference neurosis may be obscured (P. Tyson, 1978, p. 215). Once an analytic relationship is established, however, this extra-analytic transference can be recognized as such and pathological interactions, stemming from the child's behavior, can often be aborted by appropriate interpretations. Unfortunately, parental behavior may continue to be pathogenic even after a child enters analysis. Child analysts have tried a number of therapeutic interventions aimed at decreasing disturbing experiences with parents. One is parent guidance, with direct manipulation of parental behavior, concurrent with analysis of the child. Sometimes the guidance is part of a well-thought-out plan; other times it spontaneously emerges, as when I felt an irresistible urge to tell the mother of a 10-year-old girl to stop checking her daughter's body for pubic hair development. Parent guidance concurrent with a child analysis can be beneficial; however, it can also be hazardous, with the modification of the parent's behavior only temporary or with only the form of the pathogenic relationship changing.

When interactions detrimental to the child's development are fueled by both the child's and the parents' pathology, simultaneous treatment of the parent(s) by another therapist, including psychoanalysis, can prove of enormous value to the work with the child. This leaves the child's analyst free to deal with the inevitable displacements and transference split between himself and the parents within the child's analysis—intervening as indicated by the work with the child, attending both to the purpose of the split and to the way the displacement is moving (from parent to analyst or vice versa) without fearing the effect of such phenomena on the parents' support of the analysis.

Although it is helpful to be able to distinguish transference of past relationships from habitual modes of relating (Sandler et al., 1975) or displacement onto the analyst of current conflicts with the parents, such distinctions are often not clear-cut. Current conflicts with the parents may be a repetition of aspects of an earlier relationship with them, or may be precipitated by a displacement of the analytic transference or a split in the transference between the analyst and the parents. In addition, habitual modes of relating may eventually evolve into transference, as the component elements which resulted in their formation are experienced in relation to the analyst (Harley, 1971). In general, the most effective verbal interventions in these situations are those in which there is an accurate understanding of the immediate experience, in which a distinction is made, for example, between the externalization of a superego attitude and the transference repetition of the original introjections which made up the superego.

An example of a conflicted response which first began as a displacement from a current relationship with a parent but later became part of the transference neurosis comes from the analysis of Annie, the five-year-old, compliant "good" girl mentioned above, Annie came for treatment with marked separation anxiety and tremendous fear of robbers, kidnappers, and being poisoned. During an early session, she expressed some fear about touching either the split or intact geodes I had in my office. (Geodes are rocks with a rough, unattractive exterior and an exquisite crystal interior that is exposed when they are cut.) Initially, she feared that the rocks were poison and would kill her if she touched them. She spoke of her mother's injunctions not to touch things that didn't belong to her, not to take food from strangers, not to put nonedible items into her mouth. Intermittently, for many months, the geodes were the focus of her attention. Eventually, they were seen as something precious, and she feared I would hurt her if she touched, played with, or damaged them. At this time she continued to talk of her mother—moving to mother's instructions not to suck her thumb or touch herself (her genitals). Later, as she began to want to take the geodes home and to entertain fantasies of how she would get them from me, the focus was almost exclusively on me, with the geodes seen as a gift from my husband. The geodes had become, by the end of the analysis, a metaphor for my womb-baby-penis through which Annie's envy, narcissistic injury, fear of retaliation, fear, and feeling of loss of her mother's love were all explored. Although some reconstructions were made about the birth of her younger sister and the fears stimulated by her oedipal rivalries, the bulk of the work was done in the transference, with an analysis of her defensive behavior, her wishes, and her fears of my retaliation.

With Annie, as with other young children, the immaturity of ego functioning required adaptations of analytic technique. To do analysis as we know it, with a consolidation of transference manifestations around the person of the analyst, the child must have the capacity for reproducible internal self and object representations (which implies fairly intact functions of perception and memory), for symbolization and verbalization, and for repression and at least a minimum tolerance for unpleasant affect. This tolerance is often only minimal, however, and as a child's defense mechanisms tend to be more primitive and less dependable than an adult's, even interventions which address conscious material can lead to outbreaks of anxiety, aggression, or poorly modulated erotic impulses. Thus, the analyst of children *must* pay particular attention to the patient's level of arousal. In addition, with children under seven (Shapiro and Perry, 1976), for whom speaking or thinking often seems the same as doing, the analyst may need to spend considerable time addressing the very process of affects being stimulated by words, as in my telling Annie, ''When my words talk of worries, it seems like the words hurt just like the worries do. Then you don't want me to talk.'' When the child can hear that, an important step has been taken; the action of verbalizing, of interpreting, is objectified, can be talked about, and is less likely to create feelings of helplessness in the child. To counteract the sense of helplessness, the analyst can elicit the child's help with timing, saying something like, ''I'm thinking of what you just said; let me know when you want me to tell you my thoughts.'' Such a statement with an adult would be heard as condescending; with a child, being "in control" of the flow of the analyst's words, being active rather than passive, adds to his tolerance of the words. Often a child can tell me when my tact or timing is off; not in those words, of course, but as Annie did when she said, "Those words are like needles; put it in a picture first." Of course, both the content and the intent of interpreting are still subject to transference misperceptions, and these misperceptions need to be interpreted.

To my surprise, I have found that even for very young children, it is often more comfortable to talk about feelings and impulses directly in the transference than in displacement to outside objects or even toys (which can be endowed with a magical quality to retaliate). Annie, in an expression of rage stimulated by the story she was telling me about her mother's favoritism toward a younger sister, began to go on an "ant hunt" in my office using long, pointed pick-up sticks as weapons. She took pleasure in collecting the ants, torturing, and then killing them, but as she asked me if ants could talk, fear of retaliation disrupted her play. However, when she later began to blame me for not giving her powerful enough weapons, she was able to stick with her rage and to elaborate on her fantasy about the equipment I could provide my patients, if only I wanted to.

Young children do not have the capacity to abstract that is required to simultaneously experience the transference and perceive it "as if." The analytic structure with its curtailment of gratification (of both patient's and analyst's aggressive and libidinal impulses) protects the child from excessive anxiety over the consequences of his wishes and makes the expression of drive derivatives tolerable. Without analytic abstinence Annie might not have risked the full expression of her ire. Had I behaved as a benevolent object upon whom Annie had come to depend for emotional supplies (and who could withhold as well as give), this would have both distorted the transference perception *and* interfered with her comfort in "enacting the past" in the therapeutic setting.

Children and adults differ in the level of their superego and ego development; this is reflected in their differing capacity and desire to control urgent impulses and restrict discharge to verbalization. Both adult and child patients in the throes of strong affects generated by a transference neurosis find it difficult to remain within an analytic mode of exchange. With the regression in ego and superego function that accompanies the development of the transference neurosis, there is a strong tendency to "act out" or "enact" via a transference resistance. Depending on the complexity of the symbolization, these "actualizations" of the transference are often responsive to interpretation; for example, the child who reports she won't be returning because I want her to play "dirty" may be dealing with an externalization of her own drive derivatives and/or the beginning repetition in the transference of an early or fantasized seduction or primal scene experience. Whichever it is, as she struggles to find a more comfortable compromise formation for her affects, wishes, and fears, analysis with her, beginning with an exploration of her fantasies of my intent in wanting her to play "dirty," is not unlike analysis with an adult.

However, the child who throws a pillow or glass vase at the analyst, the child who tries to pinch or who repeatedly climbs into the analyst's lap or grabs at his genitalia, presents another type of problem. It matters little whether this behavior is a complex compromise formation or the primitive expression of a drive derivative via an ego that is so overwhelmed it has little ability to "force a compromise." This behavior is destructive; it destroys the analyst's and the patient's comfort with their interaction, and it makes clear that at least one member of the dyad is in no position to analyze. In addition, the very experience of being "out of control" is exciting, painful, and potentially shameful and is not conducive to the child's future participation in the analytic work.

Behavioral limits, particularly limits to the physical contact between analyst and child, are extremely important in child analysis, for immature ego functions are often weakened by the regression induced by transference. When a child wants to play doctor with me as the patient, I offer a doll as a substitute—and analyze rather than gratify or evade the issue when the doll substitution is unacceptable. Analysts often feel some awkwardness in speaking directly about the genital arousal stimulated in their patients by the analysis. This is a particularly difficult task with a child, as the initial clarification of behavior may be heard as a seduction, increasing the press of the impulse, the associated anxiety, and the push to action. Hence, there is sometimes a tendency to leave transferential sexual material unanalyzed. Although hugs or blows are rarely useful, an avoidance of physical gratification *without commentary* is liable to be received by the child as a condemnatory prohibition and may lead to a maladaptive identification. Verbalization of thwarted impulses is extraordinarily important in child analysis for both the analysis of conflicts and to protect the ongoing superego development of the child.

For example, when Annie wanted to measure me, my initial response was simply to decline. It was only when she retreated to a distant point in the room that I became aware of how hurtful my refusal without clarification had been. Overcoming my own resistance, I said I understood that she had wanted to touch me and that she had heard my "no" as saying it was wrong to want that. We needed to talk about it, because I thought her "wants" were part of her "worries." This "speech," to some extent, was heard within the transference as a challenge and led to an increase in action as well as to repeated questions about "What will you do if I do something you don't want me to do?" However, the questions and behavior led to further analysis of her conflict over impulses, analysis that would have been aborted if the erotic impulses of the transference had not been addressed directly.

Just as internal controls or the wish for controls are less well developed in the child than in the adult (even the obsessional child's rigid superego is usually more brittle than an adult's), so drive derivatives tend to be more primitive, less sublimated or well modulated in their expression, and more urgent in their push for gratification. In addition, the child has fewer resources available to deal with the frustration, feeling of rejection, and narcissistic injury that follows nongratification. This has been used as an argument for being more gratifying to the child, as if the strength of his demands or the pain of frustration would be lessened by partial or substitute gratification. Actually, I have often found the opposite to be true: partial gratification of most wishes just intensifies the push for full gratification. The child feels more comfortable knowing when and which impulses will not be gratified. Of course, limits should not be so confining that the analysis is unremittingly frustrating. Nonetheless, in child as in adult psychoanalysis, frustration is the key to understanding the unconscious wishes and fantasies (and corresponding dangers) that underlie pathology. As with other aspects of the analytic structure, the limits set by a child analyst should take into account the amount of frustration the child can tolerate, the importance of abstinence and neutrality for the emergence of the transference, and the analyst's own psychic requirements for the maintenance of an analyzing stance.

Depending on the developmental level of the child, a degree of responsiveness to requests (such as providing tissues, playing games, helping with constructions) is appropriate in child analysis. However, these "gratifications" should be part of the regular procedure of the analysis of that particular child and not increase, or suddenly become available, at times of stress or increased anxiety. As Sandler et al. (1980) pointed out, "therapists who express fear of adversely affecting the transference really mean that they are afraid of disturbing the positive transference, and their fears of refusing certain gratifications may be rationalizations they use in order to avoid the child's hostile feelings. This is a countertransference problem" (p. 197).

Abstinence neither means nor leads to the absence of all gratification; it does require the frustration of escalating demands for transference gratification. However, a child can leave an office filled with rage at the analyst, even convinced, on one level, of the analyst's malevolent intent, and return the next day and the next to continue the work of analysis.

Children do not like being overwhelmed by their impulses any more than adults do; they are simply more vulnerable to being overwhelmed because of the immaturity of their ego functions. In addition, they have less ego resources to aid in recovery of their equilibrium. When abstinence is perceived as deprivation, it can be analyzed within the transference; exciting gratification confuses the issue and renders the analyzing equipment inoperative. To repeat: consistent limits are more conducive to establishing an analytic situation than partial gratification. The only gratification that *must* be available to the child is the analyst's interest and his continual attempt to understand. Of course, patients can perceive gratification even from potentially nongratifying situations. An example is Robert, who said to me after a very difficult (for both of us) analysis in which, from his perspective, I had been quite withholding, "I know you cared because you didn't have to prove it." In spite of my abstinence, Robert had perceived me as nurturing and, like Phyllis Tyson's (1978) patient Colin, first openly demonstrated his positive oedipal longings with me as the object.

This brings me to the issue of the analyst's role as new object during an ongoing phase of development. Although development is continual in both child and adult, the intensity of the developmental thrust and the associated process of identification with important objects are much greater in the child than the adult. Consequently, the child patient makes more frequent use of the analyst as a "new object." The question is not whether this use is "analysis" but what the analyst's active participation in ongoing development should be.

Often when a child comes for analysis, he is unable to use any object in his world for successful navigation of developmental pathways; it is analysis, with the exposure and resolution of instinctual conflicts within the transference, that permits object relations to be more tolerable and development to resume.

Phyllis Tyson (1978) has suggested that when a child is "trying to cope with the upsurging drives accompanying a new developmental phase" (p. 229), the energy required for the elaboration of a transference neurosis is unlikely to be available. I disagree with this. When an analysand begins to take a new developmental step utilizing the analyst as a "real" object, his perception of the analyst will be distorted by his current needs as well as by his past conflicts—the analyst is no more "real" in this mixed utilization than he would be in the expression of transference alone. In essence, transference reactions and a transference neurosis will continue to exist even during a period of active development. Their manifestations may be different as the balance of drives and defenses changes and the relative contribution of impulses from different libidinal zones shifts. Yet the object relationship in which the drives are expressed will continue to be distorted as before—reflecting pathological interactions of the past, longed-for idealized objects of the past and present, and perceptions of the original objects that are distorted by projection of the child's own libidinal and aggressive impulses and fantasies.

A child frequently resumes or reworks (Chused, 1982) development around his relationship with the analyst. But the analyst does not need to depart from a neutral, abstinent analytic position for this to occur—the child will make of the analyst what he needs him to be. Special kindness or reassurance reflects the "benevolent object fallacy," so called because what is intended as kindness may be understood as condescending, what was meant to be reassuring experienced as controlling or intrusive. It is much better for the analytic process, and for the development that proceeds from it, if the child's perceptions of the analyst are (relatively) autonomous, both in the transference and in the transformations of transference which constitute the analyst as "new object." This does not require new technique, only a tolerance for being a passive participant rather than the active initiator of the analytic process—a tolerance for being neutral as to how the child uses analysis. Child analysis offers multiple therapeutic opportunities (A. Freud, 1965); optimally, a child in treatment will make use of those elements he needs.

When the child uses the analyst as both transference object and new object, perceptions which are not caught up in conflict need not be subject to interpretation even though they may reflect a distortion of reality (such as Robert's perception of me as nurturing). This fits in with Ritvo's point (Panel, 1980) that the analyst need work only on the identifications that are used defensively or for resistance—not the identifications and object relations that are part of the silent process of development of psychic structure and growth. On the other hand, behavior of the analyst which is misperceived within a transference framework (or just misunderstood because of lack of experience) and is liable to be used for maladaptive identifications in the development of superego and ego structure (such as my declining to be measured by Annie) needs to be addressed and interpreted.

Child analytic training does not provide a theoretical basis for responding to ongoing developmental demands with the same degree of clarity that it does for the demands dictated by unconscious conflicts. When a five-year-old repeatedly trips over untied shoes, one can wonder with him about his tendency to fall and hurt himself without taking the obvious precautions. But when a five-year-old asks you to tie his shoes so he won't trip, to interpret that his failure to tie them himself was either self-destructive or indicative of a regression to a dependent position is ridiculous if the child has not yet learned to tie. One may wonder with him why he can't tie; a missing skill may represent a neurotically determined inhibition or developmental interference, as well as reflect a constitutional delay in development. The analyst may also tie the shoe if a refusal to do so would be a senseless withholding to the child, but having done so, the analyst must monitor himself carefully for a counter-transference reaction to what the child does with the tied shoe. Does it stay tied, or does it get undone as a way to damage what the analyst (and whom he represents in the transference) has to offer? This is where the work of the analysis lies; this is the point where the transference, and later the transference neurosis, manifests itself; and this is where child psychoanalysis often fails to become analysis and remains psychotherapy.

There is another characteristic of the analytic process with children that makes work with the transference neurosis difficult. Children often do not have the interest or the psychic structure that is required for a lengthy working through. Once a conflictual issue has been resolved sufficiently so that a new piece of behavior is possible (for example, learning to read), a symptom is no longer obligatory (like a hand-washing ritual or psychogenic limp); or anxiety is diminished enough for an inhibition to be overcome (such as social isolation); action takes over, the economic balance shifts, and the conflict disappears. The conflict may reappear later in a new context but often not with the multiple repetitions that seem to be required to make transference interpretations believable to adult patients. It is not just a lack of interest or ability that keeps the child from working through. In my experience, children seem to require less repetition of conflictual situations within the transference in order to have insight result in change, perhaps because their psychic structure is less fixed and more flexible.

Some of the child analysts who question whether a child is capable of repeating with the analyst, through restricted reenactment, enough of his conflictual past experience to benefit from an analysis of transference similar to that in adult analyses, continue to believe that the child has less tendency or need to make transferences to the analyst because his primary love objects are available in his daily life for instinctual drive gratification (reported by Ritvo, 1978). However, there is abundant clinical material (Harley, 1971; P. Tyson, 1978) which demonstrates that independence from the original objects is not a determining factor in the development of a transference neurosis in children; the degree to which processes of internalization have taken place is far more important. In addition, as with adults, it is not the need or wish for gratifying objects that brings children to analysis but, rather, the unconscious conflicts over gratification, conflicts rooted not in current relationships but derived from past experiences and their incorporation into psychic structure. Potentially gratifying objects are frequently available in our patients' lives; the problem is a patient's inability to be gratified.

Another factor contributing to a disbelief in transference neurosis in children, the educational background of many early child analysts, was alluded to earlier. Educators had observed that children learned best in a positive teacher–student relationship. The combination of wishes to please and to emulate a teacher leads students to work harder and be more intellectually productive. And pediatricians were aware that a positive, nurturing mother–infant relationship was essential for optimal development of the young child. Their combined knowledge, together with the observations that, in general, a child's frustration tolerance is small and his negative responses intense, led the early child analysts to assume that a positive relationship with some degree of "real" gratification (emotional or material) was essential for the child to be an active participant in the analysis. As Kramer and Settlage (1962) stated:

> The entire technique [of child analysis] presupposes the willingness and ability of the child to communicate with the analyst verbally and symbolically, giving material which lends itself to verbal interpretations, which in turn can be understood and accepted by the child [p. 515]. . . . It is necessary that the child develop a good relationship with the analyst, because he can bear the tension associated with analysis only if he likes the analyst . . . negative feelings toward the analyst, regardless of whether they are caused by events in treatment or are manifestations of transference or resistance, are not well tolerated by the child. They usually are dealt with immediately in order to keep them from becoming a wedge between child and analyst.

On the other hand, positive feelings are encouraged to grow gradually [p. 524]. . . . Strong negative transference for any length of time does not augur well for child analysis [p. 527].

Harley (1986) sums it up: "We had felt it indispensable to maintain only a positive transference" [pp. 133f]. In this way, I believe, analysts prevented transference neuroses from developing in their child patients.

Child analysts who have had no adult analytic experience (true of many trained in England) seem to have an idealized or distorted conception of the analytic process with adults. In articles contrasting child and adult analysis (A. Freud, 1965) the adult is often presented as an active, cooperative participant in the process. I believe a more accurate description of adult analysis can be found in Bird's (1972) discussion of transference resistance: how, in the heat of the transference, the patient expresses his wish to destroy the analyst by attempting to destroy the analytic process. At this point in the analysis, regardless of the patient's original motivation, the last thing he wants is for the analysis to work. No matter how good the therapeutic alliance seemed, it has disappeared under the force of transference resistance. As Freud (1912) observed, "Over and over again, when we come near to a pathogenic complex, the portion of that complex which is capable of transference is first pushed forward into consciousness and defended with the greatest obstinacy" (p. 104).

Without intense transference resistance, reflective of a consuming transference neurosis, the analysis may remain a didactic exercise, a comforting experience—which may be therapeutic but isn't analytic. This, unfortunately, is what child analysis often becomes. It is hard to resist trying to calm an enraged or frightened child. "Poor Susie, you're so unhappy; I have all these toys and you feel you have nothing" said in response to Susie's provocative "Shut up! . . . Pretend I'm all chained up and you're beating me" (R. L. Tyson and P. Tyson, 1986, p. 36) may be accurate, but it fails to help the child understand the connection between her manifest behavior and its determinants. In addition, it presents the analyst as omnipotently knowing what the child is feeling. Even when an analyst is trying to prevent the overwhelming of an immature ego, it is counterproductive (and potentially infuriating) for a child to be told what he is thinking or feeling—it strips him of autonomy and deprives him of the opportunity to learn both to observe himself and to observe his effect on others.

Some of my observations on the development of a transference neurosis in children have also been made by others: Selma Fraiberg (1967) suggested one could see a transference neurosis in children if the analysis was conducted along the lines of the adult model

> conceding only to the use of play, free movement, and the substitution of another therapeutic contract for the analytic rule [p. 101]. . . . Increased appreciation of transference by child analysts . . . may lead to changes in technique toward minimizing supportive measures and encouraging autonomy. The very change in technique may create an atmosphere which facilitates the development of transference mani-festations. The result will be a decrease in the tendency to manipulate the transference and an opportunity to encourage the full develop-ment of the transference [pp. 102f].

On the other hand, Anna Freud, in one of her last contributions, indicated that she felt it was often appropriate to provide a child with sweets, a toy kit, or Christmas or birthday presents (Sandler et al., 1980, p. 194).

Melanie Klein, early in her work, recognized the child's capacity for transference and the development of a transference neurosis. However, the tendency of many Kleinian analysts to make early interpretations about the unconscious determinants of behavior, interpretations that seem to bypass defenses and create great anxiety in the child, may have kept other child analysts from appreciating the value of Klein's contributions and led to a discrediting of her idea that children do have the potential to develop a transference neurosis. Kleinians often seem to interpret as if the child speaks and behaves in universal symbols; his individual history and level of ego development appear to have little influence on their interventions. This, plus a seeming lack of sensitivity to the importance of the child's affective arousal remaining within tolerable limits (some Kleinian interventions sound almost like verbal rape), has led many non-Kleinian analysts in the United States to disregard the work and ideas of Melanie Klein. Although I disagree with her timetable of libidinal development and her understanding of early ego function-ing, I am impressed by her realization that the pedagogical and benevolent position advocated by Hug-Hellmuth and initially by Anna Freud interfered with the development of a transference neurosis and the ultimate therapeutic benefits of analysis (Klein, 1927).

All of the above factors contribute to the failure of child analysts to see the development of a transference neurosis in their own work with children. But also contributing is their response to the child's behavior, to his frequent progressive and regressive shifts in ego functioning, and to his rapid move to action when stressed. It is much easier for an analyst to maintain an analytic stance behind a couch than when face to face with a child. This more direct interaction continually taxes the child analyst's capacity to be neutral and abstinent.

Deviations from abstinence and neutrality occur in all analyses. Every analyst has certain preconceived notions of what is therapeutically effective; each tries to create an atmosphere in which what he believes will work has a chance to do so. An analyst who believes that the regressive transferences (most fully developed in the transference neurosis) are the major therapeutic tools of child, adolescent, and adult psychoanalysis establishes a structure in which thinking and talking are encouraged by example and, perhaps, initial education but then accepts the "actualizations" (Boesky, 1982) of the transference that inevitably occur and, where appropriate, analyzes them. On the other hand, the analyst who believes that for treatment to be effective the patient needs to be a willing, contributing participant in the attempt to understand must make a continuing effort to maintain a therapeutic alliance.

The therapeutic alliance, dependent as it is on the "basic transference," can function as a resistance (Greenacre, 1968; Novick, 1970; Brenner, 1979; Stein, 1981); when it contains an unanalyzed desire to please or is actively supported by the analyst's behavior, it may obscure the transference. Even more than with an adult, this is a danger during the treatment of a child, who, being genuinely dependent on adults, is less likely to question the roles of kind doctor and good patient. For the child, who is in the process of developing autonomous functioning with respect to both the drives and the external world, conflicts over autonomy and control, expressed through rebellion and compliance, are part of what led to a need for analysis in the first place. To the extent that the analyst contributes to the perpetuation of compliance in his patient, the compliance (or a rebellious reaction against it) is unavailable for analysis.

The "teasing out" of when and what to interpret with a child (Blos, 1979) is a difficult process—it often requires the analyst to be a silent participant in a drama which can make him quite uncomfortable. The most difficult part of child analysis is being this silent participant, eventually interpreting misperceptions yet remaining abstinent long enough for them to be fully understood by both analyst and child. When I err with a child, it is on the side of talking too much, too soon. The "real" dependency needs of all children (but particularly those children who have suffered emotional deprivation), their potential for growth, their tremendous vulnerability to external forces, and the wish to have them grow successfully with minimum suffering are all powerfully seductive forces which lead to countertransference interferences with the development of a transference neurosis.

There will be many crises throughout development for both the child and the adult. In the process of growth many wishes, fantasies, and ideals must be given up, and even children must mourn. Analysis can assist with the mourning process by making it a shared experience. But only through the transference neurosis can we learn *what* is being mourned.

In summary, there is a historical precedent for the child analyst to behave primarily as a benevolent object. Unfortunately, too much benevolence can interfere with the development of a transference neurosis. Psychoanalysis, as a therapy based on a theory of conflict-determined psychopathology, relies on the emergence of derivatives of conflict within the transference for its efficacy. When analysts begin to practice the same abstinence and neutrality with children as with adults, I believe they will see much more intense transference and full-fledged transference neuroses, have more opportunity to make experience-based interpretations, and be able to keep hypothetical genetic reconstructions to a minimum. The child patient differs from the adult—this demands changes in technique. But the analytic stance with both should be the same.

References

Abrams, S. (1980), Therapeutic action and ways of knowing. *J. Amer. Psychoanal. Assn.*, 28:291–308.

Bird, B. (1972), Notes on transference. *J. Amer. Psychoanal. Assn.*, 20:267–301.

Blos, P. (1979), Gender and its relationship to transference and countertransference in the analysis of the preoedipal and oedipal child. Panel discussion of The Association for Child Psychoanalysis (unpublished).

Boesky, D. (1982), Acting out. *Internat. J. Psycho-Anal.*, 63:39–55.

Bornstein, B. (1949), The analysis of a phobic child. *The Psychoanalytic Study of the Child*, 3/4:181–226. New York: International Universities Press.

Brenner, C. (1979), Working alliance, therapeutic alliance, and transference. *J. Amer. Psychoanal. Assn.*, 27:137–157.

Burlingham, D. (1935), Child analysis and the mother. *Psychoanal. Quart.*, 4:69–92.

Chused, J. (1982), The role of analytic neutrality in the use of the child analyst as a new object. *J. Amer. Psychoanal. Assn.*, 30:3–28.

Ferenczi, S. (1913), A little chanticleer. In: *Sex and Psychoanalysis*. New York: Basic Books, 1950, pp. 240–252.

Fraiberg, S. (1966), Further considerations of the role of transference in latency. *The*

Psychoanalytic Study of the Child, 21:213-236. New York: International Universities Press.

———— (1967), Repression and repetition in child analysis. *Bull. Phila. Assn. Psychoanal.,* 17:99-106.

Freud, A. (1927), Four lectures on child analysis. *The Writings of Anna Freud,* 1:3-69. New York: International Universities Press.

———— (1965), Normality and pathology in childhood. *The Writings of Anna Freud,* 6. New York: International Universities Press.

Freud, S. (1909), Analysis of a phobia in a five-year-old boy. *Standard Edition,* 10:5-149. London: Hogarth Press, 1955.

———— (1912), The dynamics of transference. *Standard Edition,* 12:99-108. London: Hogarth Press, 1958.

———— (1918), From the history of an infantile neurosis. *Standard Edition,* 17:3-122. London: Hogarth Press, 1955.

Furman, E. (1971), Some thoughts on reconstruction in child analysis. *The Psychoanalytic Study of the Child,* 26:372-385. New Haven, CT: Yale University Press.

Geleerd, E. R., ed. (1967), *The Child Analyst at Work.* New York: International Universities Press.

Greenacre, P. (1968), The psychoanalytic process, transference, and acting out. *Internat. J. Psycho-Anal.,* 49:211-228.

Harley, M. (1967), Fragments from the analysis of a dog phobia in a latency child. *Bull. Phila. Assn. Child Psychoanal.,* 17:127-129.

———— (1970), On some problems of technique in the analysis of early adolescents. *The Psychoanalytic Study of the Child,* 25:99-121. New York: International Universities Press.

———— (1971), The current status of transference neurosis in children. *J. Amer. Psychoanal. Assn.,* 19:26-40.

———— (1986), Child analysis, 1947-1984. *Psychoanal. Study Child,* 41:129-153.

Hoffer, A. (1985), Toward a definition of psychoanalytic neutrality. *J. Amer. Psychoanal. Assn.,* 33:771-795.

Hug-Hellmuth, H. (1921), On the technique of child-analysis. *Internat. J. Psycho-Anal.,* 2:287-305.

———— (1924), *New Paths to the Understanding of Youth.* Leipzig-Wien: Franz Deuticke.

Kennedy, H. (1971), Problems in reconstruction in child analysis. *The Psychoanalytic Study of the Child,* 26:386-402. New Haven, CT: Yale University Press.

Klein, M. (1927), Symposium on child analysis. *Internat. J. Psycho-Anal.,* 8:339-370 (and papers by J. Riviere, M. N. Searl, E. F. Sharpe, E. Glover, and E. Jones, pp. 370-391).

Kramer, S. & Settlage, C. F. (1962), On the concepts and technique of child analysis. *J. Amer. Acad. Child Psychiat.,* 1:509-535.

Kut, S. (1953), The changing pattern of transference in the analysis of an eleven-year-old girl. *The Psychoanalytic Study of the Child,* 8:355-378. New York: International Universities Press.

Novick, J. (1970), Vicissitudes of the working alliance in the analysis of a latency girl. *The Psychoanalytic Study of the Child,* 25:231-256. New York: International Universities Press.

Panel (1966), Problems of transference in child analysis, H. Van Dam, reporter. *J. Amer. Psychoanal. Assn.,* 14:528-537.

———— (1980), Conceptualizing the nature of the therapeutic action of child analysis, L. Shabot, reporter. *J. Amer. Psychoanal. Assn.,* 28:161-179.

———— (1983), Reanalysis of child analytic patients, A. L. Rosenbaum, reporter. *J.*

Amer. Psychoanal. Assn., 31:677–688.

Ritvo, S. (1978), The psychoanalytic process in childhood. *The Psychoanalytic Study of the Child,* 33:295–305. New Haven, CT: Yale University Press.

Sandler, J., Kennedy, H. & Tyson, R. L. (1975), Discussions on transference. *The Psychoanalytic Study of the Child,* 30:409–441. New Haven, CT: Yale University Press.

————— ————— ————— (1980), *The Technique of Child Analysis.* Cambridge: Harvard University Press.

Shapiro, T. & Perry, R. (1976), Latency revisited. *The Psychoanalytic Study of the Child,* 31:79–105. New Haven, CT: Yale University Press.

Stein, M. H. (1981), The unobjectionable part of the transference. *J. Amer. Psychoanal. Assn.,* 29:869–892.

Strachey, J. (1934), The nature of therapeutic action. *Internat. J. Psycho-Anal.,* 15:127–159.

Tyson, P. (1978), Transference and developmental issues in the analysis of a prelatency child. *The Psychoanalytic Study of the Child,* 33:213–235. New Haven, CT: Yale University Press.

Tyson, R. L. & Tyson, P. (1986), The concept of transference in child psychoanalysis. *J. Amer. Acad. Child Psychiat.,* 25:30–39.

12

Vicissitudes of Termination: Transferences and Countertransferences

Samuel Weiss

Interferences to the termination process may stem from one or several of the participants in the analytic process, namely, the child patient, the parents and/or the analyst. These interferences usually take the form of an action based on unconscious transference and countertransference reactions. This chapter addresses these issues and raises some philosophical questions about termination and its role in child analysis.

What Is Psychoanalytic Termination?

In formulating her four stages of the separation–individuation process, Mahler (1979) originally called the fourth stage "libidinal object constancy." She later changed that to "on the way to libidinal object constancy," recognizing that this was a process that would never be entirely completed. Bowlby (1969) departed from traditional Freudian thinking in suggesting that the need for attachment was at the level of an instinct. The ubiquitousness of alumni organizations in every field of endeavor indicates the great difficulty we have in letting go, in making separations, in fully individuating. So much of the emphasis in our lives is on establishing connections and maintaining those connections.

Considering the importance to us of our relationships, termination of an analysis would seem to go against what might be a basic psychobiological tendency. What is psychoanalytic termination? Is it a remarkable myth that we have preserved for so many years in order to support a theory, thus helping us maintain our own relationship with our analytic forebears? Freud (1937) in "Analysis terminable and interminable," addressed the question of whether one could ever completely resolve conflict. He viewed the setting of a termination date by the analyst as a way of dealing with the patient's resistances to further analysis but failed to address termination itself as a process of separation. Ferenczi, who was often quoted by Freud, believed that analysis was not, after all, an endless process but that a successful termination depended a great deal on the skill of the analyst in resolving issues of ending.

In clinical analysis, it seems to me, one of the major tasks is to reconnect the past with the present, and the unconscious with the conscious–preconscious. It has been said that in remembering the past (undoing repression) we can finally allow the past to be "forgotten"—that is, so that it no longer intrudes into the present. In other words, according to this formulation, it is possible, once the reconnections have been made, to separate from our infantile past, from our infantile imagos. Loewald (1970), on the other hand, stated that analysis provides the analysand with an opportunity for new solutions but eliminates neither· the old problems nor the old solutions; rather, analysis makes possible a reordering of priorities. Loewald (1978) went on to speculate that we would be left with frozen egos if, in fact, we could abandon our infantile past.

I think there may be a parallel to these opposing theoretical views on the function of analysis—that is, does analysis enable the patient to give up ("forget") difficult aspects of his infantile past, or does it permit him to find new solutions to the old difficulties?—in the concept of the transitional object and its evolution throughout the individual's development. Winnicott (1953) wrote that the transitional object was abandoned when it was no longer needed. Tolpin (1971), on the other hand, stated that it was not abandoned but internalized. My view is that the transitional object is neither abandoned nor totally internalized but remains external, undergoing transformation so that it continues to be socially acceptable to both the individual and those around him. The thumb and the blanket are given up, perhaps, but they are replaced by, for example, the lollipop, the ice cream cone, and—later—the cigarette, the pipe, the softness of a woman's skin or a fur coat. There are endless possibilities for transitional object transformations. The analyst himself, at some level of the analytic experience, may very well assume the role of a transitional object—an object that may not be given up with termination. It may, instead, undergo transformation and take the form of memories of the analyst that are resurrected at certain critical points in a former patient's life—memories of the analyst's style of talking or of the way he laughs or walks. Most of us do not accept identification with the analyst as an ideal solution to the analytic ending, yet we find it acceptable that the patient take on the analyst's analytic mode of thinking, presumably for the purpose of continuing a self-analysis. But can a cognitive self-analysis take place without identification, without the shadowy presence of the figure of the analyst? And is this self-analysis in the service of insight and ego expansion, or is it an attempt to be soothed by memories of the analyst, its function akin to that of the transitional object of infancy?

We all confront issues of bipolarity throughout life: the bipolarity of our sexuality, of affects, of impulse–defense constellations, of the propulsion forward towards growth and the pull backwards towards regression, of the seeking of sameness and the seeking of novelty. Holding on and letting go, staying connected and disconnecting, may also be viewed as examples of bipolarity and can be used to understand something about separations and endings. The ubiquity of bipolarity suggests that the analytic concept of termination is not at all as final a process as our clinical position would seem to suggest.

With young patients, some analysts have traditionally been less concerned with transference resolution in the process of termination. We often state that the aim of child analysis is to restore the child to the developmental track through the resolution of neurotic conflict or to assist the development of the appropriate mental structure. Anna Freud (1926) felt at first that transference neurosis in children was not possible because children are still living with the original objects. In recent years we have come to understand that there is an important difference between the infant's original perception of the object and that same object as perceived by the child of today. Some of us can even conceive of a child developing a transference neurosis to his own parent: that is, the parent of today is perceived, even with full intensity, as the parent of yesterday. In addition, it has always been accepted by child analysts that the child, because of his incomplete development, frequently seeks new objects and that the analyst, in addition to being a target of transferences, is also a new real object in the child's life. Thus, the termination of the child's analysis is, theoretically, not only a separation from the infantile imagos but also a separation from the analyst as a real person. The loss of the infantile imago is a

metaphor; neither the child nor the adult patient ever fully relin-
quishes his infantile position. He modifies his infantile attachments
and, to some extent, comes to terms with them, but the attachments
remain, even though the intensity diminishes. Not so with the
analyst as a real object. Analytic termination entails a genuine loss,
to be dealt with as genuine losses are—by mourning work (or some
equivalent) or by denial, each with its own consequences. Termination involves a real loss, not a metaphoric one. Wolfenstein (1966)
and, more recently, Altschul and associates (1988) have addressed
the many questions surrounding a child's capacity to deal with
object loss.

How Do We Terminate a Child's Treatment?

Child analysis has never clearly defined for itself what is involved in
termination. What we do in the clinical realm often reflects our
ambivalence or our dual identity—as followers of psychoanalysis,
with its theoretical positions on the origin and treatment of neuroses, on the one hand and as surrogate parents, teachers, developmentalists, and child-care specialists on the other. For example, we
may end the treatment with the child but continue an association
with the parent. Or, to be sure the child stays on the appropriate
developmental track, we avoid saying good-bye and plan a follow-
up to see the child or the parents six months or so after treatment
ends. There are even child analysts who feel that termination in
child analysis is a contaminant from adult analysis and has no place
in our armamentarium. These analysts do not hesitate to see child
and/or parent after treatment ends and rationalize this on the basis of
the fact that "the child's development is incomplete." These are
also analysts who often do not hesitate to offer advice to child and/or
parent about current and future courses of action. This approach
accepts the role of the analyst as the authority–educator and parent
surrogate to both child *and* parents and encourages a nonseparated
state for the former patient. Termination in this view is *stopping*; it
is not an *ending*. And in this approach the analyst may not hesitate
to decide unilaterally on the criteria and timing of the stopping.

  Child analysts who are more likely to follow the model of adult
analysis view termination, once the child's development appears to
be on track, as more or less final. Their aim is to achieve some sense
of autonomy for the child. This approach usually does not preclude
the parents' getting in touch with the analyst at some future date, but
the initiative is the parent's (or the child's), not the analyst's. These

analysts are also much more inclined to let the child make the decision about termination, hopefully within a framework of analyzing the resistances to remaining in or leaving treatment.

The first termination model, which supports an ending of treatment but not an actual ending of the relationship, poses no overt problems for child or parent since they continue to have access to the analyst. But doesn't this approach encourage a regressed state? Doesn't the analyst continue to exist as the surrogate parent object representation? And doesn't it preclude a resolution of transferences—those of the child and of the parents?

The second termination model, on the other hand, provides the young patient with an opportunity to deal with his own regression. During the course of the termination phase, the child has an opportunity to work over, if not work through, many of the infantile transference issues. There may be an initiation of a mourning process in an attempt to separate from the infantile imagos and the infantile wish constellations as well as, of course, from the analyst as a new real object in the child's life. The failure of this process can lead to a defensive identification with the analyst.

The parent, however, has no such opportunity to work through any of his transferences or aspects of his real relationship with the child's analyst. This means that the parent must do his own terminating, perhaps traumatically, or seek some way to continue the relationship, either openly or covertly.

The Criteria for Termination: Who Decides?

The increasing emphasis on a developmental point of view by child analysts is having an impact on psychoanalysis generally and has been extended to viewing development as ongoing throughout the life cycle. This view necessarily involves biases about what is normal development and what aspects of development we are looking at. It is within the framework of these biases, which are continually undergoing change as a result of research by developmentalists, that we define phase-appropriate development and select criteria for termination. Paulina Kernberg, in chapter 15, provides an extensive discussion of the criteria for child analytic termination.

The wish to terminate an analysis may originate with the child, the parent, or the analyst. The child's wish to terminate an analysis is frequently both a thrust toward further maturation and development and a resistance to further analysis. Most important, the wish to stop may often be the wish to *avoid terminating*. That is, stopping, without the analytic working through, can preserve the old attachments, the old configuration, the infantile fantasies.

It is here that we encounter some of the countertransference issues. My colleagues and I have struggled previously with issues of countertransference in child analysis (Kohrman et al., 1971) and have studied its history in an effort to define it and understand its usefulness, as well as the problems that it poses. We have identified three reactions of the analyst: (1) the total response of the child analyst to the patient, the parents, and the therapeutic situation, reflecting the analyst's characterological givens, both neurotic and conflict-free; (2) the spontaneously occurring, unconscious reactions of the analyst to the patient's transference; and (3) a spontaneous, unconscious, conflictual, and immaturely determined reaction to the patient as he really is (that is, a reaction to a specific patient and not part of the characteristic behavior of the analyst toward all patients).

Little has been written about countertransference issues during the termination phase of child analysis. Bernstein and Glenn (1988), in a recent review of the subject of countertransference in child analysis, provide a passing reference to the subject. For the purposes of this chapter, I define *countertransference* as the various reactions the analyst has that interfere with the orderly termination of the child's analysis. Such reactions may involve supporting or even initiating a premature termination; or they may support the child's and/or parent's wish not to terminate. They may involve the analyst's inability to face the various affects that are provoked by the termination process and/or his helping the child avoid facing those affects.

A review of my own cases and those that I have supervised over the years strongly suggests that termination is more often initiated not by analytic considerations but by outside forces:—the start of a new school year, a new school, summer camp, moving away, financial considerations, orthodontia and so on. Often, these outside forces are manifestations of the wishes and needs of parents who are confronted with issues of their own past development that may parallel the developmental phase their child is in. I am convinced that the threat of revival, of undoing repression, in the parent is a major obstacle to child analysis, not only to beginning an analysis but also to allowing for an appropriate analytic ending. The parent will be inclined to find reasons not to start the child in analysis or to interrupt the analysis once it is underway; surprisingly, the analyst may often collude unconsciously with the parent in promoting the termination.

When the wish to terminate comes from the analyst it *equally* requires analysis—self-analysis on his part. In adult analysis it is generally rare that the analyst decides on a termination date. If the patient does not deal with ending treatment, when major conflicts have been resolved, the analysis of resistances to terminating is a necessary subsequent step rather than the analyst's simply making the decision to terminate. Freud's (1918, 1937) departure from this position with patients with severe obsessive–compulsive disorders, the Wolf-Man in particular, was unique; to my knowledge, such a departure is not commonplace in traditional adult analysis today.

The termination phase in adult analysis has always been considered a significant part of the analysis. It is ushered in by the setting of the date and ends with the actual stopping. For reasons not fully understood there is often, in attenuated form, a recapitulation of the analysis, with a return of symptoms, old defenses, and old transference positions. There may be transient identifications with the analyst in an attempt to deal with the impending loss. The genetic reconstruction of the analysis itself, a history experienced by both patient and analyst, may be a most important part of the termination phase. This reconstruction, a kind of compressed history of childhood, is truly the only history the analyst can validate; the history of the patient outside the analysis undergoes endless transformations. That's why transference is hardly ever simply a bona fide re-creation of past experience. Memories of past experience undergo change over time and with each developmental phase so that the past continues to be reinterpreted, to some degree, within the framework of the present. Schafer (1982) has brought this to our attention in a number of papers. One hallmark of analytic change is the transformation of the image of the parent from one that embodies idealization and, necessarily, profound disappointment to one that reflects a more balanced view in which strengths and human frailties alike are acknowledged.

In child analysis, when contemplating termination, we consider the issues of continuing development and the child's immature ego, considerations that result in a variety of solutions to the problem of termination, some of which have been addressed earlier. And it is near termination that we, the analysts, are confronted especially with unsettled issues of our own past: problems of separation–individuation, of relationships with parental figures (the parents of the child, our analytic mentor-parents, our own parents) in myriad possibilities and involving issues of dependency, separation, autonomy, competition, and rebellion. If the parent finds it painful to deal with his own infantile conflicts, reawakened by the child who is in analysis or by the child in termination, so do we. Our own analyses only partly prepare us for these confrontations and only approximate the re-creation of our infantile past with all of its terrors. The frequency of child abandonment and abuse requires protective measures on the part of the child; that is, the child needs to protect his image of the parent. This is accomplished most often by idealization, repression, and disavowal. We—and our own analysts—have also been subject to these defenses. A kind of fiction then emerges; the analyst and patient create a narrative that is a construction more than it is a reconstruction, a narrative that satisfies the requirements of repression *and* analysis. Adult patients meet us with the same kinds of defenses we ourselves have; we can collaborate relatively easily with their narrative. Children, on the other hand, do not meet us the same way. Those of us who have strong traditional defenses probably are relatively immune to these regressive temptations and may be less likely to grasp in the fullest sense the child's affective past. But those of us who have somewhat greater accessibility to our own affective infantile past are more vulnerable to anxiety and have greater access to the child's affective past. This dialogue is ongoing throughout the analysis, but it is during the process of termination that we confront those unique issues that may have been largely academic until then—issues, for example, of separation, autonomy, and success, which are central for the child, the parent, and the analyst.

Clinical Cases

In the remainder of this chapter I illustrate some of the aforementioned termination issues and how they affect all the participants, perhaps profoundly influencing the course of the analysis.

Susie

In the analysis of Susie, a 3-year-old girl who was described by the mother's psychiatrist as overly submissive and compliant to the mother, the mother was opposed to the child's therapy, preferring that her 6-year-old, who was rebellious and difficult, go into analysis instead. With the support of the mother's psychiatrist and of the father, a decision was made to undertake an analysis of Susie. Early in treatment Susie could not separate from her mother, and both were in the consulting room for almost two months. This was seen as the mother's need to hold on to Susie, which provided a stimulus for the child's anxiety, making separation difficult for her. Shortly after Susie agreed that her mother could remain in the waiting room, the mother reported that, following the session, she felt, while watching Susie walk away from her on the street, as if Susie were walking right out of her life. The analysis continued uninterruptedly for three years, but as first grade approached there were clear pressures that this would be a suitable time for termination. The child seemed to have satisfactorily worked out her problems and seemed developmentally on track; the analyst agreed to the termination. The termination phase progressed relatively uneventfully. The child assumed that when she stopped, the analyst would then see her sister; some indirect anger was expressed and was dealt with analytically, by interpretation. After the termination of Susie's therapy there was no further contact between this family and the analyst.

Twenty years later, at age 26, Susie sought out the analyst. She had been in a second analysis, from age 15 to 22. Remarkably, she had little memory of that analysis, but she had a vivid memory of her first analysis. She reported that for a long time after the termination of her first analysis she would have the fantasy that the analyst was her father. She felt the analysis had ended prematurely.

The pressure from the mother to stop the treatment had been present almost from the beginning, but her psychiatrist and Susie's father had succeeded, at least for three years, in modifying her position. The mother's narcissism was always visible; for example, she could openly say, "Well, to be perfectly honest, I would rather be in this air-conditioned office than in that hot waiting room." This occurred during the early period, in which the child insisted on having mother in the consulting room. Susie competed with her mother on an oedipal level; the mother, however, competed with Susie primarily on a narcissistic level. Susie was able to have vivid, active oedipal fantasies in relation to the analyst, in the analytic setting, and resume a submissive role with her mother once she left the office. Now, as an adult, without her mother around, Susie continued the same life situation, finding another woman to whom she was submissive while having active sexual fantasies about men.

In retrospect, the analyst had agreed to the mother's timetable about termination in order to mollify her. In the process, the compartmentalization of the analysis as a private and protected place in the patient's life was not analyzed. The result was that Susie again submitted to a mother imago in her adult life and had become a behavioral homosexual, while her fantasies remained heterosexual. She described herself as an "uncommitted homosexual," and she had become attached and submissive to a woman who acted in the role of the mother. It was this woman who told Susie to return to her childhood analyst to see what was troubling her because she didn't enjoy sex.

The countertransference issues for the analyst had involved his having to defend against his own feelings of helplessness in relation to the mother. He had felt that he was being forced to be submissive, as were Susie and her father. The defense against the helplessness was first anger and then collaboration with the mother, a defense in which he could feel that he was taking responsibility for the case again. In support of his position the analyst could then cite the fact that Susie had attained an age-appropriate developmental level. This case illustrates not only the problem of countertransference but also how it can arouse powerful defenses so that the central issue is not always visible and accessible to the analyst. We are often at the mercy of the parent's unconscious agenda, both in starting a child's analysis and, just as often, in ending it.

Laurel

Laurel, an eight-year-old girl, had been brought for analysis because of her wish to be a boy and her poor performance in school. After three years of analysis, when much of her masculine identification had been analyzed and worked through, her father attempted suicide. The analyst then learned that both the patient's paternal grandfather and uncle had committed suicide many years earlier. (Laurel, in fact, had been named for her uncle, who had died shortly before her birth.) This appeared to be the male destiny in the father's family, and Laurel had taken on that destiny for her father. Part of her masculine identification had been the assumption of her father's burden. The father expressed concern that Laurel would grow up to be like his brother and kill herself. In her very first session Laurel played out a story in which a girl doll was in a coma and the doctor operated on her and saved her. Without knowing the full suicide history at the time, the analyst understood the fantasy as an oedipal wish, disavowed. Ultimately, it was that wish, as well as the destiny of suicide, that was elaborated and worked through in the analysis. Interestingly, the father did not sabotage the analysis. Although the vital information about the grandfather and the fantasy of male destiny in this family was lacking until the crisis occurred, enough of the other issues around Laurel's masculine identification as a defense could be analyzed so that a shift took place and the father was confronted with taking back the destiny onto himself. After his coma and crisis had subsided, he dismissed his psychiatrist and insisted that Laurel's analyst had been the one who had saved him and the family. At termination, Laurel was ready, but the mother burst into tears, somehow assuming that the analyst would continue to see her and her husband. Unwittingly, he did.

After the termination the parents would call the analyst twice a year, at first to tell him how "his" little girl was doing. But that pretense was dropped fairly quickly. Years later, on one Thanksgiving Day, the father called to ask the analyst if it was all right to go out for dinner and leave Laurel's older sister at home—she was depressed and father was worried that she might be suicidal, even though the girl's own therapist had assured the parents she was not. Laurel's analyst had never met the sister; yet he was called.

Ten years after the analysis terminated, Laurel came to see her former analyst. She said that when she left the analysis, she felt that the analyst belonged to her parents. Even this time, Laurel was unwilling to work with the analyst, and the mother immediately asked if he would see her instead.

This case illustrates some of the universal problems the analyst faces in termination. A successful child analysis requires the alliance and support of the parents. That almost always means that the "good" parent makes a narcissistic as well as an object investment in the child's analysis. The narcissistic investment helps support the analysis; it is as if a part of the parent is being cared for and helped. Laurel's parents almost never canceled an appointment in four and a half years of analysis, and Laurel was hardly ever late. But this narcissistic investment is a potential impediment as well: it can stimulate intense transference expectations in the parents. Sometimes they are visible; often they are hidden. The child's transferences can be dealt with analytically, the child's termination issues can be approached analytically, but the parent's transferences cannot be dealt with analytically. This may lead to a failure to separate, as in the case of Laurel's parents. The parents may remain attached or experience rage over feeling rejected.

Perhaps most important, the parents can unwittingly block future access to the analyst. It would be interesting to know whether this blocking also includes access to the object representations of the analyst, in terms of the real, new object he has in part represented, with its soothing, self-regulating and identificatory aspects. Do the good memories become isolated, circumscribed, inaccessible, and no longer helpful in the development and maturation of the child?

Frank

Frank was 16 when he started his analysis. His ego was that of a well-structured neurotic adolescent. He was obsessional and largely conformed to the wishes of his parents. He seemed like an ideal candidate for analysis. The analysis progressed well, with a major focus on homosexual issues, which allowed Frank increasingly to get involved with girls. The analysis had been in progress for almost a year when the issue of college arose. This had been discussed before treatment began, and it seemed clear that Frank would have been willing to remain near home now, go to a local university, and continue his analysis. Nor was there evidence that the parents would not have supported such a decision. But the analyst not only failed to analyze Frank's resistance to staying but rather subtly began to encourage Frank to terminate his analysis and go away to school. A review of this candidate analyst's cases showed they were mostly short, apparently abbreviated analyses. At matriculation years before there was concern whether he would be able to allow his patients to regress. He seemed to be fearful of any regressive trends in himself, and he therefore subtly promoted his patients' "forward" movement. The analyst's own needs for defense were threatened by the regressive pulls of his patients; his ongoing analyses did not reveal the issues as clearly as when he went about terminating his patients.

Jenny

At nine, Jenny had been in analysis for four and a half years. There was clear evidence that she was moving into latency, and she seemed developmentally on track. She had originally come into analysis because of poor socialization and academic retardation despite a very high intelligence. When she was able to attend a regular public school, perform academically, and socialize well, she was nevertheless reluctant to end the analysis. Her parents had considerable difficulty around separations and were also reluctant for her to terminate. The analyst, who had a history of early parent loss, also had a problem around separations. Since this was his final case at the institute, saying good-bye to the patient also meant saying good-bye to the institute and the supervisor. Thus, in this case, no one was willing to say it was time to stop—not Jenny, her parents, or the analyst. Jenny, whose main thrust seemed to be forward, may have been "reading" her parents and her analyst and trying to meet their needs. The analytic data clearly indicated appropriate maturation, movement toward autonomy, a resolving of oedipal transference issues, a turning outward toward friends. When the analyst tried to interpret the resistance to termination, following discussions with his supervisor, he started to badger Jenny about her reluctance to end, focusing on the conflict over her wish to leave versus her wish to stay and her parents' ambivalence about leaving. But he did not analyze his own ambivalence with the patient. His interpretations somehow lacked conviction, and Jenny was not willing to talk about ending. The analyst felt caught between his own needs and the perceived demands of the supervisor. These were discussed at length during supervision and movement began to take place. The analyst then asked to cut back his supervision from biweekly to monthly. But before a termination date for Jenny had even been set, the analyst abruptly asked to end supervision altogether. Would this be his ending without his terminating? These possibilities were discussed, and the analyst decided to continue supervision until the termination of the patient's analysis. His ambivalence emerged again as he set a termination date that followed a period during which both he and the patient would be taking their respective vacations and the analyst would be moving his office, meaning that Jenny's last appointment would be in a new office. Again this was discussed in supervision, and a more appropriate time, which allowed for greater concentration on termination issues and did not compete with other life events, was set. The analyst's ambivalence was further discussed. He revealed that in his own first analysis there had been a poor termination. And in his second analysis there had been sudden stopping when his analyst became seriously ill. He was able to verbalize that he was hoping that Jenny's termination would also afford him an opportunity to terminate.

Debbie

Debbie was 12½ years old when she terminated her analysis. She had been in analysis for three and a half years and had previously been in therapy with this analyst at age two and a half. She had originally been referred by a pediatric allergist who concluded that her asthma was caused by emotional factors. During an eight-month period of therapy when Debbie was two and a half, the analyst had acquired the magical qualities of being able to interrupt Debbie's asthmatic attacks. The therapy was then interrupted by the analyst's call into military service.

When Debbie was nine, she was in the hospital in a status asthmaticus, and no medical intervention could break the cycle. The pediatrician insisted that Debbie's mother call the analyst. He came to the hospital and interrupted the asthmatic state. The mother then revealed that she had not brought Debbie back into treatment because she felt the analyst had promised that her child would never have another attack. Although the analyst had returned from military service four years earlier, he did not see Debbie until the crisis. She then entered analysis. After three and a half years Debbie felt she was ready to terminate but had great difficulty in setting a date; finally, with great agony, she settled on the end of July. At the end of June Debbie insisted that the end of June had been the agreed-upon time. She was adamant, and so the analysis came to an abrupt end.

The analyst anticipated what would happen. He felt that the patient had stopped without adequately facing any of the separation issues. Six months later Debbie called. The first thing she said was "I don't want to come in. I am preparing for my bat mitzvah in two weeks and I have been having a lot of asthma." All the analyst could do was say, "See how things go and if they don't get any better over the weekend, let me know." Several weeks later, the analyst received a note from Debbie saying that her asthma had cleared and the bat mitzvah had gone well.

When Debbie was 16, her mother called the analyst. The parents had divorced a couple of years earlier. Debbie was asthmatic and in a chronic rage at her mother; she had stopped going out with her friends, had stopped dating, and was not doing her schoolwork. The analyst saw her once, during which time Debbie was in a rage at him, angry at being there; she didn't want to talk to him and did so grudgingly. Nevertheless, within days her asthma cleared, her rage subsided, and she began to do her schoolwork and socialize. Years later the analyst received an announcement from Debbie that she had graduated from professional school.

When she was 38 and very successful in her career, married and the mother of two children, Debbie came to see her analyst on her mother's suggestion. She had no complaints, but her mother just thought it would be interesting for Debbie to reacquaint herself with her childhood analyst. She had had almost no episodes of asthma in her adult life. She had very little to say and remembered almost nothing of her therapy; she wanted the analyst to talk and tell her about their earlier experience, and she left without wishing any further contact.

Clearly, here was an example in which the analyst had very early acquired a magical power over Debbie's well-being. Rather than face termination and the possible loss of that magical attachment, she had promoted a premature ending, thus ensuring that the attachment would remain. That, of course, also meant that the analyst retained power over her. Emancipation and autonomy were sacrificed in the service of self-preservation.

Willie

Willie was 12 when he terminated a five-year analysis. He had come into analysis because of depression, low self-esteem, and great academic difficulties compounded by a learning disability. His parents fully supported his treatment. It was only after termination that the family structure overtly broke down. The parents got an acrimonious divorce, and subsequently, each parent (at different times) was hospitalized psychiatrically. At each critical point in his life, Willie would call the analyst. He did not want to come in, but he wanted to let the analyst know what was happening in his life. He felt that he did not have parents whom he could rely on; he thought of the analyst as his parent, he said. He asked if he could call the analyst if he needed to. The analyst next heard from him when he was 23 and living in a distant city. He was seriously ill physically. Although he said he was getting good medical care, he found himself upset and anxious and wanted to touch base with his old analyst. Again he said that his own father was too unreliable for him to get any support from; Willie had lost all contact with his mother.

Given the unstable situation in which he repeatedly found himself, Willie was able to recathect the image of his analyst, probably as a real, new object in his life and possibly as a transference figure of a good, nurturing parent from infancy. The auditory contact alone was sufficient to sustain him over his various crises. His learning disability had involved visual–motor perception; his strength lay in oral and auditory skills of communication. Willie thus relied on his strength to seek out support when he needed it.

Termination Issues Represented by the Clinical Cases

These six cases focus on a variety of problems that interfere with an orderly termination process. They illustrate the conflicts of each participant in the process—the child patient, the parent, and the analyst.

Debbie could not terminate because of her need for the magical power of the analyst. Any attempt to analyze this need was met with great resistance. Clearly, these are early preoedipal issues that could not or did not get resolved. Debbie is covertly still keeping in touch with her analyst.

Willie needed a parent when his parents, in reality, failed him. Although the termination process had proceeded in a conventional manner, Willie either had not effected a separation or, more likely, was able once again to recathect the person of the analyst at times of a realistic need for a parent. This might highlight what Loewald has alluded to—that nothing is lost, nothing gets so transformed that it no longer exists in a latent state.

For Debbie and Willie, needs determined whether they could or could not terminate the analysis; they could decathect neither the analyst as a real person nor the analyst as the transference figure of early childhood. They needed him.

The problems that parents have in the termination process are especially difficult to deal with because the parents are not the patients and, therefore, problem issues cannot be analyzed. Susie's mother was enraged at the analyst because he was giving to Susie and not to her. She constantly pushed for termination. In later years, she never sought out Susie's analyst when problems arose; she went elsewhere. Her injury was a narcissistic one. Laurel's parents formed an intense transference to her analyst that prevented their turning elsewhere for help. Although efforts were made to get the parents into their own treatment, they failed. And even after the father's suicide attempt, he quickly abandoned his own psychiatrist to reattach to Laurel's analyst. It was only at termination, with the mother's reaction of crying and not understanding that the analyst would not be continuing with the parents, that it became clear how strong the attachment had been and that there had been no opportunity to help them separate.

In the cases of Jenny and Frank, the analysts brought their own problems into the analytic termination. Both analysts had sustained early parent loss; one reacted by favoring a regressive solution, which interfered with ending, while the other favored a precocious maturation by pushing for an ending. Both directions interfered with the termination process.

The Validity of Termination in Child Analysis

Should there be a termination in child analysis? Those opposed have even suggested that the analysis should be phased out so slowly that the child doesn't even know he is terminating. But Anna Freud (1965) noted that it is the patient who determines the treatment, not the analyst. Perhaps it is also the patient who determines the nature and degree of the terminating process. And one must also include the parent here as well. The child comes to analysis, stays in analysis, and ends the analysis according to the parent's needs and wishes, both conscious and unconscious. The parent's alliance with the analyst is extremely important; but his or her hidden motives and needs are often not accessible to the child's analyst to understand or attempt to alter. In that sense, the analyst and the child are potentially at the mercy of the parent's needs and wishes. Sometimes the child's cure aids the parent and makes him or her a strong supporter of the analysis, but the child's cure may also create an imbalance in the parent's psychic organization and lead to action that can be detrimental to the analysis or its ending.

The analyst provides a matrix upon which the infantile wishes and needs of the child, and often the parent, are expressed. His capacity to observe the patient as well as his capacity for self-observation are likely critical factors in the ultimate success of the analytic process. The analyst is a target of transferences, externalizations, and new real-object attachments. His reaction to the child's transference may be a countertransference response, but it may also be a counterreaction, that is, a response meant to be evoked by the transference expression. Such reactions belong in the mainstream of the analytic process and need to be shared and interpreted. If the response is a countertransference, that is, a personal reaction on the part of the analyst to the child's transference, a response based on the analyst's own infantile past, then it would burden the analysis to introduce it there. It obviously needs to be addressed, if that is possible, via self-analysis or more personal analysis. Unfortunately, as I have noted earlier, countertransference reactions are just as defended against as are transference reactions. So it is not always apparent that one is dealing with a countertransference as opposed to a counterreaction.

Externalizations, a fairly typical defensive mode of children, especially of affective states, are often a royal road to the child's internal state. When a child appears unconcerned about the termination while the analyst finds himself inexplicably sad, the analyst needs to consider externalization as a possible source of his discomfort. In one case, an 18-year-old boy, preparing to terminate his analysis and go off to college, spoke about his father helping him get into the "best" college. The analyst became aware that he himself had begun to feel unaccountably sad. As he reflected on this, he realized that his own daughter was applying to college and had no connections to get in to a good school; she would have to do it on her own. Further exploration led to his understanding the sadness as being related to the idea that he would miss his daughter and was sad about her leaving home. She was, in fact, an excellent student and would have little trouble getting into schools of her choice. This then led to appreciating the patient's defending himself against his own affects about leaving the analyst and the analysis. This insight eventually led to an interpretation and a beginning recovery of the disavowed affects.

The real relationship between child and analyst constitutes a real loss for both at termination. Again, there are affects that need to be addressed, but this must occur within a framework that does not burden the patient with guilt for the leave-taking. The shared feelings can become a very important gradient in the real-object relationship, in which one can feel acceptably sad and still leave, in contrast to the often conflictual relationship with the infantile imagos, where guilt, rage, and competition abound.

The question of whether we should have a termination phase in child analysis and the question of whether there is such a thing as a termination in any analysis are philosophical issues that eventually become technical considerations. There probably is no simple answer. Perhaps we need to appreciate the complexity of the problem, that it involves multiple layers of the personality organization, both repressed and accessible, both in the distant past and the near past; we need to realize that the child will or will not terminate the analysis, based on his own capacities and needs, provided these are not interfered with by parent or analyst. It may very well parallel the issue of transference.

Early in analytic work with children, analysts took the position that there was no such thing as a transference neurosis in children. Our technique at that time contributed to inhibiting its development and/or its emergence. We took a very active role as real people in the child's life. Our aim was to become indispensable, Anna Freud (1926) had said. We then concluded that we were right; there was no transference neurosis in children. As we adopted a more analytic posture of neutrality and ambiguity and began to interpret resistances, we found that some children were, in fact, capable of developing a transference neurosis; almost all were capable of developing analyzable transference reactions (Weiss et al., 1968; Chused, chap. 11, this volume). Perhaps we need to afford the child the opportunity to terminate if he is able to do so. If the child cannot terminate, he should have the opportunity to disengage in whatever way he has to. All of this can be effected through the ongoing analytic dialogue, without having to resort to extra-analytic or nonanalytic measures.

The alliance with the parent is no guarantee that he or she will support the child's endeavor. Parents are, of course, confronted with their own termination as well as that of the child. The developmental task for the parent cannot be aided by the child's analyst in any substantial way. It is the parent's narcissistic and object libido investment in the child that will help or hinder the process.

And, finally, the analyst has to confront his own developmental issues in relation to his infantile past and its recapitulation in the more recent past as an analysand himself. If each child affords the parent the opportunity and burden of reworking his or her own identifications with parental models and development as a child, each patient—and especially each child patient—does a similar thing for the child analyst. Hopefully, with each encounter, not only do we rework our distant and recent past but we are also enriched by the experience.

References

Altschul, S., ed. (1988), *Childhood Bereavement and Its Aftermaths.* New York: International Universities Press.

Bernstein, I. & Glenn, J. (1988), The child and adolescent analyst's emotional reactions to his patients and their parents. *Internat. Rev. Psycho-Anal.,* 15(2):225–241.

Bowlby, J. (1969), *Attachment and Loss, Vol. 1.* New York: Basic Books.

Freud, A. (1926), *The Psycho-Analytical Treatment of Children.* London: Imago, 1946.

———— (1965), *Normality and pathology in childhood.* New York: International Universities Press.

Freud, S. (1918), From the history of an infantile neurosis. *Standard Edition,* 17:7–122. London: Hogarth Press, 1955.

———— (1937), Analysis terminable and interminable. *Standard Edition,* 23:216–253. London: Hogarth Press, 1964.

Kohrman, R., Fineberg, H., Gelman, R. & Weiss, S. (1971), Technique of child analysis: Problems of countertransference. *Internat. J. Psycho-Anal.,* 52:487–497.

Loewald, H. (1970), Remarks to training analysts' workshop. Chicago Institute for Psychoanalysis, November 28.

———— (1978), *Psychoanalysis and the History of the Individual.* New Haven, CT: Yale University Press.

Mahler, M. (1979), *The Selected Papers of Margaret S. Mahler, Vol. 2: Separation-Individuation.* New York: Aronson.

Schafer, R. (1982), The relevance of the "here and now" transference interpretation for the reconstruction of early development. *Internat. J. Psycho-Anal.,* 63:77–82.

Tolpin, M. (1971), On the beginnings of a cohesive self. *The Psychoanalytic Study of the Child*, 26:316–352. New Haven, CT: Yale University Press.

Weiss, S., Fineberg, H., Gelman, R. & Kohrman, R. (1968), Technique of child analysis: Problems of the opening phase. *J. Amer. Acad. Child Psych.*, 7:639–662.

Winnicott, D. W. (1953), Transitional objects and transitional phenomena: A study of the first not-me possession. *Internat. J. Psycho-Anal.*, 34:89–97.

Wolfenstein, M. (1966), How is mourning possible? *The Psychoanalytic Study of the Child*, 21:93–123. New York: International Universities Press.

13

Deciding on Termination: The Relevance of Child and Adolescent Analytic Experience to Work with Adults

Jack Novick
Kerry Kelly Novick

In recent years analysts have acknowledged the centrality of a developmental point of view; many emphasize that psychoanalytic theory is, above all, a developmental psychology (Pine, 1985; Meissner, 1989). Psychoanalysts have studied the development of the individual mainly through reconstruction from work with adults and through direct observations of infants and children. Reconstruction with adult patients of significant aspects of the past was central to the earliest work, while psychoanalytically informed infant and child observation has a long history from Freud's own work with children (Novick, 1989) to the current explosion of infant research (Lichtenberg, 1985, Tyson, 1989). Child analysis has been a third source of data contributing to our concepts of the development of the personality. Anna Freud (1970) described the initial pervasive excitement over the potential of child analysis to confirm the findings of adult analysis and her subsequent disappointment that this early promise had not led to greater collaboration and overlap between child and adult work. Almost a century of psychoanalytic work with adults has produced a vast body of clinical material and technical precept, and analysts have tried to integrate new data from infant and child observation as it has become available. It is our impression, however, that child and adolescent psychoanalysis remains a rich but relatively untapped source of insights into psychoanalytic process and technique, at every stage of treatment.

In our previous work we have used child and adolescent clinical material to examine a variety of topics, including termination (Novick, 1976, 1982a, 1988, 1990a). This clinical focus led to a theoretical paper on the application of child and adolescent termination experience to the end phase of adult analysis (Novick, 1990b). In that paper it was noted that "three features stand out in a survey of the child/adolescent literature on termination: (1) the high percentage of premature terminations, (2) the involvement of parents in termination considerations and (3) the presence of developmental forces which gives prominence to the overarching termination criterion of restoration to the path of progressive development" (p. 433). These three features are said to differentiate child and adult analysis, but it was argued in that paper that they all may be fruitfully applied to the understanding of termination issues in adult analysis. Particular attention was paid to Anna Freud's (1965) criterion of "restoration to the path of progressive development," and it was suggested that this concept requires further refinement and elucidation. "Perhaps we can begin the refinement of this concept by saying that during the pretermination phase the balance between progressive and regressive forces along a number of dimensions is assessed and a judgment is made as to whether the stress and strain of setting a date will lead to severe regressions or will be mastered in such a way as to promote progressive development" (Novick, 1990b, p. 430). Several intrapsychic and interpersonal dimensions were suggested, including progressive shifts in sources of self-esteem. In this paper we will make use of clinical material from child, adolescent, and adult analyses to elucidate this developmental criterion and demonstrate its applicability to adults.

The Preschool Child in Analysis

Goals of analysis at any age have always included resolution of the Oedipus complex, as figured forth in the transference neurosis. Most of what we know about the course of the Oedipus complex during analysis comes from work with adults. Child analysis has played an important confirming role since Little Hans, but, as Anthony (1986) has noted, child analysis has not added much to our understanding of this phase and its resolution. The analysis of preschool children almost always involves the passage through the oedipal phase and entry into latency, so examination of the termination of preschool analyses provides an opportunity to develop criteria for judging resolution of the Oedipus complex.

Even without the accretions of later phases, the Oedipus complex of the preschool child is not simple. The normal Oedipus complex not only contains the familiar constellation of drive impulses, anxieties, and defenses but also carries with it the inevitable narcissistic insult that attends facing the reality of physical inadequacy to fulfill oedipal wishes. This humiliation echoes the child's helplessness in earlier phases to get the object to understand and gratify his wishes. In a good-enough mother–child relationship the child's inborn capacities to elicit an appropriate response provide an experience of effectance that accumulates throughout development to counterbalance feelings of helplessness. The normal passage into latency draws upon this store of competence to direct the child to sources of self-esteem in his achievements, instead of his seeking narcissistic supplies solely in his relationships to objects.

The Oedipus complex becomes traumatic when it is experienced as a continuation of an impaired mother–child relationship in which feelings of helplessness have not been offset by experiences of competence but have instead been defended against by magical omnipotent fantasies. Fantasies fill the gap between the real and the ideal, and, for the normal child, they refer usually to the self-representation—hence the surge in early latency of daydreams of glory and fame. Such daydreams can become the initiators of latency activities, and so fantasy can lead the child back to competence as a source of pleasure and self-esteem. For other children the gap is between the real and the ideal mother; then fantasy is aimed not at enhancing the real capacities of the self but at denying and transforming the pain and inadequacy of the mother–child relationship. Unable to make use of real capacities to elicit appropriate responses from mother, these children fall back on magical control of the object to maintain their self-esteem.

The oedipal and preoedipal elements in the treatment of preschool children are not different in themselves from those seen in patients of any age, but one quality stands out particularly vividly. Narcissistic sensitivity reaches a peak, and we can see most clearly in the analysis of preschoolers the importance of the termination phase to the adaptive transformation of the narcissistic economy. Let us look at material from the termination phase of a little boy who started five times per week analysis at the age of three.

By the time Robert was six and a quarter, there had been consistent good reports from home and school for some time. In the analysis there had been an extended period of fruitful work on his preoedipal and oedipal conflicts. He spoke of having few problems left and wondered what would happen when they were all gone. Termination was clearly on everyone's mind and the possibility had been raised by the parents. The analyst felt that Robert's self-esteem was sufficiently rooted in reality achievements to allow for the beginning of a termination phase. Enjoying himself as a six-year-old boy in the second grade, however, meant giving up the omnipotent idea of being his mother's oedipal partner. Robert's genuine pride in his real achievements was easily engulfed by defensive feelings of omnipotent triumph as he retreated into a magical narcissistic state in which he imagined that he kept mother alive and powerful by giving her things to do. To this end he clung to a food fad that kept him home from school at lunchtime while his mother busied herself making him special meals. His realistic appreciation of his achievements was difficult to maintain and easily slipped into a fantasy of grandiose oedipal triumph. As Robert grew tall and strong, he called the analyst a "squashed man" and "fatso"; as he experienced his own independence, he spoke of the analyst as useless. When Robert learned how to type, he gave the analyst a card with his name and address on it and said that the analyst could come to his house or telephone him if he wished to continue work. Verbalization of this pattern, where his accomplishments rendered the analyst useless, was followed by a reversal in which Robert characterized the analyst as all-knowing and himself as helpless and full of problems. The same pattern was occurring at home with his mother. Repeated interpretation of his secret oedipal fantasy that he alone kept both analyst and mother powerful and alive by being a baby with problems finally led him to confront his mother. He told her he was through with all his problems except one—her. He said that a little bit of her wanted him to stay a baby. Mother agreed that this was so but emphasized that most of her wanted him to be a big boy, and that she and Daddy enjoyed his big boy achievements.

Robert reacted with relief and a spurt of forward movement. However, he could not maintain his realistic view of himself, and he invoked magical means to deny the reality of his status as a child excluded from the parental sexual relationship and of his helplessness in controlling his mother. His magical omnipotent fantasies derived from many levels, as he imagined eating up the whole world, fooling everyone and poisoning them, strengthening his bones as the analyst's bones softened. The analyst contrasted Robert's infantile feelings of helplessness with the realistic power of his increasing competence. They understood together why Robert had felt that magic was the only route open to him, but that he could now feel good in other ways. Robert responded with renewed self-confidence and told the analyst that he had been able to put his face in the water while swimming. He alluded repeatedly to a wish to reduce the frequency of sessions, and the analyst agreed that he was ready but that he would leave it to him to decide when.

Robert worked in that very session to choose which day to drop but asked the analyst to tell mother, because "she'll be frightened out of her wits and you know what wits are. Wits are the widths in the swimming pool and she is so frightened she can't even swim a width, but I can swim a whole width with the board." When they reached the waiting room, Robert proudly announced that he was dropping a day. His mother later told the analyst she was sure that there was a clear connection between the reduction in frequency of analytic sessions and Robert's learning to swim; he did four widths that afternoon and fell asleep with a grin on his face. Soon after, it was mutually decided that the analysis would end in three months.

Termination is a reality that is hard to deny. To Robert's competent self, termination represented an accomplishment of which he could be proud. To his helpless infantile self it represented an imposition by the powerful analyst/mother that challenged his omnipotent defenses to create more powerful magic at the expense of his realistic achievements. Thus, Robert felt that he had to produce more and more problems and deny the pleasures of school, imagining that he could thereby keep the powerful analyst at his command forever. By the termination phase, however, the failure of magic did not leave Robert prey to helpless anxiety; rather, he had available alternative, reality-based sources of self-esteem.

We learn the following from this examination of the termination of a preschool child's analysis: (1) it takes the work of the termination phase to complete the work of the analysis; (2) the resolution of the Oedipus complex includes transformation of the narcissistic economy; and (3) the start of a termination phase is not when the conflicts are resolved but when the patient is sufficiently rooted in realistic pleasures to put up a good fight against the regressive pull of fantasy solutions. The same issues arise in work with adults, but appear more subtly, because of the impact of intervening developmental transformations. Therefore, we will defer our discussion of omnipotent narcissistic defense in the termination phase of adult patients until we have described some issues that arise in latency and adolescence.

The School-Age Child in Analysis

Anna Freud (1965) described the goal of analysis as the restoration of the child to the path of progressive development. The concept evokes a sense of momentum regained and implies that termination is appropriate when the child and family can continue the growth process independently of the analyst. Every child or adolescent patient ends treatment as an unfinished product; there is much development remaining. The same is true of adult patients although the stages of development may be less clearly defined and the rate of change slower. Thus, child analysts know that termination can and should occur in the midst of a dynamic growth process that has been reestablished by the work of treatment.

For patients of any age the work of analysis is aimed at resolving preoedipal regressions to allow for the resolution of the Oedipus complex. Once the patient is sufficiently established at the oedipal level, a termination phase can be started, in which working through, synthesis, and mourning can take place. This allows for consolidation at the age-appropriate phase. As one of the criteria to start termination with the preschool child we highlighted the role of the transformation of the narcissistic economy from a base in magical, omnipotent fantasy to one in striving toward reality achievements.

School-age children brought for treatment are faced with similar tasks in analysis, since typical symptom formation usually presupposes incomplete or inadequate resolution of the Oedipus complex. For instance, Erica came into analysis at eight years of age with panic attacks, fear of her parents dying, fear of using strange lavatories, fear of monsters, bedtime rituals, headaches, stomach-aches, frequent falls and accidents, difficulty in falling asleep, open masturbation, babytalk and babyish behavior, lack of friends, intense unhappiness, anger, discontent, rages, intense jealousy, constricted speech and movement, and a learning disturbance. Most of these symptoms abated or disappeared in the course of the first year of analysis. Some of this was due to structural change, but most of the improvement was a consequence of Erica's use of the analysis for fantasy gratification of her preoedipal and oedipal wishes. When the analyst interpreted Erica's use of the analysis, she wanted to stop treatment and used her symptomatic improvement as the rationale to try to convince her parents. The analyst's working alliance with the parents preserved the treatment in the face of Erica's resistance.

Two years later, when Erica was 11, the possibility of termination became apparent to Erica, her parents, and the analyst. A date was chosen and a termination phase began. As was the case with Robert, one of the criteria for deciding on starting the termination phase was that the major source of Erica's pleasure was shifting appreciably to competence and effectance. For some time it had been clear that Erica was enjoying her high-level functioning at school and with friends. One day she and the analyst talked about wishes, and Erica said that whenever she was asked for wishes, the "baby wishes," like the wish for a magic wand, immediately flashed into her mind but these were not really her wishes any more, since she knew that she couldn't make them come true. She said she would tell the analyst her "grown-up wishes" and then the baby wishes. The "grown-up wishes" were to have a yacht and that the house and garden would be finished; the "big wish" was to be a ballerina, be able to do pottery, play a musical instrument, and have four monkeys and two cats. The analyst wondered if she had the wish to be a grown-up, be married, and have babies. Erica replied, "That's a baby wish. I used to have it, but I don't any more. I had it when I was doing poorly at school and hated school. I would think to myself that grown-ups don't go to school, so I wished to be a grown-up. The baby wishes were to have a magic wand, to have wings, and to be a grown-up."

Work with the school-age child highlights the issue of postoedipal consolidation at the appropriate phase. For Erica this was latency, with its emphasis on work and play. We have already discussed the importance of the shift of the source of pleasure from the illusion of omnipotence to experiences of effectance. The school-child underscores the additional factor of change in the quality of pleasure and how to assess its manifestations.

Pleasure should become evident consistently, and we look for reports from home and school of more widespread enjoyment. Erica's parents began to envisage termination because they noted that she was frequently "beaming from ear to ear," which made father aware that she never used to smile at all. So, consistent reports of pervasive and lasting pleasure are an important factor, but external change can have many meanings and roots; a genuine analytic termination must be decided on the basis of internal criteria. This is where we must look to add substance to the abstract goal of "restoration to the path of progressive development" (A. Freud, 1965). Progressive development implies change along each of the metapsychological dimensions. We suggest that the functioning of the working alliance within the treatment relationship provides a barometer of these changes. The working alliance appears particularly vividly in the analysis of latency children, because their age-appropriate tasks include the development of the capacity to enjoy work.

At the time in Erica's analysis when everyone was aware of her much happier functioning at home and in school, she described herself as having few remaining problems and discussed the possibility of cutting down to four times a week. After some talk of the advantages and disadvantages of this, Erica produced a series of thoughts that seemed to be a working through both of old problems that had been dealt with at length and other issues that had received some attention but that she seemed to have worked through on her own.

First, Erica talked about having always been afraid of her sister Lou's jealousy. She said it didn't bother her any more. "I mean it's really up to Lou if she wants to copy her friend Jill and be someone else. I mean it's her problem. If she's jealous of me and wants treatment, then she should speak to Mommy. It's silly to make myself go down just because Lou is jealous. That won't help Lou and it won't help me." Then, of Lou's attempt to be like Jill, Erica went on to say that one shouldn't try to be like someone else, one should be oneself. "I mean there's only one Erica and Erica is not like anyone else and if I try to be somebody else then there's no Erica." She followed with the comment that she had always felt that she must be just like her mother, otherwise her mother wouldn't like her. "But I'm not like Mommy; I don't look like Mommy, I don't feel like Mommy, I'm myself, a completely different person and I want to be myself. I enjoy being myself."

The analyst wondered how Mommy might feel about Erica's being herself, and Erica talked about Mommy having been in the center of her worries but that Mommy didn't know that. Erica then wondered when her problems had started and suggested that it was when her sister Lou was born. She thought there may have been something before, "but it was just a titchy little bit and then when Lou was born I really felt they thought I wasn't good enough, that they weren't satisfied with me so they got somebody else, so from then on I had to be better than somebody else, better than Lou and I think that's when I thought I had to be better than Mommy." She took out her baby album, which she had been keeping in the treatment room, and wondered if walking at ten months was early. When the analyst said that it was a little early Erica said, "Maybe I was a little wrong to say it was just a little titchy bit of a problem before Lou was born because, you see, I'm walking early, and maybe I already felt I should be better than Mommy because I wanted Daddy's approval, you see." When the analyst wondered about getting Daddy's approval now, Erica said, "I don't know quite how it's changed but it's really not that important to me now; other things are." She said that her worries had been very important when they were there, but now they were gone and they were really not important.

In this material we can see derivatives of instinctual wishes and defenses that had appeared repeatedly in the course of the analysis, such as Erica's rivalry with her sister and mother, her wish to please the analyst as the oedipal father in the transference, and the need to deny continuing difficulties. The material also shows the significant changes that had taken place. In addition to the remaining problems and the progress, however, the level of the working alliance reflects the achievement of a new pleasure in ego functioning. This pleasure is not relief or moral satisfaction in obedience to the superego, or omnipotent sadistic triumph over envied others, but a gratification from the functioning of ego capacities fostered by the analytic work.

In the above example, Erica is making effective use of her memory, conceptual ability, reality testing, time sense, and ability to tolerate uncertainty. All of this allowed for the flowering of her creative capacity, which we can see in operation here as she arrived at independent insights about, for instance, her defensive identification with her mother. With Erica not only do we see the shift in the source of pleasure from omnipotence to achievements but also, and most important, we see that this pleasure resides increasingly in the *exercise* of ego functions, as well as in the achievements themselves; that is, the process of work becomes as much a pleasure as its product. Thus, it is in the working alliance that we may see Erica's beginning consolidation in the stage of latency. This criterion for the start of a termination phase applies to patients of all ages. Ego pleasure in the work of analysis ensures an adaptive response to the painful work remaining to be done. Application of this criterion to the timely start of a termination phase in an adult case has been described in detail in a recent publication (Novick, 1988). The way this adult patient worked on a dream closely parallels the ego pleasure we have described in Erica.

The Adolescent in Analysis

In the main, adolescents find it very difficult to leave their parents or their therapists in a mutually respectful manner that reflects a state of internal readiness and acceptance of a growth process. Most adolescents terminate prematurely, either provoking the therapist to force an ending or surprising the therapist with a unilateral termination plan. When this occurs near the end of treatment it may involve a regression from a differentiated to an "externalizing" transference, in which the therapist represents the helpless, depreciated, and rejected child discarded by the now-powerful adolescent.

In 1982 one of us (J.N.) published a detailed case example of a 15-year-old boy who attempted a unilateral premature termination. This, and many similar instances, led to the hypothesis that this adolescent form of premature termination may occur in the analysis of adults. A condition for the start of a proper termination phase with adults may be prior work on the reemergence of the adolescent form of premature leave-taking (Novick, 1976, 1982b, 1988).

If not premature, the termination of adult analysis may be unnecessarily prolonged, and here too we may use experience in the termination of adolescent patients to highlight some obstacles to the timely start of a termination phase. As we have seen, restoration to the path of normal development implies consolidation in the age-appropriate phase. This is easier to define in childhood and adulthood than in adolescence, which is normally characterized by flux and uncertainty. Compounding the appropriate uncertainty of the adolescent's life can be the analyst's counterreactions of anxiety about the patient's readiness for independent functioning. The analyst's overprotective impulses can be a formidable obstacle to starting a termination phase; the clarification of this counterreactive ingredient in the decision to start termination with adolescent patients alerts us to a similar, if more subtle, temptation to retain adult patients in a futile attempt to deal with every uncertainty and unfinished developmental line.

The Adult in Analysis

Termination of adult cases can be premature, timely, or interminable. We would like to share some preliminary thoughts on the problem of interminable analysis, an area that has thus far received scant attention in the vast and ever-increasing literature on adult termination. It is surprising that there are so few references to the issue of interminable analysis, since one of the first cases reported by Freud, that of the Wolf-Man, might be considered such a case and may have contributed to the pessimism of Freud's "Analysis Terminable and Interminable" (1937). Some of the articles that refer to the topic may be including those patients who fail to respond to analytic treatment despite lengthy and heroic efforts of the analyst with those who do respond positively but seem unable to terminate (Klauber, 1977; Anzieu, 1987; Burgner, 1988). The issue is often masked by the reluctance of analysts to admit that they have patients who have been in analysis for over ten years. Others may be concerned that they and the method may be seen as fostering a pathological dependence, so they set a time limit at the outset of treatment or force a termination of interminable patients by saying that analysis offers the patient too much passive gratification and so must end.

Mr. M[1] first came to treatment at the age of 25. He had been turned down as a training case because he was considered too disturbed. He had been diagnosed as "borderline" and at his first session he began to cry, pound the couch with his arms and legs, and plead, "I can't stand it. Please! Get it over with. Punish me . . . beat me!" Since graduating from a university Mr. M had wandered in a fog of unfocused anxiety and tension, supported himself with occasional house painting jobs, and found temporary relief in a series of relationships with equally disturbed women, who were initially allowed to play the role of a controlling mother and then driven into a state of helpless rage by his passivity and covert sadism. The initial period of work brought a beginning sense of order and meaning to his life that gave him immediate relief, since he placed the analyst in the role of the longed-for good mother who could respond to his pain and kiss away the hurt. He felt so much better at the first summer vacation that he thought he would soon be able to end his analysis. The feelings of pride, pleasure, and competence did not last long. Mr. M was soon locked in a relationship in which he saw the analyst as the powerful mother who was responsible for all his psychic and physical states of pain or relief while he felt like the innocent victim of events. Covertly, he worked to defeat all therapeutic efforts. The intense sadomasochistic transference reflected a "screaming" relationship with a severely depressed, alcoholic mother and underscored the patient's masochistic pathology and his lifelong addiction to pain.

Manifestations of these fantasies and memories were figured forth in the transference, and constant attention to the many determinants and functions of Mr. M's active pain-seeking behavior led to slow but steady progress. The patient had been in five times per week analysis for over ten years, and by all external and most internal criteria he was ready to stop. He was happily married, joyfully anticipating the birth of a child, and successful in his career; for a

---

[1]The following clinical material was first presented at the 6th annual workshop of the American Psychoanalytic Association and published in Novick (1990a). We would like to express our gratitude to the editor, Scott Dowling, and International Universities Press for permission to reprint the case material.

considerable period of time he had worked hard and fruitfully at his analysis. All that remained was to pick a date and do the working through, mourning, and consolidating of the termination phase, but this proved to be a lengthy and seemingly impossible task. The work, of course, could have ended had the analyst taken responsibility for picking the date—and Mr. M tried in every way to have the analyst do so. When this failed he became depressed, and it emerged that he lived by an 11th commandment: "Thou shalt not leave your parents or your analyst." How could Mr. M justify his lifelong need to prove that he was right to remain angry at his parents for leaving him when he was now planning "selfishly" to leave his analyst? The same situation had arisen at adolescence: when he and his friends went to Europe after graduating from high school, he broke down and had to return home. With this link to his own adolescence we will now turn to some clinical material from an adolescent case that helped the analyst understand and deal with Mr. M's inability to end his analysis.

Mary was taken into analysis following a medically serious suicide attempt. In an earlier paper (Novick, 1984) material from Mary's analysis was used to test and extend the findings from a previous study of seven such adolescents and confirmed that the suicide attempt, contrary to popular myth, was not a sudden impulsive act but the end point of a pathological regression that started in each case with the experience of failure to separate from the mother. At the beginning of Mary's analysis she never smiled, seldom spoke, and often sat with teeth clenched and legs trembling while she held in a rage that she later described as so powerful that it would overwhelm both patient and analyst and destroy everything.

At the end of her first year of analysis Mary remained totally dependent on her mother, sitting silently at meals and spending weekends and every evening in her room; other than studying, her only activity had been rearranging her furniture or trying to decide which side of the desk to put her pencils on. She was physically inhibited, looked like a prepubescent boy, and told of lifelong vows never to have boyfriends, never to marry, and never to have children. At the time the main concern was that Mary would become irretrievably psychotic or that she would kill herself. Eight years later the analysis ended by mutual agreement, with some shared sadness but mainly pride at what was achieved and confidence that she was on the path of progressive development. She had become an attractive, happy person, fulfilled in the areas of work, love, and play.

As a steady background to her many and varied conflicts was Mary's delusion of omnipotence and her desperate need to cling to an omnipotent self-image. Such fantasies defended against and compensated for lifelong feelings of helplessness, envy, jealousy, and rage. They allowed her to feel that she did not have to experience any of these painful affects since she was above it all, neither male nor female, neither child nor adult, but a being superior to all who could, if she so desired, do anything she wished to. Such fantasies can flourish relatively unchecked during latency, but adolescence brings internal and external challenges that force disturbed children, such as Mary, to even more desperate measures, such as suicide, to retain the delusion of omnipotence.

Mary started treatment helpless, dependent, and seemingly incapable of a single age-appropriate activity. Yet, quite consciously—though secretly—she felt omnipotently superior to all because she believed that she, unlike most people, including her depressed mother, could really kill herself. Like the other adolescents we studied before and since (Laufer and Laufer, 1984), Mary felt that her suicide attempt was a powerful, brave action that brought about important changes in her parents and her world. To her, suicide was a powerful, magical solution to all her conflicts and a manifestation of an omnipotent self-image.

As the work progressed, it became clear that Mary's primary pathology was not depression but an underlying severe masochistic disorder that subsumed both her depression and her suicidal behavior. The view we put forward concerning the formation of masochistic fantasies in the early school years (Novick and Novick, 1972, 1987) was confirmed in Mary's case, and our point of view that such fantasies involve omnipotence was underscored. Masochism and omnipotence are two sides of the same coin: the delusion of omnipotence can be maintained by masochistic, pain-seeking behavior such as suicide (Novick and Novick, in press). As Mary worked through the complex layers of functions and determinants of her masochism, she could experience and maintain pleasure for longer periods of time outside her analysis. The conflicts around pleasure became centered almost entirely in the analysis; she would feel happy and proud of some achievement until she walked in the door, and then would feel gloomy and bad.

There were many parallels between Mary and Mr. M. The analysis of Mr. M had also opened up the range of positive affects, and for him too these affects were kept outside the analysis. Even close to the end, Mr. M could maintain a cheerful, positive attitude no further than the threshold of the consulting room and by the time he was on the couch he was tense, confused, and depressed. As did Mary, Mr. M reacted to the end of analysis with a series of pain-seeking fantasies and actions aimed at simultaneously keeping and leaving, loving and hating, destroying and keeping the analyst safe. As with Mary, the multiple determinants and functions of Mr. M's masochism became focused on the imminence of really leaving during the terminal phase. He was terrified of facing the world alone as he once more externalized all his own functions of control, containment, and purpose onto the analyst. Mr. M idealized both the analyst and the relationship so that leaving was imbued with fantasies of unbearable pain and irreplaceable loss. In Mary's case, after working through the adaptive, defensive, and instinctual determinants of the masochism, we were left with the final motive for clinging to pain: her unwillingness to take leave of her omnipotent, magical self. It was this experience with Mary—and, by now, many suicidal and otherwise masochistic adolescents—that alerted us to the final determinant in Mr. M's interminable analysis. It took years to work through his inability to leave; finally, he could accept that he could do so without further trauma. We could then see more clearly that, ultimately, termination meant leaving his magical, omnipotent self. To leave analysis was to relinquish his omnipotent fantasy that he could have it all, do everything, and never have to choose. Because he was in analysis, Mr. M imagined that he could live an active, responsible adult life outside and still be a passive, irresponsible, angry child. Because he still experienced pain in the session, he felt entitled to live outside social expectations and even reality restrictions. He could be loving and still allow himself to be sadistic, he could be an adult man and a sulky child, he could be male and female; in sum, he could maintain the delusion of omnipotence. For Mr. M and for Mary, omnipotent fantasies were defensive responses to lifelong feelings of helplessness, especially in eliciting appropriate caretaking responses from their mothers. To both of them the converse of omnipotence was complete helplessness, blackness, and nothingness whereas the opposite of omnipotence, in fact, is competence. Competence is rooted in the child's inborn capacity to elicit a caretaking response from mother: the child's smile makes her smile, the child's cry of hunger makes her lactate and present her nipple. This is not a fantasy, a delusion of omnipotence; this is the root of competence, effectance, and self-esteem. Both Mary and Mr. M received intermittent love and care sufficient to keep them tied to people but not in a way that would enhance a feeling of confidence in their ability to elicit a necessary response from mother. Their mothers smiled only when they emerged from a depressive state and felt like smiling, not in response to the child's smile.

At least as important as a mother's empathic response to her child's signals is the capacity of the couple to tolerate and then repair the inevitable breaches in the empathic tie. Inevitable mismatches are reacted to by an "aversive response" in the infant (Lichtenberg, 1989) or by an angry response in the older child; with her love the ordinary mother can absorb and transform the child's anger into a dialectic for growth. In both Mary and Mr. M's cases these aversive, angry responses to mother's lack of empathy occasioned ever-increasing spirals of rage, guilt, and blame so that in the end these children were made to feel omnipotently responsible for mother's pain, helplessness, and inadequacy.

Mr. M described what he called a typical pattern of interaction between himself and his mother. He would come from school and put his books on the dining room table. His mother shouts that he is driving her crazy with his deliberate messiness and now she has such a blinding headache she'll have to take to her bed, they will have to make do with leftovers, and it's all his fault. He tells her that her cooking is so lousy he prefers leftovers. She collapses in tears, wails that she is totally inadequate and might as well kill herself. Terrified and guilty, he tries to make amends. He apologizes and takes his books to his room; she follows him, working herself into a fit of rage as she tells him he won't get away with it that easily, wait till father comes home. She recites a list of misdeeds that stretches back to infancy, when he was, according to her, "a whiny, demanding brat." By this point young Mr. M would become enraged and ask her why she couldn't be as cheerful and resourceful as the mother of his best friend. This remark, he knew, would devastate his mother, but the particular occasion he was recalling was one in which she had found a way of overpowering his most powerful weapon. She responded by saying that he had not only ruined her life and driven her to depression, suicide, and hospitalization but he had also ruined her marriage and she and father were discussing divorce. From that time forth he felt that he really could force them to divorce and then he would have to declare publicly which parent he wanted to be with.

Earlier, we described children, like Mary and Mr. M, for whom omnipotent fantasies serve to fill the space between the real and ideal mother. The fantasies are not aimed at enhancing the real capacities of self but at denying and transforming the pain and inadequacy of the mother–child relationship. Unable to elicit a smile with a smile, both Mary and Mr. M identified with mother's pain and imagined a special, unique relationship based on shared unhappiness. Only they understood mother's pain, and without them mother would be alone, unconnected to anyone. This omnipotent fantasy was a thread through the labyrinth of the analysis and emerged most clearly as the end of treatment approached. For example, Mary said, "When I'm happy I feel I'm not with you. To be unhappy is to be like you, to be with you, to sit quietly and depressed with the whole world right here in this room."

Mr. M said similar things many times. The analyst had learned from Mary that it is useless to challenge such fantasies directly, and Mr. M illustrated this point by saying that the analyst might not realize the unique nature of their relationship since he was probably at the peak of his health and success, but one day the analyst would get old, sick, and enfeebled and then realize that no other patient is as capable of understanding and empathizing with his pain as he is. Pain is the "open sesame" to this magical world, and through the experience of pain the omnipotent self can live on, a masochistic fantasy enshrined in the major religious systems.

Not to be omnipotent is, in Mr. M's words, "to be a piece of junk floating forever in the endless blackness of space." Any little action or interchange in treatment can be incorporated in an omnipotent fantasy to maintain power. So both Mary and Mr. M needed to stay in analysis to confirm their omnipotence, and then as omnipotent figures they carried the awesome responsibility for the well-being and survival of the analyst. They imagined that the only way to terminate was to make themselves the victim of the analyst's sadistic attack. A forced termination would actualize their masochistic fantasies, relieve them of responsibility and guilt and confirm their omnipotence, as we have seen repeatedly with adolescent patients who provoke their therapists to end the treatment (Novick and Novick, 1987).

How, then, can we bring about a growth-promoting end to a seemingly interminable situation? It would be simpleminded to propose a simple solution, especially in an analysis that extends beyond ten years. No one phase of development or set of conflicts carries the solution, and a multideterminant and multifunctional epigenetic approach, as attempted in our developmental study of masochism, is one we would recommend in order to capture the complexity of interminability. However, looked at from the vantage point of work with adolescents, the need to cling desperately to the fantasy of omnipotence stands out as an important factor in the interminability of analysis.

Our experience with adolescents such as Mary has convinced us that a major reason that termination is so frightening for adolescents is that these young people have not only the task of leaving infantile relationships with other people but must also take leave of the omnipotent self. We consider this to be a major task of adolescence; the avoidance of and regression from reality demands often seen in late adolescence relates to an inability to relinquish the omnipotent self and find pleasure and assurance in competent interactions with reality.

Mary, like everyone at the end of analysis, had to mourn the loss of the analyst as an object of desires from all levels of development and also as a real person who represented all her new-found accomplishments. But for Mary the most poignant and difficult task of mourning related to the loss of her omnipotent, grandiose self. This was the last battleground for her pathology and a final determinant for her conflict around pleasure. The experience of pleasure was a threat to her magical, omnipotent self. To have pleasure was to give up magical fantasies of control of the object and to interact in a real way with the real world. The real and the magical, the competent and omnipotent, selves became competing systems. As Mary allowed herself ever-increasing feelings of pride and pleasure, as she felt the relief and comfort of being in the real world, her omnipotent self receded proportionately.

Mary began playing basketball in the evenings, which she had done as a child. One day, after she had talked of her professional plans and the way they could be integrated with being married and her wish to have children, she said that she had decided that she didn't need basketball anymore. It turned out that while playing basketball she imagined that she was Magic Johnson, it was the final of the NBA championships, and she was putting in the winning basket. That night she dreamed of being in a championship game: she was jumping high, getting every ball, and putting in slam dunks—but she was very small, and each time she put the ball through the hoop her whole body went through. As she told the dream Mary began to cry. "That little person was wrong," she said; "that little person made me miserable all these years, but I'm going to miss her. I'm happier now but she could do things I can't do anymore. She could win championship games and she could cut her wrists." In analysis the inability to relinquish omnipotent fantasies of control over others will become manifest in either premature termination or interminable analysis.

Mary and Mr. M had not been able to shift the source of pleasure from omnipotent fantasy control of others to realistic achievements, as Robert did in the process of resolution of his oedipus complex;

nor had they achieved consolidation in the latency phase, as we saw in Erica's capacity to enjoy the exercise of her ego functions in the working alliance. Without these alternative sources of pleasure and self-esteem, Mary and Mr. M coped with the reality demands of adolescence by recourse to pain-initiated omnipotent fantasies.

The fact that termination of adult cases may require prior work on the adolescent pattern of premature leave-taking has been noted, and now, with Mary's material in mind, we suggest that the interminable analysis of adults such as Mr. M involves the patient's having to do what was not done in adolescence—take leave of an omnipotent self, give up the impossible task of controlling people magically, and find pleasure in the exercise of real skills in a real world. Omnipotent fantasies will not be relinquished easily, if at all, but through analysis we can allow for the emergence of a competing system of pleasure and self-esteem alongside the omnipotent system based on pain, avoidance of reality, and delusion. As Mr. M said near the end of his analysis: "It's my life—I have only one life and I have to choose. It's hard to admit that I was wrong, hard to admit that my pain buys me nothing but aspirin. But then I never knew that I had a choice, that I could choose to live a real life, with real pleasure."

References

Anthony, E. J. (1986), The contributions of child psychoanalysis to psychoanalysis. *The Psychoanalytic Study of the Child*, 41:61–87. New Haven, CT: Yale University Press.

Anzieu, D. (1987), Some alterations of the ego which make analyses interminable. *Internat. J. Psycho-Anal.*, 68:9–20.

Burgner, M. (1988), Analytic work with adolescents—terminable or interminable. *Internat. J. Psycho-Anal.*, 69:179–218.

Freud, A. (1965), Normality and pathology in childhood. *The Writings of Anna Freud*, 6. New York: International Universities Press.

———— (1970), Child analysis as a subspecialty of psychoanalysis. *The Writings of Anna Freud*, 6:204–219. New York: International Universities Press.

Freud, S. (1937), Analysis terminable and interminable. *Standard Edition*, 23:216–253. London: Hogarth Press, 1964.

Klauber, J. (1977), Analyses that cannot be terminated. *Internat. J. Psycho-Anal.*, 58:473–477.

Laufer, M. & Laufer, M. E. (1984), *Adolescence and Developmental Breakdown*. New Haven, CT: Yale University Press.

Lichtenberg, J. D. (1985), *Psychoanalysis and Infant Research*. Hillsdale, NJ: The Analytic Press.

———— (1989), *Psychoanalysis and Motivation*. Hillsdale, NJ: The Analytic Press.

Meissner, W. (1989), The viewpoint of the devil's advocate. In: *The Significance of Infant Observational Research for Clinical work with Children, Adolescents, and*

Adults, ed. S. Dowling & A. Rothstein. Madison, CT: International Universities Press, pp. 175–195.

Novick, J. (1976), Termination of treatment in adolescence. *The Psychoanalytic Study of the Child,* 31:389–414. New Haven, CT: Yale University Press.

———— (1982a), Termination: Themes and issues. *Psychoanal. Inq.,* 2:329–365.

———— (1982b), Varieties of transference in the analysis of an adolescent. *Internat. J. Psycho-Anal.,* 63:139–148.

———— (1984), Attempted suicide in adolescence. In: *Suicide in the Young,* ed. H. Sudak, A. Ford, N. Rushforth. London: John Wright, pp. 115–137.

———— (1988), The timing of termination. *Internat. Rev. Psycho-Anal.,* 14:307–318.

———— (1989), How does infant research affect our clinical work with adolescents? In: *The Significance of Infant Observational Research for Clinical work with Children, Adolescents, and Adults,* ed. S. Dowling & A. Rothstein. Madison, CT: International Universities Press, pp. 27–39.

———— (1990a), The adolescent process and adult treatment. In: *Child and Adolescent Analysis,* ed. S. Dowling. Madison, CT: International Universities Press, pp. 81–94.

———— (1990b), Comments on termination in child, adolescent, and adult psycho-analysis. *The Psychoanalytic Study of the Child,* 45. 419–436. New Haven, CT: Yale University Press.

Novick, J. & Novick, K.K. (1972), Beating fantasies in children. *Internat. J. Psycho-Anal.,* 53:237–242.

———— ———— (in press), Masochism and the delusion of omnipotence from a developmental perspective. *J. Amer. Psychoanal. Assn.*

Novick, K. K. & Novick, J. (1987), The essence of masochism. *The Psychoanalytic Study of the Child,* 42:353–384. New Haven, CT: Yale University Press.

Pine, F. (1985), *Developmental Theory and Clinical Process.* New Haven, CT: Yale University Press.

Tyson, P. (1989), Two approaches to infant research. In: *The Significance of Infant Observational Research for Clinical Work with Children, Adolescents, and Adults,* ed. S. Dowling & A. Rothstein. Madison, CT: International Universities Press, pp. 27–39.

14

Issues of Termination in the Psychoanalysis of the Severely Disturbed Adolescent

Marion Burgner

The content and process of termination reflect the capacity of the adolescent to become separate from the analyst as well as from the primary objects of infancy and childhood (Burgner, 1988). Becoming emotionally separate from the internal parents is, of course, one of the main tasks of the normal adolescent developmental process, a process that sometimes continues well into the individual's twenties. Other normal developmental tasks for the adolescent include assuming responsibility for the body and acceptance of the body's sexual needs; establishment of a masculine or feminine identity; assuming responsibility for feelings, fantasies, thinking, and actions toward the self and others, as well as for decisions and actions that will affect the adolescent's own future; choosing peer friendships; and developing the capacity, not necessarily realized, for finding and relating to a partner with whom the adolescent can experience a reciprocal emotional and sexual relationship.

There are, however, adolescents encountered in our analytic work for whom the prospect of psychic separation involves such primitive anxiety that it presages annihilation; for them, separation anxiety thus takes on the terror of annihilatory anxiety. Analysis reveals that such adolescents have not had adequate expectable experiences of appropriate relationships within the developmental phases. Instead, what seems to result is minimal, if any, neurotic conflict and ensuing distortions in development. By this I suggest that there have been difficulties of an impacting nature from infancy and quite often virtually no oedipal experience, conflict, or resolution, since the parents—particularly the mothers—of these adolescents are invasively and permanently present in their children's internal and external lives. In turn, these children cannot tolerate the ordinary developmental process of becoming separate and, greedily yet with overpowering hostility, have to retain the parental objects, as part of their inner world. These developmental distortions, continuing from infancy onward, culminate in stasis around adolescence, in "a foreclosure in the developmental process" (Laufer and Laufer, 1984). In fact, what appears to be a surfeit of adolescent disturbance is, in essence, a pseudo adolescence, just as the preceding developmental phases too have carried the "as if" hallmark. Disturbance is palpable in the primitive (preoedipal) nature of these adolescents' enactments to the self and others. It frequently proves impossible for them to use the analytic sessions for exploration and understanding; rather they are used for attacks on the analyst and the aims of analysis at a primary process level.

These developmental distortions become organized in the breakdown in adolescence, obviously not the first severe disturbance in the person's life, and are particularly evident in their incapacity for psychological separateness from the parents, in the chaos of their internal object relations and affects, and in faults in psychic structuralization. One of the prime analytic aims is to reopen the adolescent process—that is, to try and undo, at least partially, the premature foreclosure in development by consistent interpretation of whatever signs of conflict one may begin to discern around these issues in the transference—and eventually to facilitate a more adaptive, less destructive closure of that process.

A case could, perhaps, be made for not taking into analysis adolescents with such a degree of disturbance, but frequently analysis presents for them an end-of-the-road intervention. Most other treatments have already been tried and have been made to fail by the collusive efforts of the parents and the adolescent. Analysis sometimes seems to be welcomed by the parents, since someone else, at last, is apparently taking responsibility for their suicidal or grossly disturbed child. The parents, however, often continue to play a destructive part in the analysis, and I think one cannot really do effective analytic work until these adolescents are living apart from their invasive parents.

In this chapter I shall first briefly discuss two adolescents: one terminated treatment prematurely but, perhaps because of her one-year analytic experience, eventually accomplished some measure of closure of the adolescent process; with the second there was a mutually agreed-upon ending and an alternative closure of the adolescent process was completed within the analysis. A third case, which I shall discuss in more clinical detail, is one in which I proposed an ending, originally unilaterally, in the face of the adolescent's fantasy of an interminable analysis.

Cara

In a clinical paper (Burgner, 1989), on an adolescent who ended analysis prematurely, I have described a 17-year-old girl, Cara,[1] who spent several hours a day in a frenzied and compulsive cycle of bingeing and vomiting. I understood that the pervasive anxiety she experienced at the prospect of becoming psychologically separate was temporarily annulled by repetitive attacks on her internal objects and on the body/self. In this perverse solution, which evolved as a central part of her daily life, the fantasied destruction and revitalization of the object constantly recurred; simultaneously, Cara omnipotently kept the object always available and unseparated from the self. She ended her analysis with this central dilemma apparently unresolved; the question remained of how she could become psychologically separate from her parents without destroying them and herself in the process. *Suicide attempts seem to occur frequently in adolescents who can negotiate neither separateness nor an entry into young adulthood.*

Perhaps Cara's awareness, on leaving analysis, that she had not annihilated me was of limited but continuing help to her. She accepted my participation in her referral to an inpatient unit for anorexic patients though she discharged herself after a few weeks and then made a halfhearted attempt to return to analysis. Over the next four years Cara asked for two interviews. In the first she told me that she had moved away from her parents and had a boyfriend, but wanted admission to a different hospital to deal with her "habit," which was as compulsive as ever. Her refrain throughout the interview was on the uselessness of the many and varied treatments offered to her so far. She was in touch with her own destructiveness toward all therapy and its practitioners but was ineluctably compelled to put such destruction into operation. She struck me then as quite inaccessible to further therapeutic help, and I was certainly

---

[1]Treated under the auspices of the Centre for Research into Adolescent Breakdown, Moses Laufer, Director. The Center investigates psychological breakdown in adolescence through psychoanalytic treatment.

neither analytically nor personally comfortable with such awareness since failure was a prominent feature in her accusatory transference and in my counterresponse.

Two years later Cara came to see me again. Now age 22, she looked very different from our last meeting. Her weight and appearance were normal, and I learned that her menses had returned. Cara was neither attacking nor provocative, and she was no longer preoccupied with suicidal thoughts. Her professional success pleased her, she lived quite apart from her disturbed parents, and she was buying her own flat. While her parents were still locked together in their sadistic quarreling, she seemed more separate from them and believed that the more she stayed out of their lives, "the more they would just have to get on with it and with each other." This last comment was indeed an advance on the sexual triangulation so carefully and erotically fashioned by the three of them against their experience of my threatened incursion during her analysis. At that time Cara had characterized herself as "a pawn, as glue between my parents; without me they would fall apart"; indeed, without them she had feared her own disintegration too. She went on to tell me now of her distress at the ending of a two-year relationship and of the recent beginning of a new attachment, fearing that her "addiction" might now prove an encumbrance. She wanted me to resume therapy, though not analysis, because she still felt compelled to binge and vomit once daily (unlike the thrice-daily episodes during her analysis).

I referred Cara to a colleague, and she started therapy with him. I know little of this therapy, except that the bingeing and vomiting were reduced further to once a week; also, there ensued a stormy, promiscuous time and an abortion, which left her very depressed. But the capacity for depressive affect, that is, *experiencing feelings* rather than eruptive, unpremeditated action against the self, is an advance in the treatment of such young adults. Doubtless, this abortion was linked dynamically to the issue of her ending her analysis with me, as well as to the premature ending of her concurrent therapy. When her analyst left London, Cara decided to seek further therapy, now three times, rather than once, a week. So, nine years later she is still trying to make some order in her internal and external worlds. I do not think she could have continued with this endeavor without that minimum of separateness she had accomplished by the age of 22, when adolescence as a developmental phase was, more or less, over for her; as a result, there was for her an alternative to the foreclosure with which we had initially struggled in her analysis and which she continued to work on after she left me.

Olga

Olga, who started analysis as a self-referral and as a last resort in her late adolescence, participated in a mutually agreed-upon analytic ending (Burgner, 1988). Addicted to injectable heroin and other drugs, overwhelmed by two suicide attempts and an inpatient stay in a psychiatric hospital, and resorting to promiscuity in her despairing search for mothering, Olga presented herself as a distant and depressed, yet very needy, adolescent. She told me in our first interview that she thought she was mad: she frequently heard voices, mostly at night but also during the day; these voices, experienced as emanating from her father or from acquaintances, accused and attacked her or completed her thoughts in a more competent way, she felt, than she was able to do for herself. Our first tenuous contact occurred when I suggested to her that, rather than being mad, she was projectively expressing her own feelings about herself. Just as she had given up ownership of her adolescent body, she similarly experienced her mind as useless and without function, given over to these disembodied voices.

Two years later, by which time she had given up drugs, Olga was to talk of some of the aims of her drug taking and of her dilemma about her internal objects *as she experienced them*—that is, the invasive, devouring mother and the excited, unprotective father: drugs were taken in to subdue these internal objects, to prevent them from consuming her. Olga observed, "Taking drugs was the only way of separating myself from my mother." But it was also, paradoxically, a way of remaining at one with her parents, barely differentiated from their lack of control and incoherence. Once she felt some measure of trust in me as a person who would not invade and engulf her and with whom she could identify the sane part of herself, Olga could more safely entertain negative feelings about me and was able to report dreams about my operating on her with intricate surgical instruments—and even about my leaving her and her subsequent survival.

Olga could also, in the transference, try to engage me in a continuing, defensive, sadomasochistic battle, inviting me to take her over and direct her life, since she was ceaselessly frightened of her own success and accomplishments lest I lay claim to her achievements for myself. When she could allow herself to reclaim such control for her own use, she no longer felt herself a helpless, undifferentiated part of her parents; she could begin, probably for the first time in her life, to experience a sense of self-ownership. In effect, she was experiencing an adolescence.

By her mid-twenties, Olga considered—quite appropriately, I think—that she was ready to take responsibility for herself as an adult. She had completed a good standard university degree and needed to concentrate on her personal and professional life. She also felt that she wished to move from adolescence into young adulthood *on her own*, and this, I was sure, was a developmental step that needed my acquiescence and support. I considered that closure of the adolescent process could now be facilitated, rather than maintained as a fluid and open-ended developmental phase within the context of the analysis, and so we worked toward a planned termination a year hence, after six years of analysis. From the very occasional contacts she has with me now, I understand that Olga's life progresses well.

At the time, I reflected that such a termination, where work still obviously remained to be done, has some similarity to that of child analysis: we place the child on the path to normality; we do not complete the process in the consulting room. Anna Freud (1965) writes of the immature child's "urge to complete development"; in individuals in whom we feel analytic work has led to an alternative, more adaptive closure of the adolescent process, we can place some reliance on that urge and on the adolescents' newly acquired ego strength to continue the process on their own.

Harvey

Harvey was referred to the Centre for Research into Adolescent Breakdown at the age of 18. He spent three years in analysis with a male colleague who left; Harvey was then referred to me. His analysis ended when he was nearly 26, and I shall describe the termination phase.

I think that Harvey showed an almost intractable foreclosure in adolescent development, a fixed and virtually immutable disturbance with many perverse and delusional features. In effect, Harvey used analysis to accommodate his anal universe (Chasseguet-Smirgel, 1985) to a worrying degree, since he used the daily analytic arena and the rapidly evolving perverse transference to express his bizarre fantasies and his eruptive anal sexuality. He cherished the fantasy of an interminable analysis, with me as the transfixed and enthralled partner/mother in his fecal world. He had felt inseparable from his male analyst by virtue of his fantasy of the analyst's being inside him with his penis up Harvey's anus. Such an interminable analysis would also enable him to remain an adolescent forever, that is, an adolescent who differed little—apart from a measure of functional genitality—from the favored infant and child of his adoring, similarly unseparated mother.

I have described in an earlier paper (Burgner, 1988) Harvey's unremitting denigration of me and of the analysis and his daily threats that he would kill himself once I failed him. He had, in fact, been referred to the Centre after an overdose following the ending of once-weekly therapy, and he had effectively used threats of suicide against his mother since he was four. It emerged over the first two years that Harvey located my anticipated failure in the sphere of *change*—not in my capacity to facilitate psychic change in him but in my capacity to change him concretely into a woman. Describing the transsexual syndrome, Limentani (1979) has noted how the acquisition of a new feminine body reinforces "the illusion of being forever fused with mother" (p. 148). He desperately sought to become a woman, with me as his sexual partner, and his dreams and masturbation fantasies were replete with scenarios of two women having sex together, a woman having sex with an animal, and two prepubertal girls coupling together. One dream—and there were dozens like this—was of his watching two women prostitutes in a pornographic sex shop penetrating each other with plastic penises; he took one of their penises and inserted it into his own vagina.

To end analysis would involve Harvey in movement away from the omnipotent and primitive bisexual view of himself toward a sexual orientation that filled him with terror—homosexuality. His confusion about his sexual identity and his disavowal of his being *only* male may be traced back to early toddlerhood (12 to 18 months) when genital differences are recognized and internalized. Then, as McDougall (1989) has written, the individual is marked as belonging

> to one clan only and excluded forever from the other. It is evident that this knowledge will not be acquired without conflict, for the narcis-sistic and megalomanic child inevitably wishes to possess both sexes as well as the powers and privileges attributed to the personalities and genital organs of each parent. Much psychic work is required in order to carry out the task of mourning that will eventually allow the child to accept the narcissistically unacceptable difference and assume its monosexual destiny [p 205].

An ending would thus involve Harvey in contemplating the sort of psychic work he had been unable to begin as a small child. And an ending would also involve him in having to make a choice in the nature and quality of his relationships. As long as he remained in analysis, the transference siphoned off his indubitably perverse way of relating and postponed the inevitable decision of whether or not perverse behavior within the safety of the analysis would escalate to a real perversion enacted in the external world.

An issue of central importance in ending was, further, my own conviction that I could not, and in fact should not, accompany him in his continuing disavowal of inevitable separateness from me; further, I could not endlessly collude in his perverse use of me and of the analysis for immediate sadistic gratification rather than for acquiring some measure, however small, of understanding. The reality of experiencing an ending, of leaving and being left by me, had, I considered, to be addressed since neither analysis nor adolescence is interminable. As Anzieu (1987) has observed, "The more the analyst is cathected as an absolute and permanent part-object—whether as an object of accusations, narcissistic expectation, illusion of completeness or functional support—the more liable psychoanalysis is to become interminable . . ." (p. 15).

There were yet other issues with which I became increasingly concerned: how effectively reliable was my analytic control in the face of Harvey's relentless attempts to force me into the complementary role relationship (Sandler, 1976) of the adoring mother who passively and masochistically accepted whatever he inflicted upon me; and to what extent could I tolerate and make analytic use of my hate in the counter-transference (Winnicott, 1947) rather than enact it? Could I, in fact, continue to maintain an analytic persona that functioned adequately for this greedy and destructive infant/child/adolescent/young man, or was I, in response to his envious attempts to render me incapable and helpless as an analyst, being unduly revengeful in proposing a termination date? Was I being coerced, within a role-responsiveness context, into abandoning him, an outcome that he was terrified of throughout the analysis and yet was omnipotently convinced could never happen? Emotionally, if not perhaps also physically, invaded by his mother—and Glasser's concept of the "core complex" is of relevance here (Glasser, 1979)—Harvey did not feel capable of having a separate adult existence, a separate body and mind. As he came to understand that I claimed such separateness for myself, his destructive envy of me became intolerable, leading to his terror that I would, in retaliation, abandon him.

He accusingly declaimed in one session that his life was awful, he had no friends, and he was failing his college studies. He blamed me constantly and acrimoniously for the inadequacies in his life. (He had, in fact, dropped out of college in his first treatment, but then, with much difficulty and analytic work, resumed his studies during his analysis with me.) To this I responded that he was telling me too of his feeling that, once analysis was over, there would be no hope left in his life and that, as he had always said, he would kill himself. I elaborated on the delusional quality of this plan: that he would also kill me when he killed himself and there would be no experience of separateness for him, since we would be together forever. He went on to talk of a dream: he was kissing Jane passionately (Jane was a girl with whom he had a mythical relationship that never took place), but all he tasted was mucus. It reminded him of when he was a snotty-nosed child. Then his alarm went off, and he pressed the pause button, trying desperately to return into the dream. Following this account he went straight back to his customary ruminations—he doesn't give to people and therefore they tire of him, this had happened with Jane, his college work was at a standstill, and so on— for ten minutes. Then he lay back, well satisfied with this well-worn diatribe. I responded that I was puzzled that here was a dream in which he talked about the taste of mucus and yet he wanted so much to get back into it. This caused him to pause, and I elaborated on the dilemma he felt with me: whether to be the grown-up man feeling passionate about a woman or to continue being a snotty-nosed small boy. He agreed with this but again ruminated about his college work. I interpreted how he was doing the same to me and analysis, as well as to his studies: he was essentially claiming he would be able to *start* analysis, to *start* being a man with me, to *start* studying, once each opportunity was finished. He said that after his analysis was over he would give himself six months, and if there were no change, he would seriously consider killing himself; there was no point in living and there was no existence after death. Such suicidal thoughts were always uttered dramatically, not sadly and hope-lessly, and yet, of course, we both knew he had actively tried to kill himself when he was 17.

I think that my introduction of the issue of termination well over a year in advance, though Harvey himself eventually set and reset the actual date, brought some sense of reality into the delusional transference to which he was so complacently attached. The further issues that came up in the termination phase, some of which I shall now discuss, were, in fact, not markedly different from those in the preceding phases of the analysis, but perhaps they emerged with more anxiety and urgency, with some beginnings of conflict and shifting awareness on Harvey's part that they needed to be worked on rather than lived out endlessly and without meaning in the transference.

Following an unusually productive few sessions at the beginning of the last year of analysis, when Harvey seemed temporarily to have called a truce, he reacted with terror to personal progress and feelings of closeness with me and relapsed into his more predictable contemptuous and nullifying stance. As happened so often, he polarized our analytic exchanges—either they were dead and without affective life or he tried to suffuse them with sexual excitement. Harvey spent the first half of the session in a state of narcissistic and savage rage. Then, calming down somewhat, he talked in a rather desultory way about not studying and about how he continually feels for the "grease blocks" under the skin all over his body and squeezes them or just thinks about something else rather than his college work. He said he had a dream about a girl, Jo, but there was nothing to the dream. I eventually said that he was saying he was frightened of having got close to me and was now taking refuge in this protective, self-destructive behavior. I also tried to work with him on his rage that he could not continue always fantasying being inside me and that this understanding had prompted his retreat from the recent advances in his life. I drew a parallel between me and the myth he had of the girl Jo in the dream, somebody he saw once every two years but who remained central to his fantasy life. His rage with me at the prospect of becoming separate became very apparent in what he then said: he was fantasying that he was looking after the small brother of a dead friend when the child threw himself out of Harvey's arms and under a train. He thought he was threatening me with a similar fate if I let him go.

I think the material that follows illustrates graphically the poly-morphously perverse fragmented experiences and thoughts that flooded Harvey's mind and with which he, in turn, flooded me. He started one session with the comment that he had been thinking of "having a constructive relationship" with me but it very quickly became sexual in his mind. He then related a dream: he was sitting in the kitchen, and his mother was pregnant with a pair of legs coming out of her. At this point he confused the hymen with the placenta and went on to say that the baby was then born and that it was a girl called Georgina. He mentioned another dream, about his childhood friend George. After a long silence, I remarked that he seemed to be talking about impossibilities—whether he could have a relationship with me as a lover, whether his analyst/mother could have a baby with him, and whether he could always remain a baby for us. He did not respond directly to this and talked instead about what he had done with George as a child: they had defecated

together on the front porch and left the pile for his mother; they had
mixed up dog excrement with their hands in a bucket and played
with it; and they had been fascinated with and played in George's
cesspit. I suggested that he was attempting to escape from what I had
said about the impossibilities of his present life by trying to excite
me with anal concerns. Harvey observed that sharing this anal
excitement was something he always did with his mother, and yet
again repeated the memory of them laughing together as she talked
about catching the feces of geriatric patients in her hands when she
was a nurse. He began wildly to accuse me of not responding to what
he was saying and adroitly sabotaged the rest of the session. He
struck me as being confused and quite unreachable.

Harvey opened the next session with a dream: he was on a beach
in a landscape with deep, mysterious tunnels, watching an Asian
woman swimming; she reached the shore with her breasts and he
contrived to touch her breasts with his hand. Immediately afterward
he was in a large hotel and perhaps having sex with this woman, but
then he was next door with a different girl and arguing about a bill
she was making out for sexual services, telling her she should not
charge him for these; she agreed and gave him a deep passionate kiss
instead. But when he returned to the first woman, he found that her
breasts were no longer firm and young but wrinkled. His associations were to a small Asian girl in his holiday job in the restaurant
whose conversation he had overheard, though she did not know he
was listening. He commented that placing his hand so that it met her
breasts in the dream was like watching a pornographic video and
becoming a woman between the two women on the film. He then
debated at length whether he should leave the session early to go to
his lecture, observing that he was trying to be special, to be a woman
for the young male lecturer, who might or might not be homosexual.
He berated me for doing nothing with the session, though he had not
paused in his flow of talk since coming in. I said that the dream
seemed connected with what we had talked about the day before,
that he was confused whether he wanted an analytic relationship
with me or whether he could break out of such confines and have a
sexual relationship with me without payment. He went back to the
tunnels in the dream and thought they were "vaginal tunnels."
However, from my knowledge of his scopophilic fantasies of tun-
neling into me and of then taking up residence inside me, I
suggested that he was also thinking about his own anus and the anus
of the other person (originally, the idealized anus and fecal mess he
shared with his mother) and that he could not really bear to think
about women with real vaginas when he felt such a lack in himself.

I talked about the confusion he felt about his body, and he expostu-
lated in the form of a question: "Why can't I come to terms with my
confusion about having a vagina?" He then realized what he had
said, and I agreed with him when he observed that he still saw
himself as quite godlike and exempt from having to come to terms
with himself as a man in the real world.

As I have emphasized, a striking aspect in Harvey's analysis was
his eroding destructiveness, compounded by a primitive terror of
annihilation, and untempered by ambivalence and conflict. Almost
all sessions carried this hallmark of destructiveness, a bid to defend
himself against his feelings of need for and dependence on me.
Harvey said that if he acknowledged his need of and his liking for
me, these feelings would immediately turn to a sexual longing for
me; that would mean he was a pervert, since I was so much older
than he. Or he would be humiliated, he said, since I would refuse his
sexual advances. He spent the entire next three sessions contemptuously belittling me, his parents, and everyone else within reach.
But by the end of the week, he was more subdued, perhaps a little in
touch with his feelings of emptiness and panic. The issue became
one of how he set up his father to be stupid and incompetent, and I
interpreted that he had not allowed me and his father any masculine
autonomy and success or a secure place in his mind. He blustered
wildly in his protestations about this, but I firmly stood my ground;
I said that part of the trouble was surely that his parents had always
allowed him to treat them in a cruel and denigrating way (I think
they were probably frightened of him), that they had never been able
to say to him, "No, that's enough." Three times Harvey, despite my
pointing out the mistake, repeated this as "No, not enough." I
consistently took up his feeling that he had never had enough
opportunity to express his sadism and his conviction that his parents
had invariably and masochistically to accommodate him. I talked
too about his panic that I was, in effect, proposing an end to the
analysis by saying, "No, that's enough" and that contained within
his despair was a growing awareness of his dependence on me.
Finally, in that session, Harvey began to become somewhat aware of
his feelings about the analysis ending and my saying that it was time
for us to stop.

As the issue of ending became a reality (in fact still many months
ahead but for Harvey as if it were tomorrow), the panic, the suicidal
threats, and the degradation of me and of the analytic work became
even more unremitting. He seemed determined to kill off that which
he could not permanently possess, thus protecting himself against a
growing awareness of loneliness and depression.

Harvey's conviction about my daily enslavement to him (as he experienced his mother's behavior toward him and his father) was germane to the analysis, as was his destruction of what I gave him and his triumph at getting such a bargain. In his mind I was the Jewish prostitute, forced to tolerate his perverse treatment of me while he paid the Centre a parsimonious donation for my services. (He was—defensively—imbued with racist prejudice, against Jews particularly but against other minorities too, and was convinced I was Jewish.) This bargain seeking reflected how Harvey greedily, but secretly, took whatever he could from others (the analyst, parents, lecturers at college, girls he met for an evening) yet was terrified of giving in return; as long as he evaded mutuality, he avoided acknowledging his need of the other. Acceptance of the possibility, let alone the pleasure, of learning from the analyst and others would interfere with fantasies of his godlike omnipotence. He reflected that he had always been like this, recalling a photograph taken when he was one year old, "sitting with staring, triumphant eyes as if I am even then emperor of the world." The emphasis was on his narcissistic specialness for me, either in various superhuman guises or in the sense of being so maimed and damaged that I would feel morally bound to keep him in analysis forever. Then he would be able to fulfil his fantasy of becoming me so that he would be both analyst and analysand, permanently and inextricably unseparated from me. I think this is a similar phenomenon to one described by Segal (1988) of a patient with an underlying fantasy that caused him to stay in treatment for a long time. She writes of her patient's conviction that "analysis was, or would end in, a marriage between us—a marriage in which he would fuse with me and eventually would become me" (p. 168).

Harvey defensively tried to deal with his increasing homosexual panic by renewed degradation of women. He dreamed of women in their nakedness but dressed up as chickens ready for the oven, dancing in front of him. I interpreted how he felt that the analyst, in fact all women, were trussed-up birds ready for him, for the plucking and the eating. He talked of a girl who, he thought, was wasting herself by working with mentally and physically handicapped children when they all ought to be immediately killed off. He wished to pursue an eugenics policy of killing the handicapped, just as the Nazis had done, and I interpreted his own feelings of being handicapped and monstrous and afraid I would find him equally so. He then recalled a comment I had made a long time before, namely, that there was something about his older brother that frightened him and therefore he rarely mentioned him. He knew, he continued, that the Nazis sent homosexuals to the concentration camps, and he talked more freely than before of intense sexual play between him and his brother from latency until he was about 14. He added that, like himself, his brother had also tried to have sex with horses. He related a fantasy elaborated during their sexual contacts of mutual masturbation and fellatio: they were both strapped down on an immobile rack and in front of them was a revolving rack of women who were also strapped down; they had sex with each of the women in turn in order to impregnate them and create their own master race. I thought silently that this fantasy was chilling, as indeed I had experienced the whole tenor of the session. I interpreted that he was telling me how difficult he found it to think of himself as a warm-blooded man wishing for a mutual relationship with a woman and that he felt, instead, compelled to fill his life with such mechanical fantasies, which not only degraded me and other women but himself as well. This, I went on, was very much his dilemma in analysis: whether to tie me down and bash away at me while he felt equally tied down by me, or to allow a more mutual interaction to occur.

In the closing sessions of the analysis Harvey brought a number of dreams, which he was unusually prepared to work on with me. Perhaps by this time the ending of the analysis had assumed some reality in his mind. Arising from one dream, he observed that he had "no history of self-restraint," an issue for him of setting limits, which, as I have described earlier, had become important. He linked this lack in himself with what he surmised he had done to me throughout his analysis. He swung between feelings that analysis had helped him and that he had destroyed it completely. He also noted the external gains: he had been living away from home for one and a half years and he was in the final year of college.

Harvey observed that he had not made love to a woman for over a year (he had had a relationship lasting three months with a visiting student from another country) and that perhaps the trouble was that he did not really want a relationship; he was impotent when he started analysis with me. However, he continued, he did want a relationship, he did want real friends, but only after the analysis was over, after he was independent of me; in fact, he looked forward to the ending with some relief since this would actually be the first time in his life that he would be independent. He went on to say that the previous night he had tried to excite himself with the fantasy of a woman having sex with a dog but he found it did not work and he wasn't really interested. He thought his fantasies were much more heterosexual than they had been. He said he knew he had insisted on stopping the analysis early (four months early, in fact) and that I would have gone on to the arranged date but he felt he had to assert himself over this. I accepted this wish in him, and I also acknowledged the shared feeling we both had that it was indeed time to stop.

In the last session Harvey felt safe enough to talk again about his homosexual attachment to his brother and we were able to go back to their fantasy of fathering a master race together. He said—rather too compliantly—that he hated to think he was attracted to evil. I responded that this was a dilemma for him; he had been immersed in his sadistic fantasies, and it was important for him to be in touch with his conflict, of what he had been so irresistibly attracted to and yet now perhaps was beginning to repudiate. He seemed relieved by this. He talked of being optimistic about the future and hoped he would be able to use what he had gotten from analysis. He thanked me when he got up to go and we shook hands. He said he was sorry he had made it such a hard and difficult analysis for me, and I replied that I thought it had been thus for him as well. I was interested that I had no anticipated feeling of relief that this was my last session with him. Rather, I beguiled myself into wondering whether he might *now* use analysis, though I knew this was something of a counterresponsive illusion on my part. Harvey had to be given the opportunity for more appropriate closure of the adolescent process and the chance to try to live without analysis.

Summary

The three adolescents I have described were not able to use enough positive and pleasurable experiences of infancy and childhood to move forward into and through a developmental adolescence. Their inner worlds were, in the main, desolate and lonely, inhabited by objects who—as they experienced them—threatened any progress they might make toward independence. It was safer, then, to remain in the delusionally invulnerable world of primitive affective enactment toward the self and internal objects (bingeing and vomiting; taking drugs; frenetic, perverse behavior) than to undertake the much more hazardous and inherently painful tasks of gaining autonomy and establishing the relationships of young adulthood. I have suggested in this chapter that unless such adolescents can be analytically helped toward an *alternative, more adaptive closure of the adolescent developmental process*—that is, alternative to the *foreclosure* with which they presented—they remain marooned in their primitive, dispossessed worlds and they cannot contemplate a separate internal life for themselves, a life that encompasses the emotional loss of the primary objects. Another way of characterizing such an analytic process would be in terms of attempting to lessen the pervasive pressure of primitive anxieties, fantasies, and enactments and to facilitate development of a psychic organization that has a more oedipal emphasis, an organization in which the terror of and overwhelming wish for the mother have receded and the father is recognized as having a more active yet protective internal role.

Of the three adolescents it was only Olga who accomplished such an alternative closure within the analysis. Cara was enabled to proceed, after her premature termination, to some measure of alternative closure. And Harvey moved in the analysis from delusional and perverse fantasies and primitive functioning toward a closure that would perhaps allow him more choice in his sexual orientation and relationships and that could also enable him later in his adulthood to seek further analytic help.

References

Anzieu, D. (1987), Some alterations of the ego which make analyses interminable. *Internat. J. Psycho-Anal.*, 68:9–19.

Burgner, M. (1988), Analytic work with adolescents: Terminable and interminable. *Internat. J. Psycho-Anal.*, 69:179–187.

———— (1989), Cara: The destruction of an analysis—treatment of an adolescent with bulimic and vomiting symptoms. In: *Developmental Breakdown and Psychoanalytic Treatment in Adolescence*, ed. M. Laufer & M. E. Laufer. New Haven, CT: Yale University Press, pp. 43–54.

Chasseguet-Smirgel, J. (1985), *Creativity and Perversion*. London: Free Association Books.

Freud, A. (1965), *Normality and Pathology in Childhood: Assessment of Development*. New York: International Universities Press.

Glasser, M. (1979), Some aspects of the role of aggression in the perversions. In: *Sexual Deviation*, ed. I. Rosen. Oxford: Oxford University Press, pp. 278–305.

Laufer, M. & Laufer, M. E. (1984), *Adolescence and Developmental Breakdown*. New Haven, CT: Yale University Press.

Limentani, A. (1979), The significance of transsexualism in relation to some basic psychoanalytic concepts. In: *Between Freud and Klein*. London: Free Associations, 1989, pp. 133–154.

McDougall, J. (1989), The dead father: On early psychic trauma and its relation to disturbance in sexual identity and in creative activity. *Internat. J. Psycho-Anal.*, 70:205–219.

Sandler, J. (1976), Counter-transference and role-responsiveness. *Internat. Rev. Psycho-Anal.*, 3:43–47.

Segal, H. (1988), Sweating it out. *The Psychoanalytic Study of the Child*, 43:167–175. New Haven, CT: Yale University Press.

Winnicott, D. W. (1947), Hate in the counter-transference. In: *Collected Papers: Through Paediatrics to Psychoanalysis*. London: Tavistock, 1958, pp. 194–203.

15

Termination in Child Psychoanalysis: Criteria from Within the Sessions

Paulina F. Kernberg

Termination is a critical phase in psychoanalysis; its importance is underscored in work with children, in whom issues of separation and attachment are of particular developmental significance.

In this chapter I discuss some criteria for planned termination in child analysis, that is, termination that is considered timely and appropriate by patient, analyst, and parent. In this context the entire process of treatment could be considered a kind of planning for termination. Weekend interruptions, vacations, and illnesses all present opportunities for exploring attenuated forms of termination, especially with children, for whom the sense of time may be undeveloped and in whom developmental issues of attachment and separation may be particularly sensitive.

The termination phase itself should give the child or adolescent a chance to examine issues of separation and loss, to draw connections to past experiences of separation, and to prepare for future ones. Thus, the process of ending treatment can have long-range benefits for the child. When the treatment allows for the full exploration of these issues, the experience of future separations from important people, such as those occasioned by going away to college or getting married, may benefit from resonance with the termination stage of treatment, which may have occurred years earlier. Indeed, there is no other situation in which the child can so fully explore the experience of separation and loss in all its genetic and current aspects and be aided by someone who is close yet objective.

What are the signs that a child is ready to enter a phase of termination and is prepared developmentally and intrapsychically to deal with specific issues of ending treatment? I will explicate some criteria based on clinical experience. A brief review of the well-known phenomenology of termination will underscore the importance of having such criteria, and a clinical vignette will illustrate how the psychoanalytic sessions themselves can provide the data that the analyst, the patient, and the parents need in order to plan and prepare for ending treatment. The criteria I discuss require simply that the analyst systematically observe the child in the analytic sessions and compare the child's symptoms, behavior, and developmental level with those of earlier stages of treatment. After discussing the derivation of these criteria and their current clinical and research applications, I conclude with a brief summary of some technical considerations for ending psychoanalysis with a child.

The Phenomenology of Termination

Most analysts recognize the characteristic reactions that may ensue once termination appears as a dominant theme in treatment. Frequently, in spite of careful plans for termination, the confrontation of the reality of an actual end to treatment results in the child's using denial. Denial may be expressed in various wishes to "forget" about these plans. Instead of acknowledging sadness, a child may talk of celebration. One boy, for instance, described how he was going to get a full array of the most expensive toys for Christmas, although he clearly knew his parents could not afford them. Another boy suggested celebrating the termination with a special lunch party and in this way denied his sense of grief. Denial of dependence with reaction formation or displacement may also appear.

At other points during the process of termination the patient may appear passive, letting the analyst determine the date and even the final move in the last session. This kind of reaction is illustrated by a 15-year-old patient who, when the time was up in her last session, waited for the analyst to indicate closure and ask her to stop. To the very last second, the analyst interpreted her need to have the analyst "push her out" of treatment in spite of their having talked about termination for a couple of years. Indeed, an important theme in this analysis had been the patient's fear that nobody really cared for her and that people wanted to get rid of her.

Related to passivity may be a sense of consternation. Why does treatment have to end? Isn't it possible to continue for a longer time? No matter who initiates the termination, the patient may unconsciously feel that he or she is being thrown out. There may be a sense of not having been a good enough patient. Or we may find the fantasy that the analyst brings the patient home and provides a protective umbrella forever. Alternately, we may find the attempt to turn passive into active, by missing appointments, for example.

Anxiety may arise about the durability of the achievements attained during the treatment, and this needs to be explored fully. An 11-year-old patient who had broken many toys in the initial session (and had threatened to shoot darts at the analyst) engaged in a similar activity at the point of termination. At that point, however, he tore pieces of paper into bits. When the similarity was pointed out to him, he said firmly, "Shut up. I want to make sure I went through everything." Other patients, as if rehearsing, may play out their need to distance themselves. One patient created a game with various cars going around tracks and coming back to be refueled at a gas station. The cars traveled along circuits further and further away from the gas station, with less and less need to come back. Also in this game the patient's car competed with the analyst's car, often with a tie of victories and losses.

A sense of disillusionment may enter into the evaluation of what has been achieved in treatment. As this disillusionment comes out, the patient may convey ambivalence toward the therapist. One child declared that he hated the therapist; at the same time he made sure his fingers were crossed, thus undoing his communication. Or the child may express sadness and grief at losing the relationship with the analyst and at the same time may communicate a sense of relief at having more free time for other interests—specifically, sublimatory activities such as sports, artistic endeavors, and also friendships with peers—which have emerged in the course of treatment.

Transitory fears of the analyst may surface, with the analyst perceived as seeking revenge and potentially spoiling good things for the patient. With this reaction we may find that the child experiences leaving as an act of aggression toward the analyst. On the other hand, a young patient may express gratitude. A 12-year-old boy mentioned that although the analyst had never given him candy or tangible gifts, she had given him "attention and friendship." He felt that she in turn deserved a present from him, and he offered a model of an airplane that had explored and guarded the coastline during World War II (in which members of his family had fought).

I have written elsewhere that "during termination the task of consolidation in the stage on the way to object-constancy may be replayed. Positive and negative object-images and self-images are further integrated" (Kernberg, 1980, pp. 272–273). Following the criteria of Mahler, Pine, and Bergman (1975), separation (the distinction between the subject and the external object) and individuation (differentiation between the self-representation and the object representation) are finally achieved. This move toward object constancy can be seen in the remarks of a 10-year-old during the last session of his successful analysis. He indicated that he knew every corner and every object in the analyst's room so well that if he were to return in a few years for a visit, he would recognize every part of the office and every object, even if they were "turned around." A 9-year-old boy with a diagnosis of depression with borderline features stated on termination that he would always recognize his analyst, even if he were to "shave his beard" or "get very old." In other words, he had confidence in the continuity of his internal object and felt assured of his analyst's ongoing psychological presence even though he anticipated functioning away from this important person.

Such reactions to termination in psychoanalysis are admittedly familiar and frequently discussed. By themselves, though, their presence or absence does not tell the analyst much about the patient's readiness for termination. The vignette that follows illustrates more fully the manifestations of such reactions in child psychoanalysis and also suggests the importance of systematically weighing these reactions in the broader context of the treatment history and the patient's overall adaptive defenses, affects, insights, perceptions, and communications in the current situation.

A Clinical Vignette

James was an 8-year-old boy who suffered from depression, difficulties with peers, and poor academic performance. The family planned to move to another city but postponed their date of departure in order to wait for James's treatment to reach termination. The following sessions occurred several months before the actual termination date.[1] Before the first session to be described, I received a call from James's father, who wanted to meet with me. James had cajoled his father into helping him set a termination date by having him ask me if we could decrease the frequency of sessions from four times weekly to twice weekly.

---

[1] Material from Lawrence Shaderowsky, M.D.

James arrived 15 minutes early for his next session and brought a small book on minerals. He promptly chose some minerals in my office, tried to look them up in the book, and asked for my help in trying to identify them by name. I mentioned to James that his father had called. "Yes," he replied, "I want him to come help me. It took a month to settle the stopping date. I want to cut down to one time a week. Also, the stopping date is March 12." (The tentative termination date was in June.) I pointed out that he had a lot to say about stopping and that recently he had not come to some of his scheduled appointments. James agreed but made an excuse, claiming that he could not come by himself. He then shifted to complaints about how the treatment interfered with his friendships, leaving no time for them. Finally, he admitted that he had skipped a few sessions because he wanted to see what it would be like to cut back; now he wanted to come to his sessions more often or less often, as he chose. When I brought out a calendar so that James could visualize the months as we spoke, he indicated that he wanted to stop on that very day. Immediately afterward he decided to postpone his *decreasing* his sessions to March 12. Then he showed me on the calendar when he and his family would move to Boston (in the spring), and he said that he would visit the school so that he could meet some of the new kids.

James arrived promptly for the next session and announced that he had overheard his father talking to me on the telephone. He said that he wanted to come to a session with his father and since it was *his* treatment, he should be allowed to do so. In fact, he continued, he *would* do so or else he would blow open the door to my office with batteries that he would take from the playroom. James then tore a piece of paper from a pad and wrote a contract, which he wanted me to sign, in which he would agree to stay until March 12. When he became insistent that I sign, I said that it seemed that he wanted me to *force* him to stop, that maybe he would feel better if his therapy ended that way. "Shut up and sign," he exclaimed. Then he repeated the process, this time indicating that he wanted to decrease the frequency of sessions. Again James wanted my signature. I told him that perhaps we could leave the matter unsettled and continue to talk about it.

In a later session James entered the office smiling and announced, "Today is the last day because I am going to cut down on Monday, and Friday is my day off." He showed me a wooden boat that he had made and called it a "last day boat." After playing with the boat for a while, he dropped it in water and the anchor dissolved, allowing the boat to float freely. James then wondered why no one had used the Play-Doh since his last visit. "You should encourage them to," he said. I told James that I understood how uneasy it made him feel to be moving some place where everyone and everything would be new and yet how eager he was to make the move quickly and get it over with. I said that he must have similar feelings about stopping treatment—wanting to get it over with and not wanting to have to wait and think about his feelings. James agreed and then asked how many people use the Play-Doh. I translated this into a question about whom else I see and whom I would see when James would no longer be coming to the office. He said that I had better get another patient to pay me when he leaves. Then he asked if I still had notes from his first session. "Will you keep the notes until you rot?" he asked. Then he wondered if he could contact me after his treatment ended. We talked about this and James became somewhat anxious.

At the end of one session James lingered, unable to find his pencil. Finally, he left the office but soon returned to say that he had mixed up my pencil and his pencil. He said that he felt that he had left something behind. "Me," I replied and James departed, laughing.

Criteria for Termination

Anna Freud (1970) states that since the aim of child analysis is "to promote normal redevelopment, the aim is fulfilled when the previously held up development proceeds again" (p. 243). Smirnoff (1971) has succinctly outlined the criteria for termination: symptomatic improvement, development of fantasy life, sublimatory activities, autonomy from fantasy, improved adaptation, and such structural features as flexible defenses and ego mastery. Certainly all of us would agree that symptom improvement is an important criterion for termination. Yet this improvement has to be in the context of true growth and not simply an escape into health. Aspects of the child's personality should be viewed from dynamic, structural, genetic, and adaptive perspectives. In this respect Anna Freud's (1963) psychoanalytic profile serves as a useful guideline for comparing development at the beginning, middle, and end of treatment.

In assessing the appropriateness of termination, the analyst needs to look at the patient's level of defenses and ability to modulate affect. How spontaneous is the child's expression of feeling? Does the child show an increased sense of pleasure with a real capacity for humor? Another aspect to be evaluated is the balance between progressive and regressive drive and ego forces. Does regression, for instance, take place "in the service of the ego?" Is phase dominance appropriate? Libido distribution, the development of sublimatory channels, object relations (including the management of aggression), and self-esteem must also be assessed. Superego integration is revealed in the child's ability to express grief and concern and to have an autonomous sense of values. A major consideration is the child's relationships with teachers, with authority, with parents and siblings, and, especially, with peers. One needs to look at the ability to make and keep friends, the number of friends, the frequency with which friends are seen, and, in the preadolescent years, the beginnings of love relationships (Kernberg and Richards, 1981). Questions that arise at this point include the following: To what extent will the patient be able to progress through subsequent developmental stages given an average expectable environment? If the patient were to be seen for the first time at this point, would treatment be recommended?

Using examples from analytic sessions, I will examine 10 criteria that serve as useful guidelines that have both clinical and research applicability.

1. Statements About the Therapist

Once an ending date has been established and a reworking of feelings about the meaning of separation has begun, children typically comment on their sense of having been listened to or helped to find connections. Part of this is the internalization of the analyst's function and the pride taken in the new ability to find hidden meanings. Abrams (1978) mentions a patient who talked about "the figuring out partner" (p. 464). For this to occur, a positive relationship with basic trust must have been established in the analytic situation. The child's ability to use humor in the presence of the therapist and to make observations indicating an awareness of the therapist's personality may indicate emergence from transference neurosis. A sense of individuation within the context of a trusting relationship is also illustrated by the child's capacity to talk about the analyst's traits and to use his or her observing ego.

The child may begin to anticipate comments by the therapist or to make statements reflecting an identification with the therapist or the therapist's role. James, the patient in the foregoing vignette, once showed his identification with the analyst by mistaking the analyst's pencil for his own. This parapraxis was one way in which James attempted to deal with separation and loss. In another example, a 12-year-old boy remarked that when he grew up he would have a room in his house and "invite other kids in the neighborhood to drop in and talk things out." A patient may describe thinking about the analyst or imagining that the analyst, if he or she had been present at a particular moment, would have asked, "What do you think about it?" or "What could be the connection between how you are feeling and what you are doing?" These examples reflect an internalization of the analyst's function.

2. Therapist's Interventions

Toward the latter part of treatment the therapist's interventions may be more interpretive, with confrontations, transference and genetic interpretations, and reconstruction predominating. By contrast, in the initial or middle stages of treatment, clarifications and, to a lesser extent, confrontations and setting statements are more often used to facilitate the patient's communication (Lewis, 1974); the proportion varies with one's technique and the child is psychological-mindedness.

An excellent example of an interpretive intervention given during termination is offered by Abrams (1978):

> I told Martin he must have had some idea that a penis had something to do with sex for a long time. He could remember excited feelings even when he was very little. He probably decided that pee came out of the penis during sex, pee was dirty for him. That may have been harder to imagine, grown-ups making love. He could only imagine his mother was being peed on, that his father was making bubbles in her. The reconstructions gave him pause. It was an idea that did not evoke a dramatic and immediate response. Instead, Martin became reflective. It was sensible. Why shouldn't he have been confused about such matters when he was little? It was nice not to be so mixed up! [p. 457]

3. Perception of Treatment

As termination approaches, the patient's exclusive investment in the treatment will begin to decrease. This is to be distinguished from resistance and is seen in the context of all the other criteria listed here. One indication of this shift is the child's introducing more material from current reality, a departure from the typical fantasy-play of children engaged in the treatment process. We can expect to hear about future plans (following termination) with anticipated pleasure and some sadness at the loss of the analyst. Van Dam and associates (1975) cite a patient who "left with the wish that she could be around when the next patient discovered that she was no longer in treatment" (p. 466).

An important change in the patient's perception of the treatment is a sense of the passage of time within the treatment situation, a sense of meaningful history. The child may spontaneously reminisce about past events in the therapy, an activity that represents the wish to remain important to the analyst (e.g., "Will you keep the notes from my first session until you die?"). The sense of the passage of time is also typically projected into the future, as in the question "Can I still see you if I have more problems?"

All of these criteria involving the perception of the treatment reflect a more integrated self-concept. The child's ability to relate to the analyst as a separate person and to view the treatment experience within a total life context suggests a growing strength in his or her observing ego.

4. Quality of Communications

Although conflicts may remain in the terminal phase of treatment, their resolution proceeds at a faster pace, with more rapid response to interpretations. The quantity of verbalization may increase, and reflectiveness in general may be more apparent. During the terminal phase of his treatment, for example, a ten-year-old boy with a behavior disorder announced for the first time, "Wait a moment, my brain is beginning to think about the reasons," as he assumed the pose of Rodin's The Thinker.

Abrams (1978) raises several basic questions that relate both to changes in the patient's communications and to the therapist's interventions and are highly significant for anyone who studies termination in children. These questions can be used as a guideline for assessing the thoroughness of the treatment and may help the child analyst to determine whether the initial goals have been achieved: (1) Are dynamic issues dealt with, positive and negative oedipal issues as well as preoedipal determinants? (2) Have specific drive derivatives become manifest? (3) Is the direction of treatment moving toward development of age-appropriate ego and superego structure? (4) Has the resolution of past conflicts led to more adaptive pathways through sublimation or neutralization?

5. Play and Dreams

As treatment progresses, play is used as a vehicle for the expression of fantasy and the resolution of conflict. There is an increasing absorption and pleasure in play, the quality of which changes as the ending approaches. For example, a child who used to play cops and robbers with his analyst would get so excited with his play that he would have to leave the room in a hurry to go to the bathroom. Upon his return, he would repeat the themes aimlessly and with anxiety. Toward the end of treatment, this child played differently. He and the analyst would make two parallel roads in the sandbox. Potential crises would emerge, such as cars going full speed in opposite directions and boulders falling off cliffs. Nevertheless, the child's car and the analyst's car arrived at their destination safely. The child left sessions in a joyful mood by the end of his treatment. While the early play of the aforementioned James had often entailed chaotic and hopeless games with dinosaurs, in the last session James brought a boat that could float freely without an achor, a metaphor for his own increased confidence to function independently.

Dreams, too, may be useful in assessing the child's readiness for termination. Their content may encompass the wish to terminate as well as the anxieties that arise with this wish.

6. Affects

The child's modulation of affects should increase, and there should be an appropriate range, intensity, and content. Shifts in affects should fit the situation, and the child should spontaneously talk about what he or she is experiencing on a feeling level.

Discussion of possible termination inevitably provokes feelings of sadness, but a sense of relief also comes to the foreground. Speculating on how it would feel not to have regular appointments, one girl explained that she "would never really know until it actually happened, [but she] imagined that talking about it would give her at least some idea!" (Van Dam et al., 1975, p. 463). Implicit here was a recognition of the mix of feelings, both positive and negative reactions, which the patient first rehearsed in thought.

Expressions of gratitude and concern are also indications of readiness for termination. These high-level affective responses, when present, imply a deepening of object relations with a modulation of aggressive components. Gratitude and concern may reflect the patient's capacity for deeper relationships within the family and for future investments in others.

7. Sublimatory Behavior

Within an analytic session, sublimatory behavior can be seen in the patient's bringing in and sharing new interests, whether these involve new toys or games, or reports about achievements in the arts or sports. James showed his sublimatory capacities in the "last-day boat" he built and in his new abilities with numbers.

8. Insight

Insight is revealed in patients' capacity to express humor about themselves and to laugh about "silly" mistakes without denying them.

Empathy with peers can be an indirect expression of insight. The comment "Johnny is in trouble at school—maybe he should see somebody like you" reveals an attempt to understand others through an understanding of oneself.

9. Defenses

As termination approaches, the analyst can examine the predominant defenses used and assess their flexibility and adaptiveness. James gradually acquired the ability to turn passivity into activity. Since the initiation of termination is anxiety-producing, James had asked his father to help him in setting a date, and he also suggested a decrease in the frequency of the hours in an attempt to wean himself from therapy. Moreover, in a counterphobic way, James set a date a few months earlier than estimated by the analyst. Then James skipped a few sessions "to find out what it is like to cut back," as if he wanted to rehearse not coming and to assess his capacity to master the termination of the treatment. James also tried to coerce the analyst to sign a contract for settling the termination date, attempting to transform passivity into activity and to protect himself from the anxiety about deciding on a date on his own. The ability to assume responsibility for oneself and one's actions is observed in such comments as "I think I provoked that reaction from my brother by teasing him."

Related to assuming responsibility for one's own actions is the absence of externalization. Another sign of growth is the application of the analyst's interpretations to other areas of the child's life. A good example of this is the following remark: "If I see you as strict with me when you really aren't, that may mean I see my teachers as stricter, too."

10. Appearance and Behavior

Finally, the child's behavior during analytic sessions should point to a decrease in acting out and a decrease in symptoms or pathological character traits in comparison with the initial assessment. Age-appropriate behavior should predominate, indicating an age-appropriate sense of identity. Body posture and manner of dress may provide further clues to an objective self-image and positive self-esteem.

Clinical and Research Applications of the Termination Criteria

The criteria presented in the preceding paragraphs were developed from the discussions among 10 child psychotherapists and 15 child psychoanalysts. I shall briefly review the clinical and research implications of these criteria.

Applied clinically, these operational criteria can serve to guide, reinforce, or assess a decision about termination. Not infrequently, a child will appear better outside the sessions, either at home or at school or both, than within the sessions. The criteria provide a systematic framework within which the child's behavior and affect during therapy sessions can be more thoroughly evaluated. Along with data from outside the sessions, the observations based on these criteria can help eliminate the pitfalls of either prolonging the treatment or ending it prematurely without the benefit of a full termination stage. Moreover, therapists generally need checkpoints for making objective decisions, since judgments of change and improvement tend to become inaccurate because of various countertransference factors (Kohrman, 1969). Particularly in terminating with children, such factors as idealization, disillusionment, and envy may influence the therapist's judgment. Finally, these operational criteria can aid clinical supervisors and consultants in their reviews of the appropriateness of termination.

The research implications of the criteria rest on their application to behaviors in the child that can be assessed and compared at various points throughout the treatment. The criteria correspond to important dynamic and structural developments that are analyzed in detail in the following paragraphs.

1) Statements about the therapist reflect the dissolution of transference distortion, an increased capacity to test reality, and the existence of an observing ego. Both a positive basic relationship and the use of humor indicate the presence of basic trust and its corollary, namely, the absence of paranoid ideation.

The presence of selective identifications with the therapist and especially of identifications with the therapist's function attest to the child's capacity to use the newly acquired ability to work through his or her own conflicts and issues. Statements from the child about keeping the relationship in memory point to the child's capacity to maintain an object representation despite separation or aggressive impulses, another positive sign of progress toward the attainment of solid gains.

2) The therapist's interventions operationalize our definition of a well-conducted treatment. One would expect a progression during the course of treatment toward more use of interpretation in an attempt to bring meaning to the child's communications. Thus, the interventions not only reflect a well-functioning therapeutic alliance but should also signal ongoing progress in the child's capacity to receive such interpretations, that is, in his or her self-understanding.

3) The child's perception of treatment represents the trend toward the resolution of transference paradigms and/or transference neurosis as the child's interests expand to the outside world. At the same time, these developments are echoed in the child's willingness to bring material from current reality into the analytic sessions. Statements about the history of the treatment reflect the child's sense of continuity of the self throughout time and the ability to synthesize different aspects of the self in a cohesive self-representation. Statements concerning the anticipated termination similarly indicate an expectation of continuity of the self in a future without the therapist and signify a capacity for autonomy and age-appropriate independence.

4) The quality of communications reflects the child's greater capacity to put needs into words rather than into action. More broadly, what is represented here is the capacity to delay, to contemplate alternatives through thinking, and hence to master conflicts more efficiently.

5) The quality of play reflects globally the capacity to derive pleasure, to sublimate drives, to invest and resolve conflicts, and to

adaptively master anxieties and such other affects as aggression and depression. The quality of play, of course, will also give an indication of the capacity to interact with peers. Indeed, it is a global measure of ego strength. Similarly, the manifest content of dreams will reflect these capacities as well as the flexible use of defenses. The child may remember dreams without anxiety and recognize that dreams too are part of oneself. In other words, the child comes to experience a continuity of the self between awake and sleep states.

6) Affects are a "barometer" of change. Their variety, modulation, appropriateness, and verbalization reflect the capacity for tolerating frustration and anxiety, for integrating superego functions, and for the ability to differentiate self and other: The integration of ambivalence allows for a modulation of affects. High-level affects, such as gratitude and concern, reflect more sophisticated object relations and the resolution of greed and envy into a sense of trust and empathy.

7) Sublimatory behavior reflects the opening of new expressive channels for drives.

8) Signs of insight indicate the capacity for self-monitoring and for assessing oneself in changing circumstances. The ability to function more adaptively intrapsychically and in the world offers the possibility of avoiding endless repetitions of maladaptive behaviors.

9) A flexible use of defenses signifies a position of strength and the possession of equipment for directing one's life.

10) The last group of criteria relate to appearance and behavior which correspond to the level of self-exteem and social appropriateness.

The preceding criteria reflect freedom for the child from cumbersome symptoms. With the disappearance of the helplessness associated with being impulse-ridden, secondary social complications are no longer evident. Enhanced by improved appearance and more mature, self-directed behavior, the child can enter peer interactions more advantageously and proceed with development.

The further quantification, reliability, and validity of these operational criteria for termination warrant the attention of researchers and clinicians alike. Properly applied to a wide variety of cases, the criteria could provide rich data on the development of personality and object relations and their changes through the course of treatment. Moreover, with third-party payers concerned about the length of treatment, a reliable instrument based on these criteria could serve as a rational basis for judging the merits and the costs of continuation or termination.

Technique of Termination

Given the importance of the termination stage, the treatment should end at a point where the full impact of the process can be explored, without the intermingling of outside contingencies. An upcoming vacation or other plans may provide rationalization and blur the effects of the separation and loss on the patient (Abrams, 1978; Sandler, Kennedy, and Tyson, 1980). Similarly, a termination date that coincides with the end of the school year would not be ideal. When termination occurs independently of vacations, the patient has a real opportunity to experience what ordinary life is like without the analyst while knowing that any difficulties can be explored with the analyst should the need arise.

The date of termination should be agreed on by the parents, the child, and the analyst. It is, however, best that the patient set the date and assume an active stance in the decision. The patient should also be able to change his or her mind and postpone the date if there are things that still need to be worked through.

The child must have ample opportunity to explore "what if" situations. With younger children, a calendar may help to make the passage of time more visible and concrete. Depending on the patient, however, the amount of time needed will vary. An adolescent patient once mentioned to me that she had been preparing for termination ever since the beginning of the analysis. Some patients spend several months working out issues of termination.

Anxieties about separation should be explored. The patient may feel that the termination signifies either that he or she is being abandoned by the analyst or that the analyst is being abandoned by the patient. This feeling needs to be clarified. Ideally, the patient will reach the conclusion on his or her own that the analyst has a commitment to the patient and will be available if the patient should ever want further contact. At the same time, the patient needs to know that the analyst can let go, that if the patient chooses not to contact the analyst again, this will also be acceptable.

Many analysts attempt to wean the patient from four to two times to one time a week, but this should not be necessary (Sandler et al., 1980). It is an illusion to think that the analyst–patient relationship and the analytic process are the same if the frequency of sessions decreases; in my experience, the quality of the relationship changes quite drastically, and the reduction in frequency of the sessions may mean that the patient and the analyst, though still in the same psychoanalytic setting, cannot explore the issue of termination. Furthermore, the fact that the setting continues while the frequency of sessions decreases may obscure changes in the relationship and the meaning of these changes to the patient.

Another danger during the termination phase is that the analyst may try to step out of his or her role as psychoanalyst. It is very important that the analyst remain in this role for the duration of the treatment, for it is in this role that the patient has come to know, accept, and identify with the analyst. To be inconsistent with the patient (and even with the parents) at the end of an analysis may well undermine analytic work.

Termination also brings a high risk of countertransference reactions in the analyst (Kohrman, 1969). Succumbing to the temptation to adopt the role of "regular friendly adult" may appear directly in behavior toward the patient or indirectly in attempts to manipulate the environment through the parents (Sandler et al., 1980). The analyst also risks sharing the disillusionment experienced by the patient and feeling, with self-criticism and self-devaluation, that the initial goals have not been fully achieved.

Another risk in the termination stage is prolongation of the treatment. The child may be thought of as "an ideal patient." Here, more than ever, the therapist's self-analysis is crucial and is needed to help avoid a particular "countertransference misunderstanding" that may occur with adolescents. Since adolescents normally have a natural developmental tendency toward the dissolution of object ties with the parents (and hence with the analyst in the transference), the analyst must differentiate these normal wishes to end treatment, on one hand, from those attempts to terminate that, on the other hand, represent ways of clinging to, rather than disengaging from, infantile ties. Clearly, it is important to consider, in addition to all dynamic factors, as many life areas as possible (school, peers, family, syndrome improvement, resumption of development, and changes within the session) in order to become convinced that we are dealing with a termination process and not with resistance.

A final point to emphasize is that the parents also experience a process of termination to which the analyst must be attuned. The analyst needs to support the parents in their anxieties about resuming full responsibility for the child and to explore their fears of possible relapse. One mother, whose 10-year-old son ended treatment successfully, became quite anxious; for his last few sessions she gave the boy food to eat during the hour, since she felt he must be hungry. At the same time, she developed somatic symptoms that were understood to be signs of anxiety over her loss of the child's analyst and over her resumption of the role of mother. Obviously, the analyst needs to deal tactfully with the parents so that they too can complete the process of termination.

Conclusion

Termination provides an opportunity to enhance the child's ongoing process of separation–individuation, particularly the stage that Margaret Mahler has called "on the way to object constancy." In assessing the child's readiness for termination and progress during the termination phase, it is useful to look at the interactions within the sessions in addition to such external criteria as school and family adjustment and peer relationships. The criteria outlined in this chapter provide a means of evaluating ego development, maturity of object relations, and strength of self-concept, as well as the ability to handle anxiety, depression, and frustration. During the process of termination, the analyst must also remain aware of any deviations of technique or specific reactions that may interfere with a complete exploration of termination issues.

References

Abrams, S. (1978), Child analysis and therapy. In: *Termination in Child Analysis*, ed. J. Glenn. New York: Aronson, pp. 451–469.

Freud, A. (1963), The concept of developmental lines. *The Psychoanalytic Study of the Child*, 18:245–265. New York: International Universities Press.

Freud, A. (1970), Problems of termination in child analysis. *The Writings of Anna Freud*, 7:3–21. New York: International Universities Press.

Kernberg, P. (1980), Origins of the reconstructed psychoanalysis. In: *Rapprochement*, ed. R. Lax, S. Bach & A. Burland. New York: Aronson, pp. 262–281.

Kernberg, P. & Richards, A. (1981), Love relations in pre-adolescence. Presented at the Meetings of the Academy of Child Psychiatry, October, Chicago.

Kohrman, R. (1969), Annual reports: Problems of termination in childhood and adolescence. *J. Amer. Psychoanal. Assn.*, 17:191–205.

Lewis, M. (1974), Interpretation in child Analysis: Developmental considerations. *J. Amer. Acad. Child Psychiat.*, 13:32–53.

Mahler, M., Pine, F. & Bergman, A. (1975), *The Psychological Birth of the Human Infant*. New York: Basic Books.

Sandler, J., Kennedy, N. & Tyson, R. (1980), *The Technique of Child Analysis, Discussions with A. Freud*. Cambridge, MA: Harvard University Press.

Smirnoff, V. (1971), *The Scope of Child Analysis*. New York: International Universities Press.

Van Dam, H., Heiman, M. D., Heinicke, C. M. & Shane, M. (1975), Termination in child analysis. *The Psychoanalytic Study of the Child*, 30:443–474. New Haven, CT: Yale University Press.

16

Termination in Psychotherapy with Children and Adolescents

Robert D. Gillman

Termination in psychotherapy follows the same general principles that govern termination in psychoanalysis. The shift from an open-ended therapy to a phase in which there is a definite time of ending sharpens the focus on certain special issues of ending, separation, loss, and mourning. There is a final working through of conflicts that takes place during a formal termination period.

Psychoanalytic principles of termination serve as an excellent model for psychoanalytic psychotherapy, even though the time frames of psychotherapy may be much condensed. Even once-a-week therapy lasting only a few sessions requires an awareness and sensitivity to the problems mobilized by ending the treatment. To deal with these issues in a meaningful termination requires, first, that a definite ending date be set to permit sufficient time to focus on the ending and, second, that the therapist address termination issues as they emerge in direct or displaced form.

In contrast to psychoanalysis, the subject of termination in psychotherapy has not been granted special interest and study and it lacks a unified body of knowledge. In the practice of psychotherapy, the conduct of a termination can be widely variable, depending on the training of the particular therapist. This is especially true in the psychotherapy of children and adolescents, in which there is the

I want to express appreciation to Joan Lieberman, M.D., and Eric B. Cohen, M.D., for contributing clinical material to this chapter.

additional factor of "childism," a tendency to avoid the enormous significance of the therapist to the child. "Childism" is a result of ignorance, countertransference, and the child's relative inability to verbalize his feelings.

While many analysts emphasize the qualitative similarity between the process of termination in psychotherapy and that in psychoanalysis, there are certain differences that stem from differences among the patients themselves. On one hand, patients in psychoanalysis are a relatively homogeneous group in their ability to undergo, respond to, and complete a formal termination phase. In contrast, patients in psychotherapy vary widely with respect to presenting problems, diagnostic categories, and treatment experiences. Cooper (1989) has divided psychotherapy patients for whom analysis is not recommended into three groups: (1) those who lack the psychological capacity for deep exploration, (2) those whose areas of difficulty are limited so that limited goals can be set, and (3) those whose emotional difficulties make it impossible for them to tolerate the deep explorations of analysis.

The group of patients with more severe pathology may never have as complete an experience of termination. They may have intermittent treatment and "face limited separations with the knowledge that there can be a resumption of contact or treatment when it is appropriate" (p. 5). This is as true of borderline children and adolescents as it is of adults.

Cooper describes the termination of adults who are "regarded as lacking psychological capacities for deeper self-exploration," that is, as having specific conflicts for which the ultimate understanding and resolution are unavailable to them:

> The danger in these patients is that termination may be falsely smooth. The patients experience more than they are able to convey or realize consciously and the therapist should be alert to the nuances of the powerful attachments that these patients often form and of the painful termination stress that they often experience [p. 3].

Cooper's description of the patient who has a limited capacity for psychological thinking can also be applied to the child in psychotherapy, for the young patient "has had limited experience in translating his complex feelings into abstract verbal communications" (p. 3).

An important contribution to the study of termination in the psychotherapy of children appeared almost 50 years ago in a book by Allen (1942). Deriving his theoretical position from the work of Otto

Rank, for whom separation was the basic experience, Allen wrote, "The values of the therapeutic experience emerge in part around the fact that this relationship is begun with the goal of its eventual termination. From the first hour this is the basic goal of the therapist" (p. 265). Allen calls the ending phase "an integral part of the whole therapeutic experience" (p. 268).

While we need not embrace Allen's theoretical orientation, as when he says, for example, "Ending is understood as starting actually in the early phase of treatment, with the first awakenings of a separate self which the child discovers" (p. 273), we can value his understanding and descriptions of the vital importance of the termination process to the child. He sees ending as a new separation experience for which the child must be prepared in advance. When both the child and therapist are aware of the child's readiness to end the treatment relationship, the child must be an active participant in the plan. Readiness for ending is assessed by observing the feeling tone of the hour, changes in the child's verbal content, and changes in the child's outside relationships. Of course, the parents are always participants in any plan of ending with a child. While this chapter primarily addresses the nature of termination for the child, it is clear that parents may exert pressures for premature ending, an ending that ignores the child's need to work through the problems of termination, or for prolongation of treatment beyond the optimal point, either for their own goals of greater perfection for the child or for reasons of their own dependency on the therapy and the therapist.

Children need an opportunity to experience the problems evoked by termination through some of the conflicting feelings that are aroused by the step of setting an ending date. They experience new anxiety over the impending separation and fear that their gains will be lost and that the therapist's support will end. Some children want to end right away in order to avoid the anxiety, and some feel that they will never want to leave. The therapist helps the child express not only the anxiety and struggles but also the feelings of satisfaction over ending.

The case of a nine-year-old boy illustrates some of these points. Jules had made considerable gains in once-a-week psychotherapy over a period of two years. He was now able to concentrate in school, have a mutual relationship with a best friend, and get along fairly well with his younger brother. The subject of termination was raised by his parents, and lately Jules himself often seemed to be hinting about ending. When I addressed the subject directly with him, he said, "I'm not sure I want to stop." Despite my frequent admonitions to myself to be aware of such feelings in children, I was once more taken by surprise. Jules had never verbalized any positive feelings toward me or the therapy; on the contrary, at the end of each session he seemed especially eager to be done with it. He was a relatively nonverbal child who, except on rare occasions, expressed his feelings in dramatic play with dolls, puppets, and games. Jules discussed termination with his parents, eventually deciding to proceed with it, at which point his parents became reluctant for him to end treatment. When we finally set an ending date with a four-week termination phase, Jules said at the start of the next session, "This is our last time, isn't it?"

This case illustrates two of the points mentioned above. First, there was Jules's hidden transference dependence and the fear expressed by his parents that Jules would not be able to make it on his own. Second, there was Jules's ambivalence about ending and his anxiety over the termination process itself with its attendant transference feelings, which led to his saying, "This is our last session, isn't it?" despite our going over several times the need for a longer termination period and our actual ending schedule.

Goals in Psychotherapy

Termination, and its appropriate timing in psychotherapy, cannot be considered without reference to therapeutic goals. Unlike the aims of psychoanalysis, the working through of resistances and the resolution of transference, more limited goals are envisioned by the therapist, patient, and parents for many, if not most, children and adolescents in psychotherapy. Limited goals are set even for those children, treated in psychotherapy, who are eventually treated in psychoanalysis. Reasons for this include the fact that it is often difficult to assess at the beginning whether a treatment with limited goals will suffice to permit the child to go forward with normal development. Also, it is often difficult to convince parents to begin a psychotherapeutic endeavor with formal psychoanalysis; a trial of psychotherapy is usually the first step.

Shane (1989) has contrasted the goals in psychotherapy with those of psychoanalysis.

> In contrast to psychoanalysis, the termination of a psychoanalytically-oriented psychotherapy does not involve such thoroughgoing resolution of transferential aspects; while transference is inevitably and importantly part of such therapeutic work, it is usually less central to

the process and, in any case, is not the foremost consideration in the decision to end. Another major difference between the decision to stop in psychotherapy, versus the decision to stop in psychoanalysis, concerns symptomatic improvement versus structural change. . . . It often happens that psychotherapy is terminated when symptoms are relieved, whereas analysis proceeds in its own unique course generally uncoupled from symptomatic change. . . . The achievement of life goals does influence the decision to terminate more often in psychotherapy than in analysis [p. 3].

It is often a problem for analytically-oriented therapists to restrict themselves to the limited psychotherapeutic goals that are complementary to the needs and developmental stage of the child or adolescent. Psychoanalytic theory can be used to help the therapist understand a dynamic formulation of the problems the child presents, but it should be used with flexibility in recommending a treatment plan. The same theory must be used to embark on a therapeutic regimen that is distinguished as much by knowledge of what is not going to be explored as of what is going to bear scrutiny.

The therapist must be sensitive to the situation of a patient who is reacting to therapeutic accomplishment. A child or adolescent who slows the pace of treatment, shows limited continuity in therapeutic work, experiences the usual increased anxiety over thoughts of terminating, and misses treatment hours may be showing increased signs of resistance to uncovering new areas. On the other hand, such a patient may be reacting to a therapeutic accomplishment, may have reached his or her therapeutic goals, and, for a variety of reasons, may be ready to stop. The therapist must be sensitive to this and certainly avoid prolonging a treatment that is antithetical to the treatment arrangements and the goals of the patient or the patient's parents. This does not mean, of course, that psychotherapeutic goals are always determined at the beginning of therapy nor that we accede to every request to end treatment; in the course of therapy further goals may emerge that were not evident at the start.

Mann (1973) and others have attempted to solve the problem of limited goals in psychotherapy by setting a time limit to the therapy itself. Mann states, "Too frequently, long-term psychotherapy dribbles to an unspoken end, . . . a chronic impasse between patient and therapist that relates to a transference-countertransference situation which is neither understood nor resolved" (p. 31). The artificial imposition of a time limit (in Mann's work, a limit of 12 sessions), as opposed to therapy in which the goal is symptom relief or attainment of life goals, brings termination issues into sharp focus. Mann concentrates on the central issue of current problems. Termination-oriented psychotherapy is especially useful for those late adolescents whose circumscribed developmental conflicts over dependency, autonomy, separation, and loss are mobilized.

Samuel

The problem of therapeutic goals and the timing of termination is illustrated in the treatment of 9-year-old Samuel, who was brought in for evaluation because of worries, self-doubts, and unattainably high standards. He told me that he heard voices, meaning that when he was tense, obsessional thoughts occurred to him that were nonsense. For example, when taking a timed test, the thought "Go sit in that far chair" intruded and interfered with his concentration. Samuel did his homework and practiced his violin as early in the day as possible so that he wouldn't worry about them for the rest of the day.

Samuel was a boy with superior intelligence, although he was not as gifted intellectually as his older brother. He excelled in sports, was popular with his friends, and was artistic like his artist mother. From the beginning I considered the possibility that he would benefit most from psychoanalysis. However, as things turned out, Samuel's symptoms were so relieved after 32 sessions of weekly therapy that he and his parents were convinced that no further psychotherapy was indicated. I concurred with this view.

Samuel was in the third grade, the highest grade of his school. When it was necessary to choose his next school, his parents favored the academically rigorous, prestigious school that his brother attended. Samuel preferred a school with a more relaxed environment that would provide opportunities for his study of art. He wanted to know my opinion, and I interpreted that he saw me as he did his parents, with a definite point of view. (His parents also wanted me to express a firm opinion.) Samuel responded to my neutrality by talking openly about the strengths and weaknesses of the programs at both schools, particularly the negative features of his brother's school. Whenever he spoke of the advantages of his preferred school, he would also present the counterarguments. I interpreted that although he could tell his thoughts freely to me, it seemed as if he had to accede to his parents' arguments, as if he were unable to express his feelings firmly to them. I wondered, since he had never told his parents exactly how he felt about the schools, what he feared. Samuel pondered this, and began to express himself more freely with his parents, at first only with his mother, to whom he was quite attached. His parents listened to his preference and eventually enrolled him in the school of his choice. He immediately relaxed and his obsessions disappeared.

Six months after the end of therapy his mother wrote, "We know you will be happy to learn that Samuel has made a fine adjustment to his new school. He has made many new friends. We've been pleased with the school as well and do feel it is the right choice for him. None of the compulsive behavior has returned." While no one would pretend that the resolution of symptoms in this case was comparable to the outcome of analytic work, Samuel was able to use analytic psychotherapy in order to exert some autonomous behavior, resolve a crisis, and make therapeutic gains that permitted him to proceed with his development.

Susan

In the case of Susan a once-a-week therapy of only a few months, which focused on a prepubertal girl's awareness of feelings that were previously warded off, led to a meaningful termination experience even though the goals of therapy were limited by the patient's and her parents' unwillingness to explore the fullest meaning of the dramatic symptoms that originally brought her to treatment.

Susan was almost 11 when she was referred for outpatient psychotherapy after a 30-day hospitalization for paralysis of her legs following a respiratory illness that had been treated with antibiotics. Diagnosis was conversion reaction with astasia-abasia. At home Susan had crawled crabwise and was mostly confined to a wheelchair; physical therapy had been ineffective. In the hospital she improved with psychotherapy. She walked first with a walker, then unaided.

Susan was a gymnast, who had recently failed to make the team. She was now in conflict over whether to return to her gymnastics practice. Because of her recent illness she had also failed in her bid to be elected vice president of her class.

Susan was a middle child, with brothers 14 and 7. The older brother was in repeated battles with the father, a rigid, volatile man who was unusually preoccupied at this time since he was attending night school to find a more satisfactory career. Mother, a passive woman, had submerged her own interests for her husband's sake. Theirs was a troubled, isolated marriage.

Susan was seen twice-weekly for about six months; her parents were seen in collateral couples therapy. Her mother welcomed the chance to work on her problems while her father felt forced into it. Susan seemed indifferent to her recent difficulty and was ready to stop treatment now that she could walk. She had difficulty expressing feelings, customarily submerging them under her role of family peacemaker, but shortly after therapy began there was an outbreak of rage at her therapist, whom Susan blamed for ruining her vacation by continuing therapy.

In therapy Susan tried to model herself after her mother by proclaiming, "Everything is fine." Yet conflicts emerged soon and took the form of worries about whether to return to gymnastics and whether to become a crossing guard, which the family considered too stressful an activity for her. Also, Susan revealed her difficulty in integrating a relationship with her two best friends at the same time. She seemed unable to tolerate the competitiveness, the favoritism, and the potential anger involved.

Susan approached therapy as if it were a school performance test, as if she would be put back in the hospital for getting a bad grade. Good performance involved putting a good face on family interactions. However, on one occasion Susan told her therapist how angry she had felt at the consulting family therapist, who had confronted her parents during a meeting attended by the whole family. She accused him of trying to break up her family, because he had called attention to her father's anger. In this context she recognized that she was too frightened to be angry at her father for fear of his retaliation. She even wondered if her difficulty with anger could be the basis for her paralyzed legs.

Susan delayed showing her therapist her outstanding report card for fear of being called a perfectionist, a term her mother used to describe her father. This discussion led to her first admission of an interest in boys. With reluctance she revealed her fear that boys would dislike her if she showed an interest in them. She decided against resuming gymnastics because that would prevent her from being "the kind of girl that goes with boys."

The anxiety associated with her interest in boys led to Susan's renewing her efforts to end treatment. After four months of therapy she said, "I'm walking, I'm talking about feelings, I don't need to come here—though I do need help with boys. I'm afraid you'll make me stay. You're like my friends who make me do things I don't want to do. Let's at least cut down to every other week."

In response to Susan's pressure to end treatment and in light of her considerable gains, the therapist encouraged a discussion of termination. Eventually a date was set four weeks hence and Susan felt immediate relief that she was not "being made to come forever."

In response to her relief she spoke more freely, telling for the first time about her crush on a boy.

In the first meeting after the termination date was set, Susan revealed that she was able to talk to the therapist in special ways, unlike the ways she talked to everyone else. She denied that she would miss the therapist but admitted, "You have taught me to express feelings." She contrasted the therapist with her father, "who doesn't want to know"; with her mother, who refused to let her have a skating party, ignoring Susan's point of view, and with a critical art teacher, who Susan felt was too judgmental.

In the next session both therapist and patient were relieved at the news that Susan's parents would continue their couples therapy after Susan stopped her treatment. But she was angry that her therapist talked about termination, complaining, "If I knew that I would have to talk about leaving, I would have left weeks ago." Despite her protest, her associations were to other leavings: breaking up with friends and possibly transferring to a school for talented children, a move that would take her away from all her friends (and one for which she was currently taking admission tests).

Susan sparred for the moment with her therapist in a discussion about mixed feelings and anger and then said, "I have something to say. I'll miss you. You helped me." When her therapist replied, "I wouldn't have known," Susan said, "I thought you knew." She then remembered moving from a childhood home where she had lived for six months and where she had felt "safe and free." "Like therapy," the therapist suggested. Susan answered, "It's been a long time here, half a year. Can I call you. I will lose the hospital,[1] the nurse—can I visit?"

In the final session Susan smiled broadly for the first time and showed her therapist pictures of several friends, including Bill, the boy she liked so much. Again she talked of leaving friends, and she recalled a childhood move from Europe to her current place of residence, where she initially found herself excluded. She added, "This year I felt comfortable and included. My friend Terry has no friends. She stopped her therapy, but she only played. She still can't express feelings." After telling her therapist about some arguments with friends and with her mother, Susan ended by saying, "I know now I'm really a nice, good person. When I first came in I worried that you had a gun. Now I can trust you."

As in the case of Samuel, the therapist, recognizing that sufficient work had been accomplished to permit the child to resume normal

---

[1]Susan's outpatient therapy took place in the same location as her hospitalization.

development, was willing to respect the limited goals of the patient and the desire to terminate treatment. In Samuel's treatment there was some attention to transference and a corrective emotional milieu, permitting him greater freedom and autonomy, which translated into improved communication with his parents. In Susan's case there was a working through of some of her defenses against feelings that had been isolated, particularly anger, which for her had been ego-dystonic. Again, there was some work with the transference and a corrective emotional experience that permitted greater freedom to explore her thoughts and feelings. These gains made it possible for Susan to experience a full range of feelings of loss during the scheduled month of the termination phase.

June

June, a high school senior, was referred at age 17 after a self-inflicted burn that followed two years of increasingly dysfunctional behavior at school. In her home there was marital tension and a failure of parental modeling. June, hoping to mobilize her parents to function more appropriately, typically related to them in a style of excessive reaction. Her father's anxiety interfered with his setting reasonable limits, and her mother openly encouraged maturity while covertly encouraging dependence. From June's description of it, the therapist felt that the home environment was permissive to the point of chaos, with great tolerance for psychopathological behavior in both the immediate and extended family.

June saw her self-inflicted burn as a cry for help; she was not suicidal, but she felt she had been depressed since age ten. She recognized her fears of growing up and the threat represented by the end of high school in six months. June was seen in dynamically oriented psychotherapy for the next one and a half years, and terminated when the therapist left town. In the course of this therapy, June worked on problems of adolescent development: her struggle for autonomy, separation from her family, concerns over sexuality, and the fulfillment of her responsibilities as a student and worker. She was able to graduate from high school, following which she at first took a job, instead of applying to college.

June formed an early alliance with her therapist that was motivated by the wish to entertain and be liked. As she began to view the therapist as a savior and protector, she became more and more curious about his personal life. In the course of the first year she developed a mostly positive erotic transference, within which, along with her increasing self-observation and tolerance for anxiety, June began to relinquish her flaky exterior as she discovered and explored her previously hidden capabilities. Despite the intensity of her curiosity about her therapist, viewing him in dreams and fantasies as an omnipotent savior, she was able to tolerate analytically oriented responses to her questions. Through this work she gradually saw the therapist as a more realistic helper. She was able to express her anger when at first he failed to recognize her accomplishments at work and her new ability to take responsibility for herself.

When her therapist gave her six months' notice that the therapy would be terminating when he left town, June reacted with a wide range of feelings: she was being wronged, she was being abandoned, her "obnoxious" behavior was forcing the therapist to flee. In the session following the therapist's declaration of his intention to leave the area, June stated that she was convinced she'd seen him in the street prior to that declaration, seen him "disappear into the mist. I know it wasn't you. It's amazing how I'd know it was about to happen." She began to wonder if she had precipitated his departure by this fantasy. Even though she seemed able to observe her ideas more objectively, she became more regressed, lying on the floor provocatively and begging the therapist not to leave. And while June accused her therapist of making her condition worse and expressed rage that he was cruelly abandoning her, she nevertheless recognized her inner and outer gains. She fantasied about being the therapist's child and leaving town with him, and asked if the therapist took his child with him to the supermarket (while unknowingly assuming the position of a child in a shopping cart). She asked, "How can I function with no one to help me?" When the therapist interpreted her anger, she retorted, "I'm disappointed—not angry, stupid!"

June began to work through her anger during the next session, scolding the therapist for abandoning her and refusing to gratify her sexual fantasies. "I'm very upset with you today. I was talking with my father about it, slamming doors. But now I don't feel angry. I had the whole thing prepared, and now I can't talk about it. I'm just frustrated, not angry with you. Why didn't you try behavior modification? It probably wouldn't have worked, but why didn't you try it? I know I'm headed in the right direction, but you've made little mistakes that sometimes upset and confuse me. What is going on here? What *are* we doing?"

The therapist responded, "I think you've answered many of your own questions. It seems that you needed to repeat behaviors in here that you used in earlier times in order to try to mobilize your parents.

Hopefully, by working though these conflicts here, you can be freed from having to repeat these behaviors again in future relationships." To this June said, "There have been so many crazy people in my life, and you're so normal." The therapist suggested that his leaving brought up earlier feelings of disappointment and loss. June replied, "I guess, but I'm still confused. Are you angry with me? Am I being obnoxious? I'm not really angry with you, just frustrated."

In the next session June declared, "There's no structure here. I'm worse. I need to go somewhere else to fix what was done here. I'm going to a behavior therapist. You'll be glad to get rid of me." Yet in the same session she reported more assertive and responsible behavior on the outside. Three months before the end of her treatment June demonstrated her growing independence by traveling to a distant college for an interview. Despite her own threats, she resisted her mother's wish that she stop therapy at once and resume with a different therapist chosen by her mother. She was now more able to acknowledge the therapist as a real person. "Will I ever see you again? I'm afraid I'll see you in San Francisco where you're moving. I don't like that you have a life outside of here. It's not fair that you're not just a figment of my imagination."

In the last few sessions June felt sad, recognizing that therapy was "unfulfilling" and "not fun." She reviewed her progress and saw the difficulties surrounding the therapist's departure from a more mature perspective. In a poignant final session she brought, as gifts, symbolic objects from childhood that "I don't need anymore." As the session drew to a close, she added, "You know what? I'm not crying. I don't know why. Should I be? I graduated from high school and felt so depressed and horrible, but it turned out OK, and I guess this is working out the same." The therapist said, "I hope you can give yourself credit for the progress you've made. You've changed in many ways." June replied, "I don't know, I guess. You know I'm really going to miss you. You're so levelheaded. You're really special." When the therapist thanked her, June presented her gift articles from childhood and said, "I don't like to say things when I am on my way out, but I have to tell you a few things you know already. You know I've had a crush on you the whole time, right? I mean it's normal stuff when you see a shrink. There's a name for it. And you know I want to marry a man like you some day."

About eight months later June telephoned to say that she would be traveling abroad with friends for the summer and planned to attend college away from home in the fall.

In this analytically oriented exploratory psychotherapy of an adolescent girl, conducted at a frequency of twice a week for one and a half years by a male therapist in his early thirties, there was an intense erotic transference that was largely worked through. Many adolescent developmental issues were worked on, with successful resolution. The termination phase of six months, much like a termination phase in psychoanalysis, permitted the working through of a wide range of feelings, including the anger of being abandoned, the transferential and then real sense of loss, and a true awareness by the patient of her therapeutic gains. Even if the therapist were not leaving town, it is likely, as in the case of so many adolescents, that the patient would have chosen to leave town to go to college as an expression of the newly won autonomy and independence of a new developmental phase.

Peggy

There are patients with serious pathology for whom one might never consider terminating treatment, who undergo intermittent psychotherapy with the expectation that they will return to the therapist or have additional therapy with a different therapist. In some instances the therapy may continue over many years with the same therapist with no thought of termination. For example, an adolescent boy whose illness was characterized by severe social anxiety and withdrawal from people began psychotherapy with me at age 17. A psychotic break with reality early in college required hospitalization for one and a half years. Upon his release from the hospital, outpatient therapy was resumed and continued for 32 more years. During this time he completed college and graduate work and embarked on a successful career that lasted 21 years. At age 52, after several years of early retirement, psychological problems again intervened, and he moved from the area and began therapy with a new therapist.

The case of Peggy (Parsons, 1990) illustrates intermittent psychotherapy in a young patient whose early life was marked by deprivation and chaotic parenting. Each phase of her therapy ended with the expectation that there would be another phase of therapy later on. Peggy was the only child of disturbed parents. Her mother, an orphan who had been reared in an institution, was a depressed, alcoholic woman who was intermittently suicidal and at times abusive to Peggy, and to neighbors who sometimes called the police to interrupt the fights. Peggy's father had been hospitalized for depression; he both physically abused and spoiled Peggy. The parents' relationship was turbulent, and Peggy's father left the house before she was four.

Peggy entered the Anna Freud Centre nursery at two years ten months, at which time she was charming and precocious and seemed to be developing normally. Development came to a standstill a year later when her mother attempted suicide and her father left the home. At four and a half Peggy began intensive psychotherapy. She made good use of this therapy, working in an intense transference on feelings of rage, worthlessness, and deprivation. However, therapy was interrupted after a year, when her therapist left the area. Following this loss of therapist, Peggy's nursery school teacher entered into a long-term supportive therapeutic relationship with her. The therapist provided help with problems of living and also tutored her in her school work.

At age 11 Peggy entered dynamic psychotherapy again. At this time she was sad, silent, and stubborn. She was superficially compliant, but after a few months she precipitously ended treatment, in which she had been experiencing early memories of her father.

At 14 there was a crisis in Peggy's life: her mother's divorce proceedings against her father. Peggy reacted to this event with shoplifting and truancy. Intensive psychotherapy was begun with a new therapist, and significant work was accomplished around her fear of aggression, her mistrust of adults (based on fears of abandonment), and her truancy. She returned to school but feared adolescence and growing to adulthood. As she began to recognize her love for her father, Peggy quickly became sexually involved with an older man. With analysis of oedipal derivatives she became more depressed and recovered many memories of deprivation and abandonment in her early childhood.

In the transference, Peggy feared her rage would destroy her female therapist. As she gradually began to trust that she would not be abandoned by her therapist (as she had been twice previously), Peggy began to be aware of and appreciate some of the positive aspects of both of her parents.

In presenting thoughts about termination, Parsons (1990) suggested that not only would Peggy need to be fully involved in any termination process but she would need to know that she could return to her therapist at any time if difficulties arose. At the time Parsons's paper was presented, after a little more than two years of psychotherapy, Peggy had plans to enter college.

Parsons concluded that with children and adolescents whose chief problems are developmental, structural, and characterological, rather than neurotic, the therapist functions as much as a *new* object as he does as a transference figure. Such a process has no moment of termination, but an ending more like an interruption.

Summary

In this chapter I have shown both similarities and differences between termination in psychotherapy and in psychoanalysis although, in general, the theoretical principles are the same. The systematic, close attention to termination phenomena that is characteristic of psychoanalysis should be applied to psychotherapy as well. Many psychotherapists tend to underestimate the importance of the therapist and the therapy to a child or adolescent and to give insufficient attention to the meaning of termination. The focus on and special meaning of termination in the works of both Allen (1942) and Mann (1973) are especially instructive in their emphasis on separation and loss, even though the theoretical viewpoints of these authors differ.

The termination phase that is characteristic of psychoanalysis is a model that psychoanalytically oriented psychotherapy would do well to approximate. A careful study of cases with an analytic termination can provide the psychoanalytic psychotherapist with guidelines and direct attention to specific crucial aspects of termination that are typically overlooked in psychotherapy.

However, in briefer psychotherapies with more limited goals, and, hence, limited working through in the transference of core conflicts, the timing of a termination will depend more on symptom relief and achievement of external life goals. The termination phase in such therapy will be briefer and less likely to involve further working through of conflict in the transference. And while more extensive exploratory psychotherapy will have a termination phase comparable to that in psychoanalysis, there are those psychotherapies, with children and adolescents who exhibit borderline psychopathology, where treatment is intermittent, continuous without clearly defined termination, or includes a termination that resembles an interruption.

The ending of a psychotherapy is one of the many losses patients will experience, beginning in earliest childhood and extending throughout life. Patients cannot handle the loss inherent in termination without preparation and help by the therapist. Without such help the patient will inevitably defend against full awareness of the conflicts and feelings that accompany this new separation experience. This defensive posture will become the model the child or adolescent will use to cope with future separations and losses, leading to inhibition of feelings and the failure to resolve developmental conflicts. When the therapist is an ally in helping the patient face the termination of psychotherapy, the patient will gain an understanding of his ambivalence, anxieties, satisfactions, anger, and sadness over the loss of his therapy and therapist. This working through in the termination period will provide a freeing of the patient from an unhealthy attachment to the therapist, and the new understanding gained will serve to provide the means to face future separations and losses.

References

Allen, F. (1942), *Psychotherapy with Children*. New York: Norton.

Cooper, A. M. (1989), Paper presented at Panel on "The Difference Between Termination in Psychotherapy and Psychoanalysis," fall meeting of the American Psychoanalytic Association, New York City.

Mann, J. (1973), *Time-Limited Psychotherapy*. Cambridge, MA: Harvard University Press.

Parsons, M. (1990), Some issues affecting termination in the analysis of a high-risk adolescent. *The Psychoanalytic Study of the Child*, 45:437–458. New Haven, CT: Yale University Press.

Shane, M. (1989), The decision to terminate in psychotherapy and psychoanalysis. Paper presented at fall meeting of the American Psychoanalytic Association, New York City.

Author Index

Subject Index

libidinal impulses toward, 93
loss of, fear of, 32
narcissism, 273
oedipal, 166
oedipal aggression toward, 8, 9
omniscient, 39
phallic, 59
positive attachment with child,
235
preoedipal and oedipal relationship with, 127, 205
reaction to child's analysis, 273
termination and, 104–105
pressure for, 373–274
transference, See Maternal transference
traumatic sexual exploitation by,
203–204
Mother-analyst relationship, helplessness feelings in, 274
Mother-child relationship
fantasies and, 300
good enough, 287
impaired, Oedipus complex and,
287
Mourning process, 161, 212
adolescence and, 228
initiation of, 269
Multiple terminations, 181
Mutative interpretation, 243
Mutual termination, 181
Mutuality, 208
evasion of, 317
Myth, personal, 142
Mythology, x

N

Narcissism, mother's, 273
Narcissistic injury
in late latency child, 73
in midadolescence, 145
vulnerability to, 38
Narcissistic insult, 287
Narcissistic sensitivity, in
preschool child, 287
Negative maternal transference,
213

Negative oedipal conflicts, 212
resolution of, 228, 229
Negative Oedipus complex, 141,
228
Negative transference, 15, 18, 89,
106–108
in adolescence, 127
in children, compared with
adults, 238
resolving of, 136
strong, 259
transference neurosis and, 136
Neglect, during infancy, 6
Neurotic conflict, origins of, termination and, 115
Neurotic symptoms, childhood,
142
Neutrality, 62
analyst's, related to termination,
179–180
analytic, 214
departure from, 22, 123, 242,
261
importance of, 247
transference and, 254
New object, analyst as, 245, 255,
256, 353
Nongratifications, 254
Nonincestuous dreams, related to
termination, 219
Nonincestuous object, 211
dreams of, related to termination,
226, 228–229
Nonincestuous women, feelings
toward, 200
Nurturing figure, ideal, 197

O

Object
child's perception of, 267
fantasied destruction and revitalization of, 307
Object-constancy, 323–324
Object of desire, analyst as, loss of,
301
Object relations

For Product Safety Concerns and Information please contact our EU
representative GPSR@taylorandfrancis.com
Taylor & Francis Verlag GmbH, Kaufingerstraße 24, 80331 München, Germany

www.ingramcontent.com/pod-product-compliance
Ingram Content Group UK Ltd.
Pitfield, Milton Keynes, MK11 3LW, UK
UKHW021114180425
457613UK00005B/78